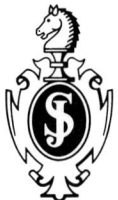

Duplex Sonography

Edward G. Grant   E. Maureen White
Editors

Duplex Sonography

With 459 Illustrations, 22 in Full Color

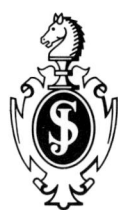

Springer-Verlag
New York Berlin Heidelberg London
Paris Tokyo Hong Kong Barcelona

Edward G. Grant, M.D.
Professor of Radiology
Department of Radiological Sciences
UCLA Medical Center
Center for the Health Sciences
Los Angeles, California 90024, USA

E. Maureen White, M.D.
Assistant Professor of Radiology
Georgetown University Medical Center
Washington, District of Columbia 20007, USA

On the front cover: Fig. 4.13. *Normal hepatic veins*, p. 144.

Library of Congress Cataloging-in-Publication Data
Duplex sonography
   Includes bibliographies and index.
   1. Diagnosis, Ultrasonic.   I. Grant, Edward G.
II. White, E. Maureen.
RC78.7.U4D87 1987   616.07'543   87-13128
Printed on acid-free paper.

© 1988 by Springer-Verlag New York Inc.
All rights reserved. This work may not be translated or copied in whole or in part without the written permission of the publisher (Springer-Verlag, 175 Fifth Avenue, New York, NY 10010, USA), except for brief excerpts in connection with reviews or scholarly analysis. Use in connection with any form of information storage and retrieval, electronic adaptation, computer software, or by similar or dissimilar methodology now known or hereafter developed is forbidden.
The use of general descriptive names, trade names, trademarks, etc. in this publication, even if the former are not especially identified, is not to be taken as a sign that such names, as understood by the Trade Marks and Merchandise Marks Act, may accordingly be used freely by anyone.
While the advice and information in this book are believed to be true and accurate at the date of going to press, neither the authors nor the editors nor the publisher can accept any legal responsibility for any errors or omissions that may be made. The publisher makes no warranty, express or implied, with respect to the material contained herein.

Typeset by Publishers Service, Bozeman, Montana.
Printed and bound by Arcata Graphics/Halliday, West Hanover, Massachusetts.
Printed in the United States of America.

9 8 7 6 5 4 3

ISBN 0-387-96564-5 Springer-Verlag New York Berlin Heidelberg
ISBN 3-540-96564-5 Springer-Verlag Berlin Heidelberg New York

Introduction

The use of diagnostic ultrasound has expanded tremendously during the last 10 years. Major technologic advancements of this decade have changed the nature of the modality from a medical curiosity to one of great diagnostic importance. As recently as 1975, simple bistable display was still relatively common in many centers. With improvement in amplification and transducer design, gray scale sonography emerged, enabling parenchymal organ detail to be clearly displayed. Although gray-scale imaging represented the advancement that gained ultrasound its place in modern diagnosis, it was the proliferation of real-time technology that allowed it to keep pace with other modalities.

Duplex sonography seems to represent a further "break through" in ultrasound imaging. Although duplex scanning is opening new frontiers in sonographic diagnosis, it actually represents little more than the union of two basic forms of preexisting ultrasound technology. These two basic forms of ultrasound are, of course, real-time imaging and Doppler. In the pursuit of noninvasive vascular diagnosis, each modality has serious limitations when used alone. Together they seem to compensate for one another's weaknesses; the diagnostic ability of duplex ultrasound far outweighs the sum of its parts.

As a successful diagnostic modality, duplex ultrasound owes much to the pioneering spirit of Dr. Eugene Strandness and his co-workers in Seattle, Washington. Dr. Strandness recognized the usefulness of coupling pulse-gated Doppler to real-time ultrasound some years ago. It is only recently, however, that duplex scanning has begun to receive widespread recognition. The reasons for this are many. Some physicians stated ultrasonic vascular diagnosis would soon become obsolete as venous digital angiography was the ultimate answer. Other hinderances to the acceptance of duplex sonography included difficulty in mastering the technique, its extreme operator dependence, and early on, the limited availability of equipment and educational facilities. Finally, a problem well-known to most sonographers, is the general distrust by referring clinicians of a modality that yields images that they cannot easily interpret themselves.

Sonographers have been capable of evaluating blood vessels almost from the start. Fibrous vessel walls are excellent specular reflectors and were readily visible even with bistable display. Although sonographic images of veins and arteries are useful, they are very limited in their ability to assess hemodynamic events. The real-time sonogram gives little indication if there is flow in the vessel or if flow is in the proper direction. Duplex technology gives life to the sonographic void inside of blood vessels and for the first time allows the sonographer to derive truly useful information about hemodynamic events.

Duplex technology has radically changed the approach to noninvasive vascular diagnosis. Noninvasive vascular evaluations have typically been approached from an indirect standpoint using plethysmography, strain-gauge evaluations, pressure measurements, and other methods of inferring vascular compromise by identifying abnormal physiology. Drawbacks to such an approach are numerous. Although many diagnosticians have achieved relatively good results using these techniques, the fact that indirect diagnosis only implies disease rather than identifying it directly leaves much to be desired. It is the unique ability to provide conclusive and specific information about important vascular abnormalities that makes duplex sonography so attractive. The ability to directly diagnose and quantify stenotic lesions in the carotid, iliac, or femoral arteries, to identify reversal of blood flow in the portal system, or to conclusively evaluate for complex vascular events such as renal transplant rejection has become possible noninvasively only since the advent of duplex scanning.

For many readers, duplex sonography is a relatively foreign subject. Many radiologists, although familiar with real-time ultrasound, have little experience with Doppler and noninvasive vascular diagnosis in general. Conversely, many vascular diagnosticians are more familiar with Doppler than the workings of real-time ultrasound. The marriage of the two components, needless to say, creates complexities of its own. Because duplex sonography is unique in so many ways, we shall begin with a chapter on basic principles. The emphasis of this important section will be on practical application.

The remainder of the book shall be devoted to diagnostics and consists of six chapters. Technical considerations will be included in each chapter as scan technique varies considerably from one part of the body to the next. The first chapter will be devoted to duplex evaluation of the cerebrosvascular system and of the arteries supplying the brain, the carotid is by far the most important. The carotid artery is accessible in almost every patient and its bifurcation has been extensively scrutinized using duplex ultrasound. This chapter is, therefore, quite detailed and hopefully assists the sonographer to achieve the highest possible degree of diagnostic accuracy.

Like the carotid arteries, the heart has been the subject of much duplex investigation. Because color flow imaging has been found to provide unique information in the heart, examples of this new adaptation of duplex are emphasized. In the third clinical section, we discuss the uses of duplex sonography in the abdomen. Abdominal duplex is still rapidly evolving and its eventual role in abdominal disease remains to be further investigated. The present uses of duplex in the abdomen range from relatively simple tasks, such as establishing the vascular or nonvascular nature of cystic structures or providing qualitative information about the portal venous system, to the evaluation of blood flow in transplanted organs, various tumors, and a host of disease states with underlying vascular abnormalities. Although still technically within the abdomen, obstetrical duplex is sufficiently unique to warrant a separate chapter. The use of pulsed Doppler in the fetus remains somewhat controversial yet represents a fascinating and challenging area which will undoubtedly expand in the future. The final chapters are devoted to the use of duplex in the (noncarotid) peripheral arteries and veins. Peripheral arterial disease is primarily taken to mean atherosclerosis in the legs, and the greatest part of the chapter is devoted to this subject. Duplex evaluation of peripheral atherosclerosis is challenging using today's equipment. Such evaluations are not routine. On the other hand, duplex evaluation of the deep venous structures of the legs may become the primary investigative tool in thrombotic disease.

This text has been designed to impart to the reader an overall working understanding of duplex sonography from its physical principles through to its various clinical applications. The technique is difficult. Beyond reading, the mastery of duplex scanning requires hours of hands-on experience. Those familiar with duplex scanning, however, would probably agree that the diagnostic results are well worth the effort.

Edward G. Grant
1987

Contents

Introduction
EDWARD G. GRANT v

Color Plates xii

1 Technical Considerations, Equipment, and Physics
   of Duplex Sonography
   FREDERICK W. KREMKAU 1

2 Duplex Sonography of the Cerebrovascular System
   EDWARD G. GRANT 7

3 Cardiac Doppler
   FREDERICK J. DOHERTY and KEVIN P. MCINERNEY 69

4 Duplex Sonography of the Abdomen
   E. MAUREEN WHITE and PETER L. CHOYKE 129

5 Duplex Evaluation of Fetoplacental and
   Uteroplacental Circulation
   MICHAEL C. HILL, IAN M. LANDE, and JOHN H. GROSSMAN, III . . 191

6 Duplex Sonography of Peripheral Arteries
   EDWARD G. GRANT 211

7 Duplex Sonography of the Lower Extremity
   Venous System
   E. MAUREEN WHITE 239

Index 261

Contributors

PETER L. CHOYKE, M.D., Assistant Professor of Radiology, Department of Radiology, Georgetown University Hospital, Washington, District of Columbia, USA.

FREDERICK J. DOHERTY, M.D., Assistant Professor, Radiology, Director of Ultrasound, Department of Radiology, New England Medical Center, Boston, Massachusetts, USA.

EDWARD G. GRANT, M.D., Professor of Radiology, Department of Radiological Sciences, University of California Los Angeles Medical Center, Center for the Health Sciences, Los Angeles, California, USA.

JOHN H. GROSSMAN III, M.D., PH.D., Professor of Obstetrics and Gynecology and Microbiology, Director of the Division of Fetal Maternal Medicine, The George Washington University, Washington, District of Columbia, USA.

MICHAEL C. HILL, M.B., Professor of Radiology, Director, Cross-Sectional Imaging Section (Ultrasound/CT), The George Washington University, Washington, District of Columbia, USA.

FREDERICK W. KREMKAU, PH.D., Professor and Director, Center for Medical Ultrasound, Bowman Gray School of Medicine, Winston Salem, North Carolina, USA.

IAN M. LANDE, M.D., C.M., F.R.C.P. (C), Assistant Professor of Radiology, The George Washington University, Washington, District of Columbia, USA.

KEVIN P. MCINERNEY, Division of Echocardiography, Department of Cardiology, Tufts-New England Medical Center, Boston, Massachusetts, USA.

E. MAUREEN WHITE, M.D., Assistant Professor of Radiology, Georgetown University Medical Center, Washington, District of Columbia, USA.

Color Plates

Fig. 2.17B. Color flow image depicts effect of vessel narrowing and irregular surface of plaque on flow. Various colors are seen as blood travels through the lesion. Differing colors (*arrowheads*) reflect an increase in flow velocity beyond an area of stenosis (*arrows*) and marked turbulence. Courtesy of Dr. Eugene Strandness, University of Washington Hospital, Seattle, Washington.

Fig. 2.20E. Color flow image shows areas of blue (*arrows*), confirming flow reversal in boundary separation zone. Courtesy of Quantum Medical Systems, Inc., Issaquah, Washington.

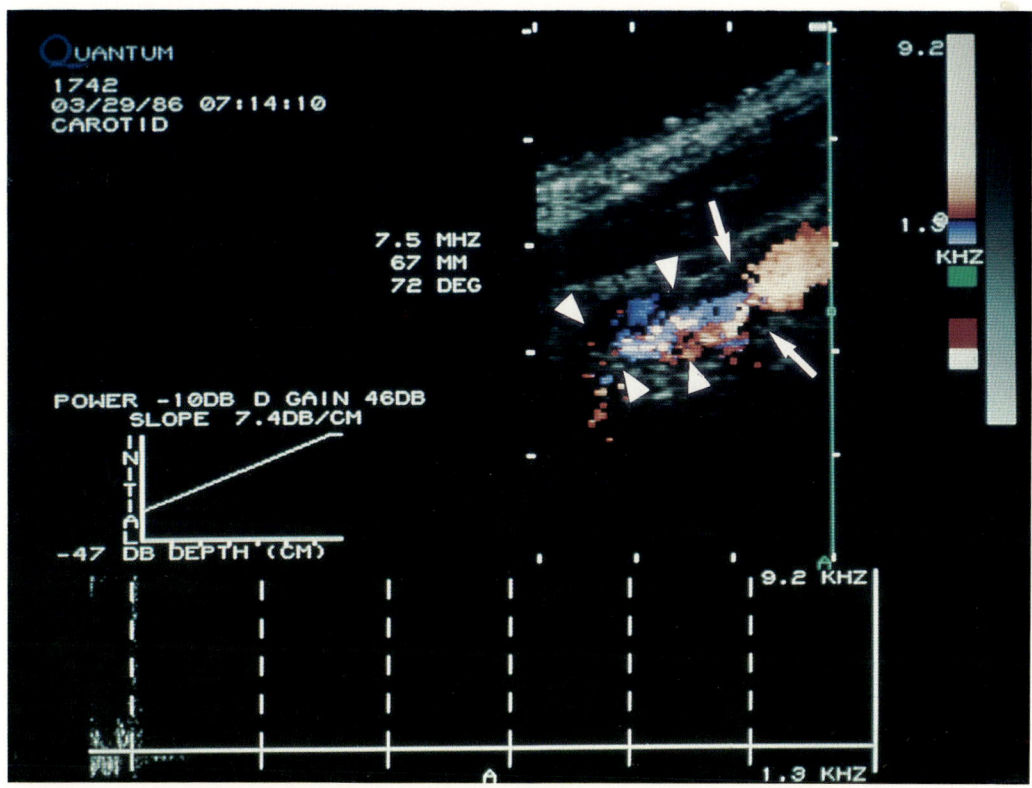

Fig. 2.17B.

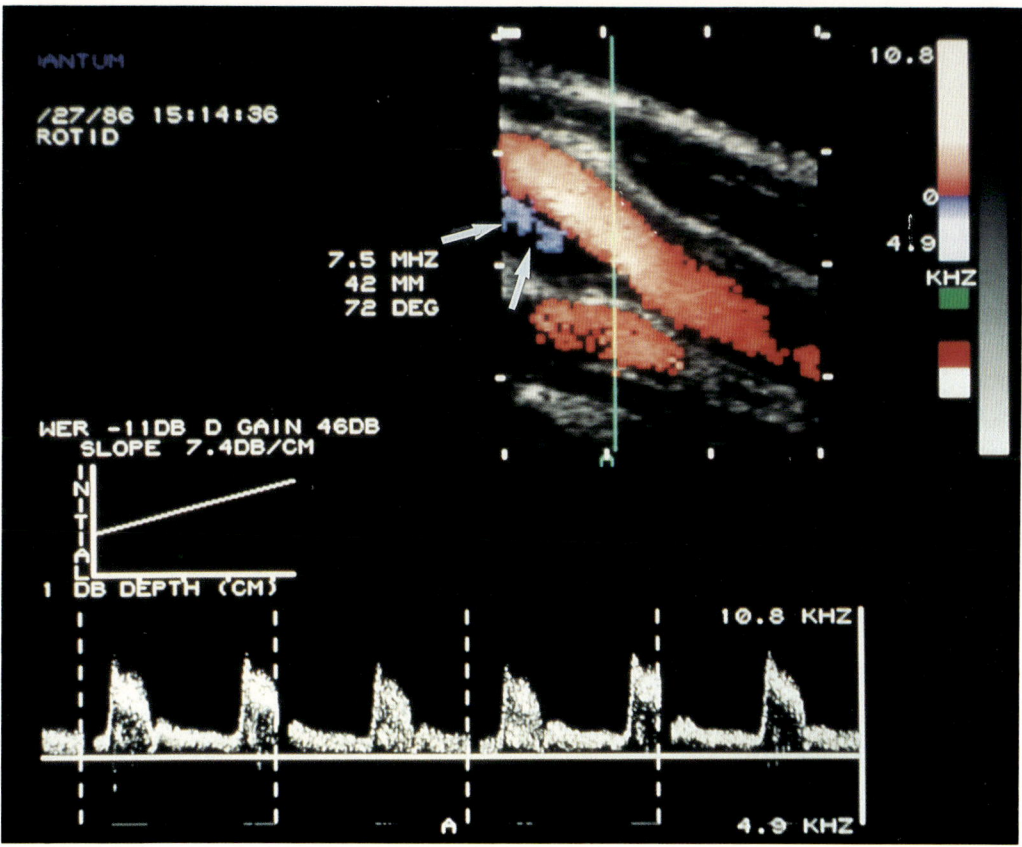

Fig. 2.20E.

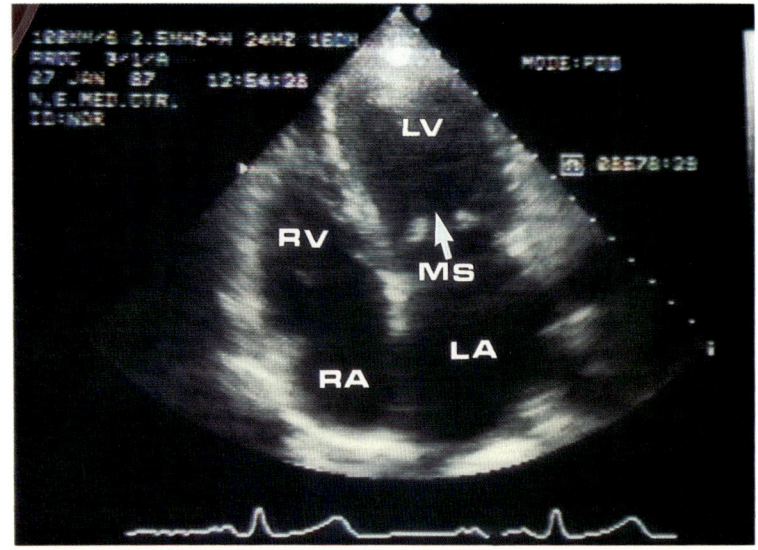

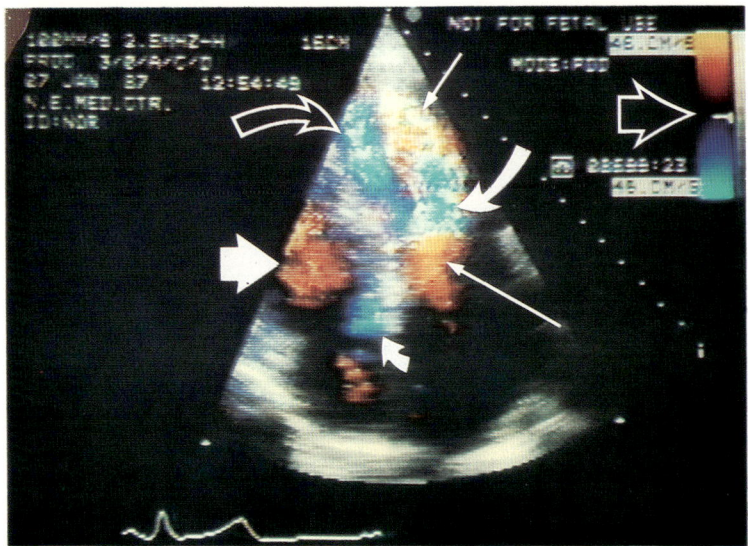

Fig. 3.7A,B. Typical color Doppler illustration. **A.** Black and white apical four-chamber view in a patient with mitral stenosis. Both the left atrium and left ventricle are enlarged; thickened, restricted mitral leaflets are seen (LA, left atrium; LV, left ventricle; RA, right atrium; RV, right ventricle; MS, stenotic mitral orifice). **B.** Color Doppler image in diastole in the same apical four-chamber view as in Fig. 3.7A. Positive flow toward the transducer is displayed in shades from dark red through orange to bright yellow-orange. This is shown on the color scale in the upper right-hand corner of the illustration. The darker red colors correspond to slow flow and the brighter yellow colors to fast flow (*broad open arrow*). Negative flow away from the transducer is displayed in shades of deep blue, for slow flow, through blue-green to bright light green, for fast flow (*broad open arrow*). The fastest flow detectable becomes so intense as to be displayed as white, and aliased flow is seen as a mosaic of colors. Because both positive and negative Doppler signals are displayed in aliased flow with pulsed Doppler, color Doppler likewise displays both positive and negative information, and the mosaic of intense multiple colors is obtained. In this example, forward flow in the left atrium is seen in red, being darker in the middle of the atrium, and going through orange to yellow as the blood speeds up as it goes through the narrowed mitral orifice (*long thin arrow*). The jet of blood curves somewhat laterally as it goes into the left ventricle. A large high velocity jet is seen, accelerating through the mitral orifice toward the apex (*short thin arrow*), which is an intense mosaic of colors primarily in white, bright yellow, or bright blue-green. The jet through the mitral valve into the apex is displayed as a mosaic of color because it represents aliasing of high-velocity flow. The intense blue-green flow just inside the valve is not reversed flow, but aliased flow (*long closed curved arrow*). A normal vortex of negative downward flow toward the aortic valve is seen in blue shades, hugging ▶

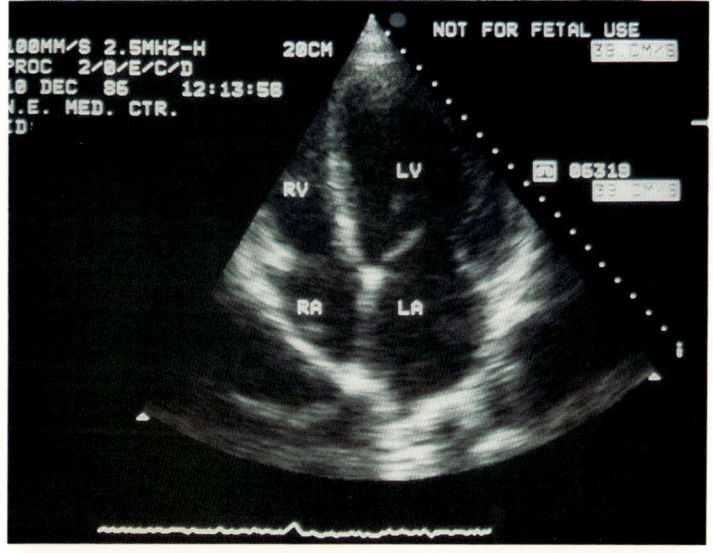

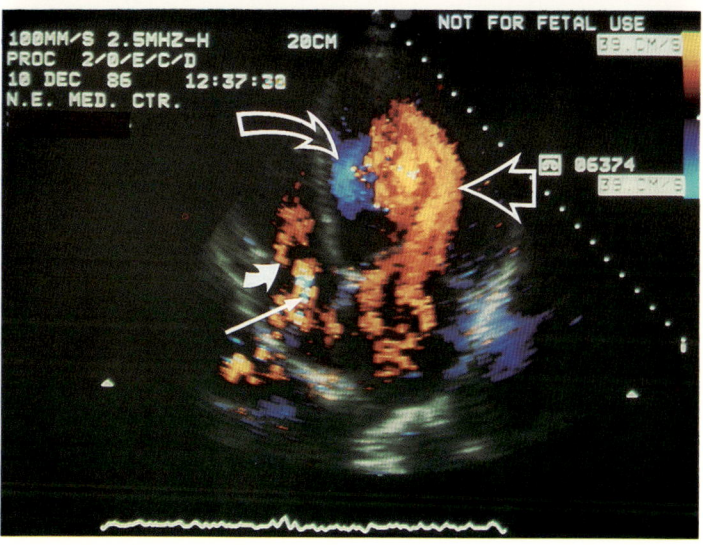

Fig. 3.14A–D. Normal left ventricular color Doppler images. **A.** Black and white apical four-chamber view of a normal heart. **B.** Early diastole. Normal forward positive flow is displayed in red and orange extending from the back of the left atrium toward the apex (*broad open arrow*). Areas of slightly higher velocity are seen in this jet in the left ventricle as areas of yellow to white. The normal downward vortex toward the aortic valve is seen along the septum in blue shades (*curved open arrow*). Right-sided forward flow is shown in red and orange (*short curved arrow*). The patch of blue (*thin arrow*) within this orange in the tricuspid area is partial imaging of normal downward flow out of the adjacent ascending aorta. (*Continued.*)

the ventricular septum (*long open curved arrow*). Higher flow velocities in this area are seen as light blue-green to white. Normal forward flow into the right ventricle from the tricuspid valve area is displayed as a red-orange jet (*broad closed arrow*). The small patch of blue on the right side of the atrial septum (*short closed curved arrow*) is partial detection of downward aortic flow, because of its close proximity in this view.

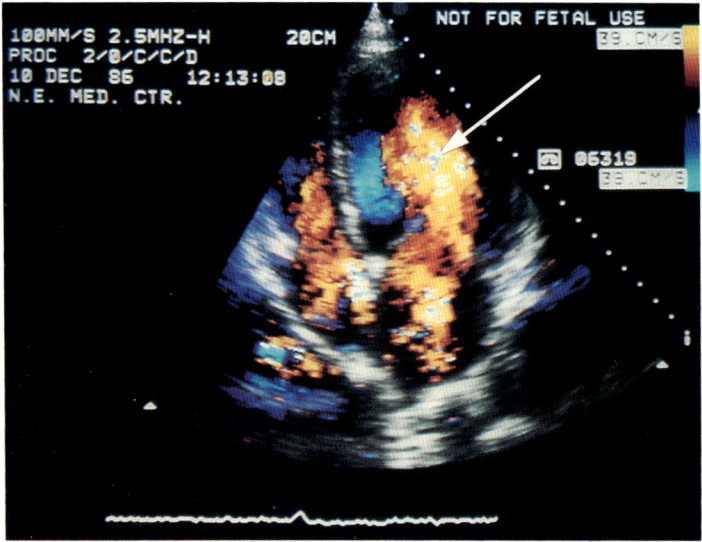

C

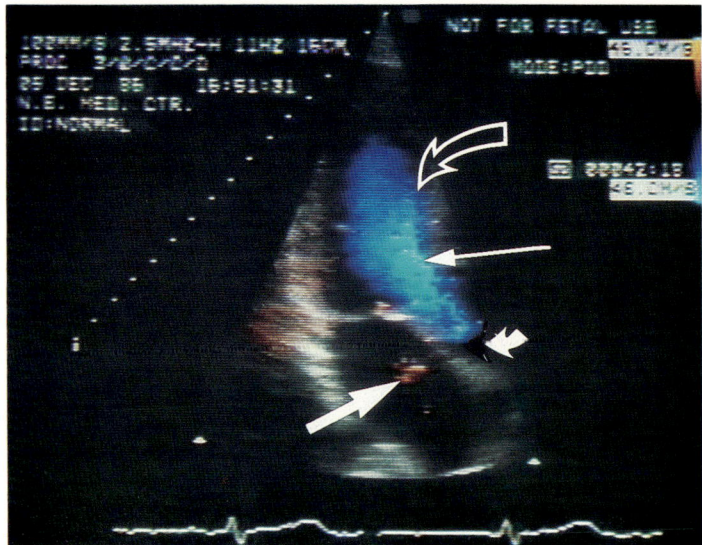

D

Fig. 3.14C. Later in diasole. All the flow patterns shown in part **B** are again shown here. The velocities have all increased. The orange forward flow on both sides of the heart is now displayed with more yellow and white, indicating higher velocities. Note the higher velocities on the left side compared with the right. The patches of blue with the yellow-white areas of the left ventricular inflow represent aliasing (*arrow*). Note the acceleration in the downward vortex along the septum as blood approaches the aortic valve. This pattern is now displayed with brighter blue-green than in **B**. **D**. An apical long axis view of the left ventricle and left atrium in the same individual. The transducer has simply been rotated 90° at the apex. It offers a Doppler approach identical to the four-chamber view. A small patch of red is seen in the left atrium (*closed straight arrow*) probably representing pulmonary venous emptying, whereas the mitral valve leaflets are closed. Normal left ventricular outflow is demonstrated. Negative downward flow is shown in most of the anterior portion of the left ventricle in shades of blue (*open curved arrow*). This pattern extends through the aortic valve into the proximal ascending aorta. Note the increase in velocity in the subaortic region, hugging the upper septum and extending through the aortic leaflets. This is displayed as bright blue-green (*long thin arrow*), and shows the blood accelerating through the valve and actually outlining one of the sinuses of Valsalva (*short closed curved arrow*).

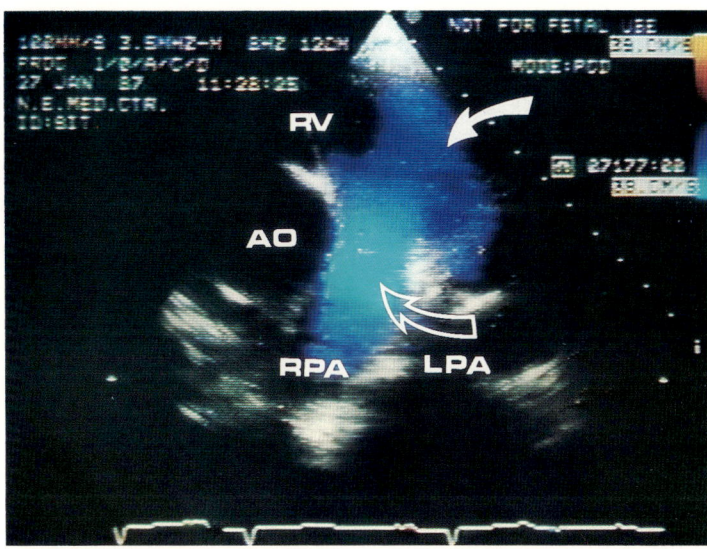

Fig. 3.18. Normal pulmonic flow. This is a short axis view of the right ventricular outflow tract obtained from the left parasternal approach. Normal downward negative flow is displayed in shades of deep blue, for slow flow in the right ventricular outflow tract (*closed curved arrow*), to shades of bright blue-green, showing the blood flow as it accelerates through the pulmonic valve into the main pulmonary artery (*open curved arrow*), and down into the right pulmonary artery. No flow is shown in the left pulmonary artery in this illustration (AO, aorta; RV, right ventricle; LPA, left pulmonary artery; RPA, right pulmonary artery).

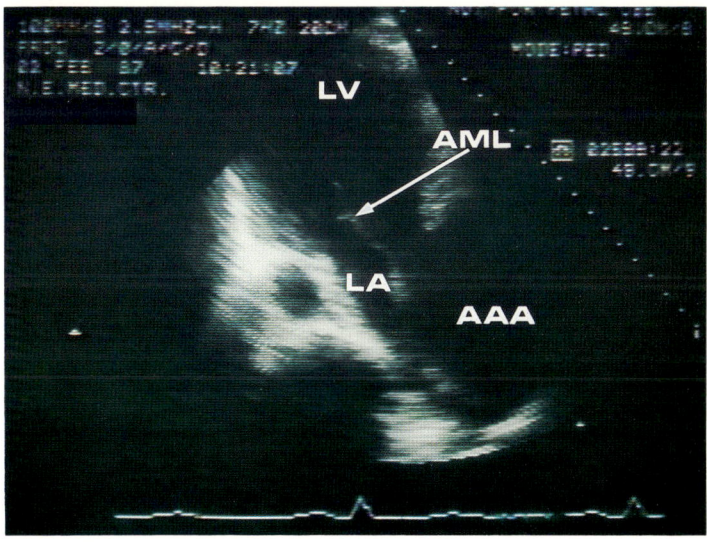

Fig. 3.24A–C. Aortic insufficiency. **A.** Black and white apical long axis view of a dilated left ventricle and massively dilated ascending aorta. This patient, with an aneurysm of the ascending aorta, had severe aortic insufficiency (LV, left ventricle; AML, anterior mitral leaflet; LA, left atrium; AAA, ascending aortic aneurysm). (*Continued.*)

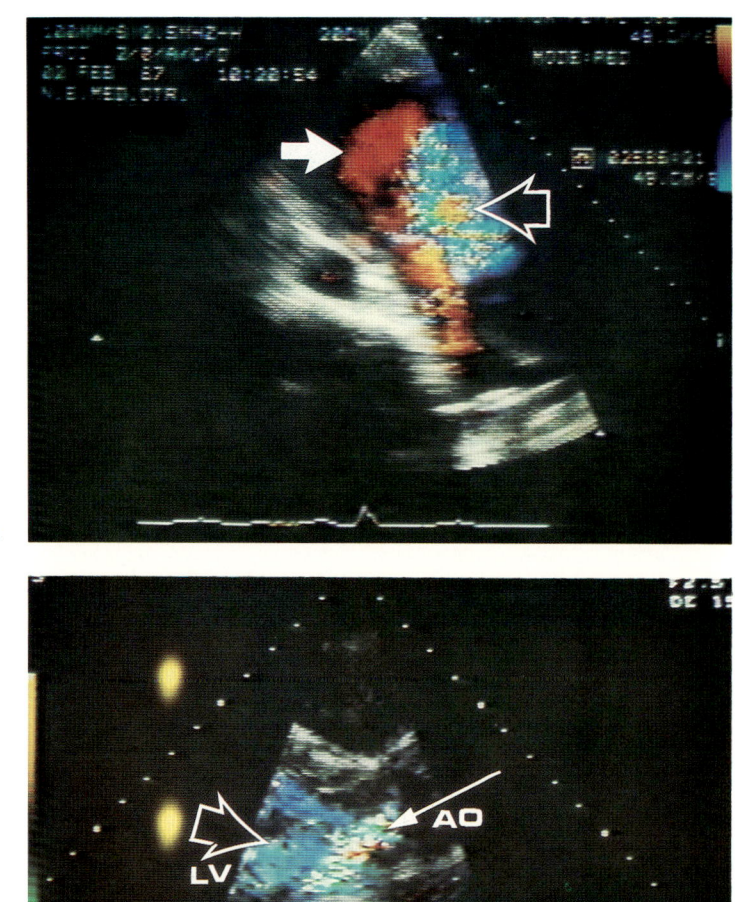

Fig. 3.24B. Color Doppler image in diastole. Normal mitral inflow is seen in the left atrium extending into the posterior portion of the left ventricle, and is displayed in red to yellow-orange shades (*closed arrow*) corresponding to the positive forward motion of blood. The coincident jet of severe aortic regurgitation is displayed in the anterior portion of the left ventricle adjacent to the septum. It is displayed in a mosaic of blue-green, yellow, orange, and white (*open arrow*), representing turbulent high-velocity aliased flow, and not downward negative flow. **C.** Mild aortic insufficiency. This illustration is from a different patient with a small jet of aortic insufficiency. In this long axis parasternal view, the sector angle has been narrowed to increase the line density and image quality. The regurgitant aortic jet in diastole is shown as an area of blue and blue-green (*open arrow*) in the subaortic region of the left ventricle. A small discrete high-velocity jet is shown as a bright mosaic of color (*long thin arrow*), indicating aliased high flow originating from the center of the closed aortic valve leaflets (AO, ascending aorta; LA, left atrium; LV, left ventricle). For a color reproduction of this figure see frontmatter.

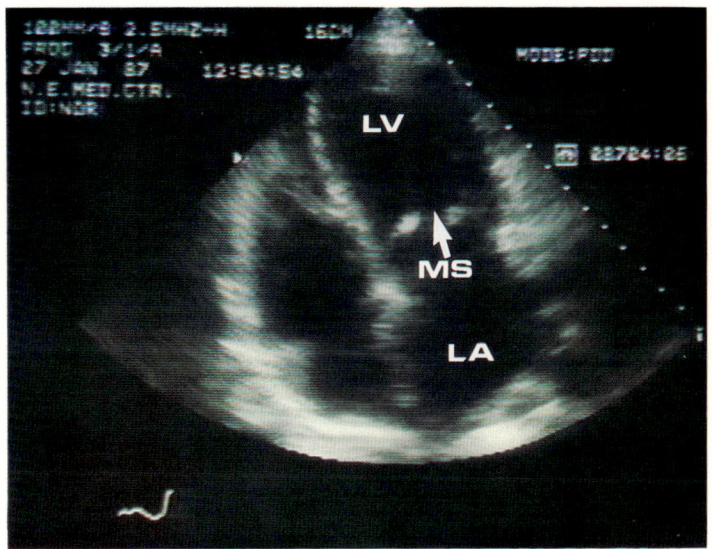

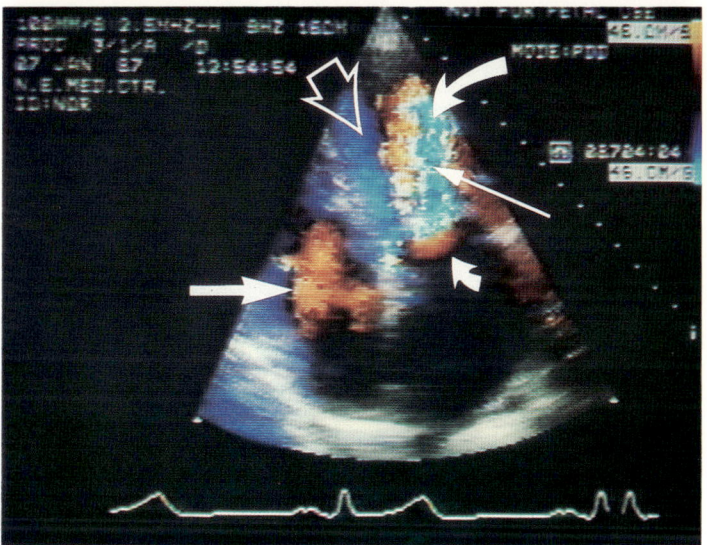

Fig. 3.28A,B. Mitral stenosis. **A.** Black and white apical four-chamber view in a patient with mitral stenosis. Both the left atrium and left ventricle are enlarged, and the mitral valve leaflets are thickened with restricted motion (LA, left atrium; LV, left ventricle; MS, stenotic mitral orifice). **B.** Color Doppler image of mitral stenosis in diastole. Normal forward right atrial flow is shown in red and orange (*straight closed arrow*). The normal downward diastolic vortex adjacent to the septum is seen in shades of deep blue to a slightly lighter blue (*straight open arrow*). The high-velocity jet of mitral stenosis is seen in the lateral aspect of the left ventricle, extending from the mitral orifice close to the apex (*long curved closed arrow*). It is displayed in a variety of colors but is clearly distinct from the normal negative vortex against the septum. Here, the bulk of the stenotic jet is displayed in bright orange to bright yellow. The central portion of the jet shows the fastest velocities, and is displayed in a bright mosaic of yellow-blue-green shades (*long, thin arrow*), representing very high velocity aliased flow, bordered by white, representing the highest flow properly recorded in this pulsed-Doppler system. Note the slowdown and backup of blood on the atrial side of the mitral valve as blood piles up here before it is squeezed through the narrowed opening (*short closed curved arrow*). Also note both the similarity and the difference of the appearance of the normal downward vortex adjacent to the septum and the aliased abnormal high-velocity jet of mitral stenosis going in the opposite direction. Both patterns are displayed with much blue. The normal blue flow is more homogeneously deep blue to blue-green. The abnormal aliased blue flow is brighter, yellower, and less homogeneous.

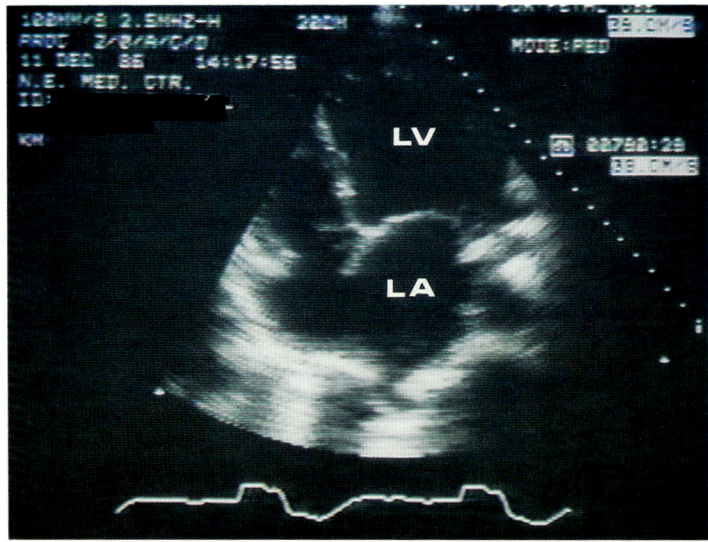

Fig. 3.30A–D. Mitral regurgitation. **A.** Black and white apical four-chamber view of a patient with mitral regurgitation. An enlarged left atrium and left ventricle are seen here (LA, left atrium; LV, left ventricle). The right-sided chambers are normally sized. The mitral valve leaflets appear normal. **B.** Color-Doppler image in systole. Normal downward negative left ventricular outflow is seen extending along the left side of the ventricular septum up to the immediate subaortic area (*closed straight arrow*). This is displayed as deep blue with some normal acceleration of flow shown by the lighter blue-green closer to the aortic valve and septum. The abnormal high-velocity regurgitant jet (*open straight arrow*) into the left atrium, through the closed mitral leaflets in systole, is shown as a bright mosaic of blue, green, yellow, and white traveling along the lateral aspect of the left atrium all the way to its posterior aspects. When the jet reaches the back wall of the left atrium, it appears first to turn medially and then it turns forward along the atrial septum (*long thin arrow*) going toward the mitral valve. It changes from aliased blue-green to yellow, and then to red as it finally slows down in the left atrium close the mitral valve.

Color Plates

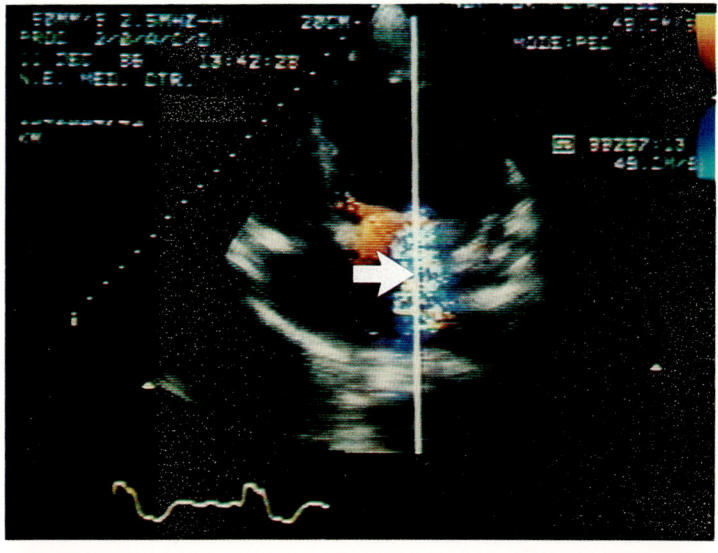

C

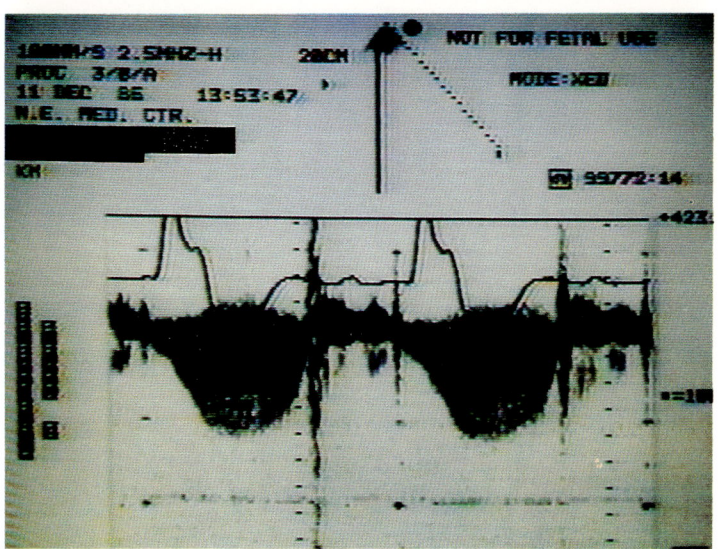

D

Fig. 3.30C. Another color Doppler image in systole, showing how easily color flow mapping can be used to guide the placement of the Doppler cursor if one wants to do a tracing of the flow velocity profile. In this example, the Doppler cursor is directed exactly through the center of the jet of mitral insufficiency (*short broad closed arrow*), which extends to the back wall of the left atrium. **D.** Continuous-wave Doppler tracing obtained along the path shown in part **C**. Severe mitral insufficiency with a V max of 4.3 m/s is measured (calibration marks, 1 m/s).

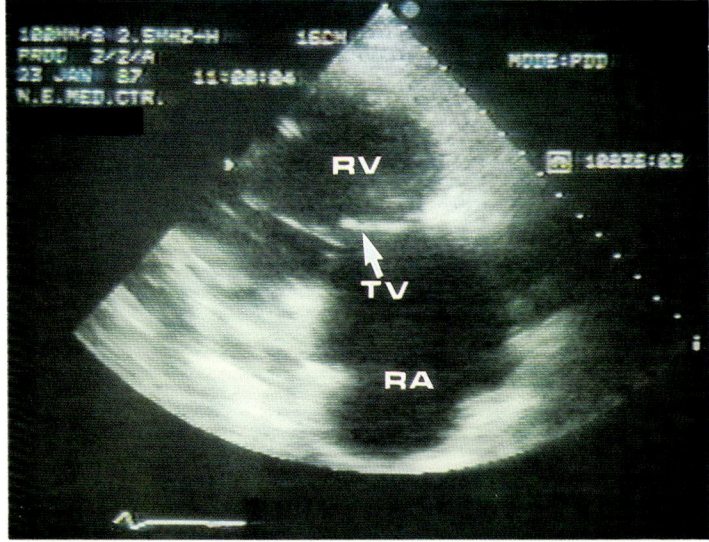

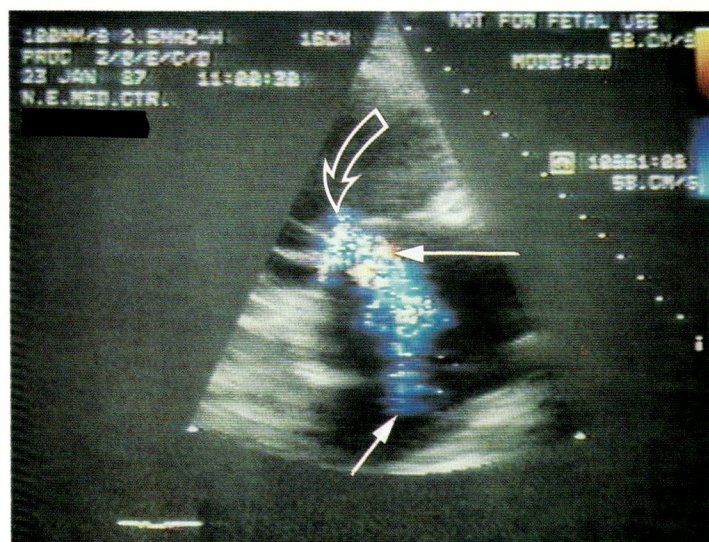

Fig. 3.36A,B. Tricuspid insufficiency. **A.** Black and white parasternal long axis view of the right atrium and right ventricle. Both chambers are enlarged in this patient with severe tricuspid insufficiency (RA, right atrium; RV, right ventricle; TV, tricuspid valve). **B.** Color Doppler image in systole, with sector narrowed, showing negative downward high-velocity flow in the right atrium. The blue regurgitant jet (*curved arrow*) through the tricuspid valve reaches the back of the right atrium and is classified as severe. The portion of the jet from the tricuspid valve to the midatrial level is displayed as a bright yellow-blue-green mosaic, with some red, indicative of high-velocity aliased flow in this area (*long thin arrow*). Note that the most aliasing and the brightest mosaic pattern is closest to the tricuspid valve. The regurgitant flow slows down to a normal shade of blue as it gets deeper into the right atrium (*short thin arrow*).

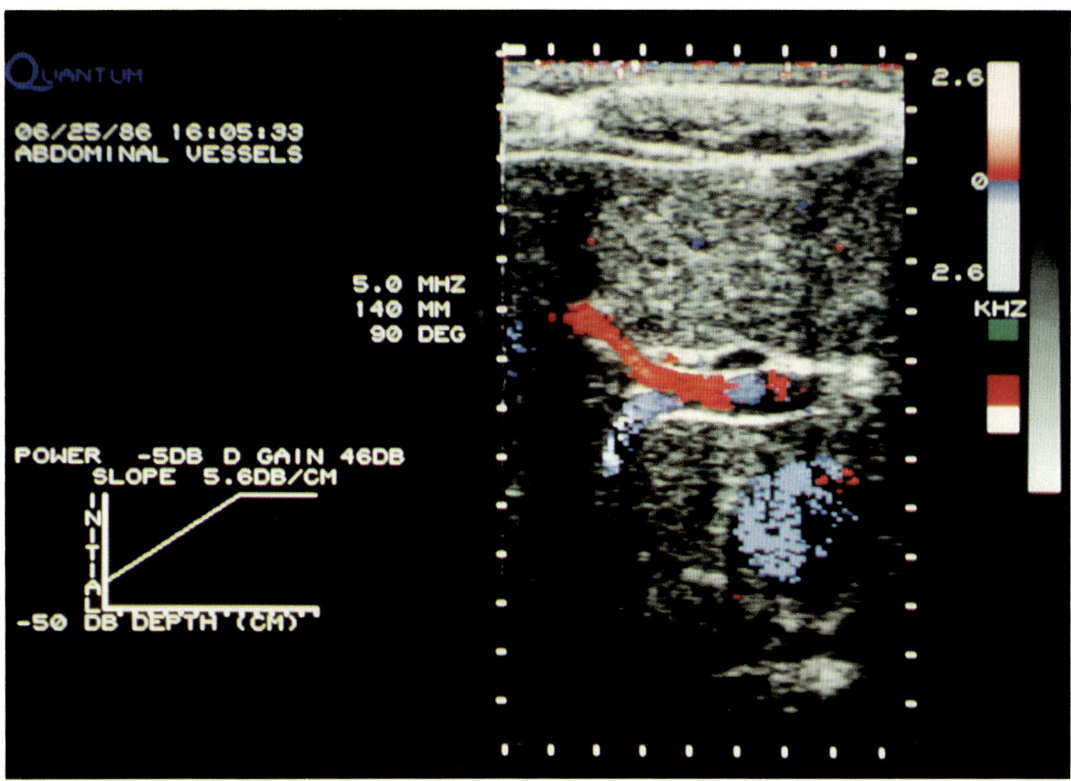

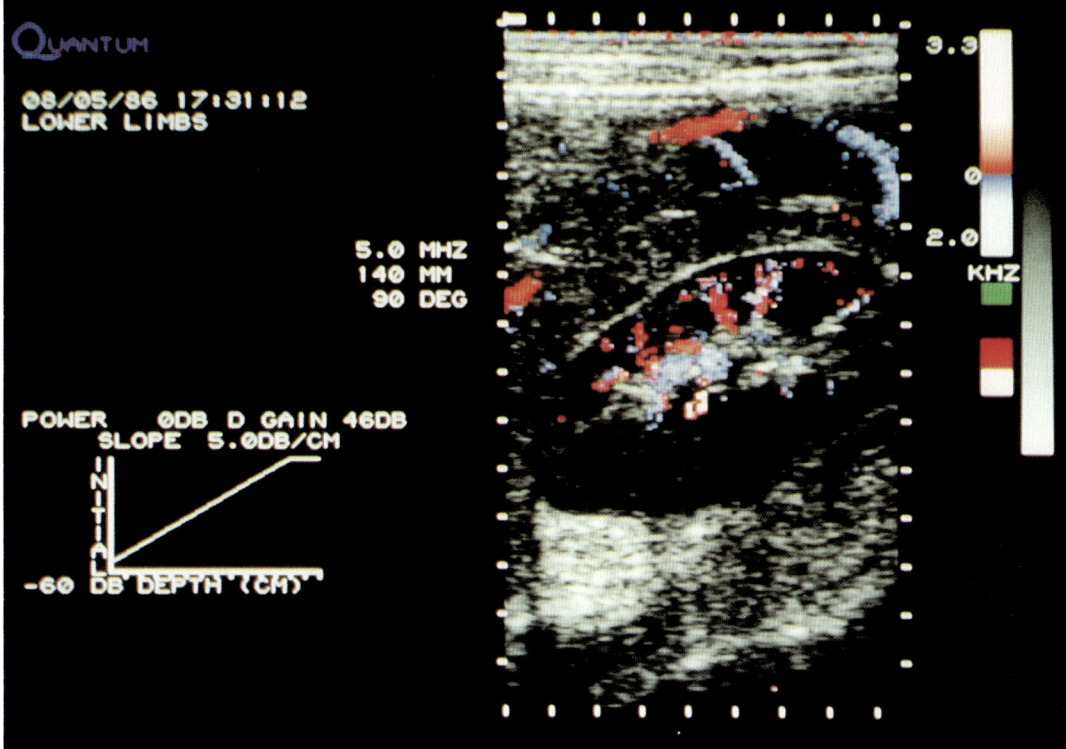

Fig. 4.39A,B. Color-flow imaging in the abdomen. **A,B.** Clinical work is in progress to evaluate the potential role of color-flow imaging in evaluating the abdominal vasculature. Images of the portal venous system (**A**) and right renal vessels (**B**) are courtesy of Quantum Medical Systems, Inc., Issaquah, Washington.

1
Technical Considerations, Equipment, and Physics of Duplex Sonography

FREDERICK W. KREMKAU

Duplex sonography involves the combined use of real-time pulse-echo gray-scale ultrasound imaging and pulsed-Doppler ultrasound. Imaging provides anatomic information, whereas Doppler provides physiologic information in the form of blood flow data. Pulsed-Doppler instrumentation provides the ability to detect and measure flow at specific anatomic sites. To intelligently use this capability, it is necessary to know the anatomic origin of the flow information. This is achieved by combining Doppler ultrasound with imaging. The principles and instrumentation of Doppler ultrasound are presented in this chapter. Principles of real-time ultrasound imaging (1–6) and Doppler principles and instrumentation in greater detail (7–8) are described elsewhere.

Doppler Physics

The Doppler effect is a change in frequency of a wave resulting from motion. The motion may be that of the wave source or wave receiver or, in the case of a reflected wave, the motion of the reflector. The Doppler effect is used in many ways including police radar speed detectors, home burglar alarms, and automatic door openers in public buildings. For each of these uses, reflector motion generates the Doppler effect. The first example uses electromagnetic microwaves and the latter two use airborne ultrasound. In medical applications, the source and receiver (ultrasound transducer) are stationary, and the Doppler effect is, likewise, generated by reflector motion. Medical Doppler ultrasound is used for detecting and measuring blood flow and, thus, the dominant reflector is the erythrocyte in circulation. If motion is toward the transducer, the echo frequency is greater than the frequency of the transmitted pulse. If motion is away from the transducer, the echo frequency is less than that of the transmitted pulse. The Doppler equation provides a quantitative relationship between the flow speed and the change in frequency:

$$f_D = \frac{2\,fv\,\cos(a)}{c}$$

where f_D is Doppler shift frequency (echo frequency minus transmitted pulse frequency), f is transmitted pulse frequency, v is reflector speed, a is the angle between reflector motion and transmitted pulse direction, and c is sound speed. This equation can be rearranged to solve for reflector speed:

$$v = \frac{f_D\,c}{2\,f\,\cos(a)}$$

When the speed of sound (1540 m/s) is inserted we get:

$$v\,(\text{cm/s}) = \frac{77\,f_D\,(\text{KHz})}{f\,(\text{MHz})\,\cos(a)}$$

Figure 1.1 shows the relationship between the ultrasound beam, blood vessel, and the Doppler angle, a. Table 1.1 give examples of Doppler shifts for various transmitted pulse frequencies, blood flow speeds, and angles.

The Doppler effect is applied in medical ultrasound blood flow measurement as follows. An ultrasound pulse is emitted by the trans-

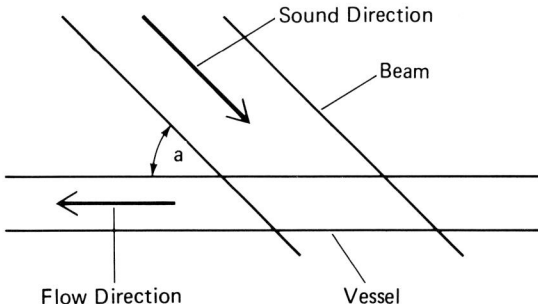

Fig. 1.1. Angle a is the angle between the direction of flow and the sound propagation direction.

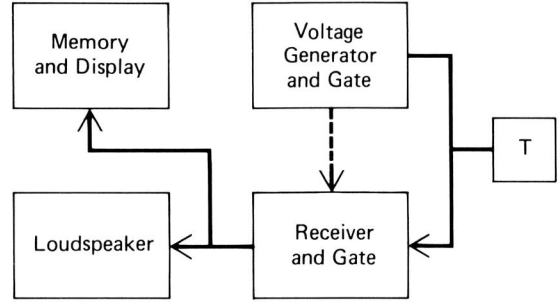

Fig. 1.2. Block diagram of a pulsed-Doppler ultrasound instrument; T, transducer.

ducer. The pulse travels through tissues interacting with them in such a way that echoes are produced. As these are received by the transducer they are used for generating an anatomic image of the tissues. As the pulse encounters moving blood cells in a vessel, Doppler-shifted echoes are produced. These are also received by the transducer, but are processed differently by the instrument so that the Doppler shift is calculated and presented audibly or visually to provide flow information. The duplex instrument provides a means for intelligently selecting the anatomic location from which the Doppler information is obtained and means for dealing with the angle between the transmitted pulse and flow directions. It is a combination of a pulse-echo imaging instrument and a pulsed-Doppler flow detection instrument. A block diagram for the pulsed–Doppler portion of the instrument is shown in Figure 1.2. The gated voltage generator produces sinusoidal voltage bursts of several cycles in length. Pulses used for Doppler flow detection are longer than those used for imaging because accurate detection of the frequency shift cannot be done with pulses of only two or three cycles' length. The voltage bursts are applied to the transducer, which responds by producing ultrasound bursts of several cycles' length. Generator frequency is matched to transducer operating frequency to maximize efficiency. Returning echoes from the anatomy are received by the same transducer and converted back into electrical voltages that travel to the receiver. The receiver compares the frequency of the returning echoes with that of the voltage generator (and thus the transmitted pulses) and derives the Doppler shift, the difference between echo frequency, and transmitted pulse frequency. The Doppler shift frequencies of the returning echoes are applied to a loudspeaker for audible presentation and analysis and to a memory and display for visual presentation and analysis. As in ultrasound imaging, echo arrival time can be used to determine the site (depth) of echo generation. Thus, Doppler-shifted echoes arrive at times after the generation of the transmitted pulse that correspond to the depth from which they interacted with the moving blood cell. Later echoes come from deeper vessels. The relationship between time and depth is 13 µs/cm. This comes directly from the speed of sound (0.154 cm/µs), taking into account round-trip travel time. The receiver

Table 1.1. Doppler Frequency Shifts (f_D) for Various Frequencies (f), Reflector Speeds (v), and Angles (a).*

f (MHz)	v (cm/s)	a (degrees)	f_D (KHz)
2.5	50	0	1.6
5.0	50	0	3.2
7.5	50	0	4.9
2.5	100	0	3.2
5.0	100	0	6.5
7.5	100	0	9.7
2.5	150	0	4.9
5.0	150	0	9.7
7.5	150	0	14.6
5.0	50	30	2.8
5.0	50	60	1.6
5.0	50	90	0
5.0	100	30	5.6
5.0	100	60	3.2
5.0	100	90	0
5.0	150	30	8.4
5.0	150	60	4.9
5.0	150	90	0

*Flow is toward the transducer (flow away would yield negative Doppler shifts).

gate provides a means for selecting Doppler information from a given depth (vessel). The gate opens at a time corresponding to the arrival time of the echoes from the desired depth and closes subsequently. Therefore, echoes from shallower and deeper vessels are not permitted to pass through the receiver and are eliminated. The gate can be adjusted so that the flow from the desired vessel can be received. The location of the center of the gate as well as the length of the gate can be adjusted by the operator. Indication of the gate location and length is superimposed on the cross-sectional ultrasound image so that the operator knows the vessel from which the Doppler information is being obtained and what portion of the flow within the vessel is being monitored (Fig. 1.3). Table 1.2 indicates the relationship between echo arrival time and corresponding depth. Table 1.3 presents the relationship between the spatial gate length and the time that the gate is on. For example, echoes from the center of a vessel located 3 cm from the surface would arrive 39.0 μs after pulse generation. To monitor the central 2 mm of flow in the vessel, the gate would open at 37.7 μs and close at 40.3 μs. If the vessel diameter is 4 mm, the gate must open at 36.4 μs and close at 41.6 μs in order to receive echoes from all the flow across the vessel. However, no echoes from outside the vessel would pass through the receiver.

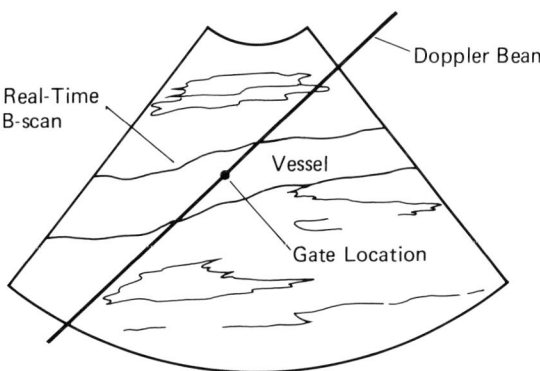

Fig. 1.3. The display of a duplex instrument combines the anatomic image with Doppler beam indicator and gate location. The Doppler receiver gate depth can be located visually inside a vessel. (From Kremkau F: Diagnostic Ultrasound: Principles, Instrumentation, and Exercises. Orlando, Grune & Stratton, Inc., 1984. Reprinted with permission.)

Table 1.2. Echo Arrival Time (t) for Various Reflector Depths (d)

d (cm)	t (μs)
0.5	6.5
1.0	13.0
2.0	26.0
4.0	52.0
8.0	104
15.0	195
20.0	260

Equipment

Duplex instruments of three types are available — mechanical, phased array, and linear array. The mechanical type uses a rotating group of transducers for imaging but must stop the transducers in order to use one of them for acquisition of Doppler information. The phased array type produces a sector scan for imaging by electronically phasing the voltages applied to the transducer array. A Doppler pulse can be transmitted from the same array in any desired direction by proper phasing. Thus, Doppler pulses can be interspersed between groups of imaging pulses producing apparent simultaneous acquisition and display of both anatomic and flow information. The linear array transducer assembly has a separate Doppler transducer mounted at the end of the array such that the Doppler pulses travel across the image plane. Again, because no mechanical motion must be interrupted, apparent simultaneous (ie, interspersed pulse) presentation is achieved.

Because the blood cells are not all moving uniformly (at the same speed) in vessels (particularly smaller ones; Fig. 1.4), several Doppler shift frequencies are found in the returning echoes. The sounds heard from the loudspeaker

Table 1.3. Spatial Gate Length (L) for Various Temporal Gate Lengths (T)*

T (μs)	L (mm)
1.3	1
2.6	2
6.5	5
13.0	10

*Time from gate turn-on to turn-off.

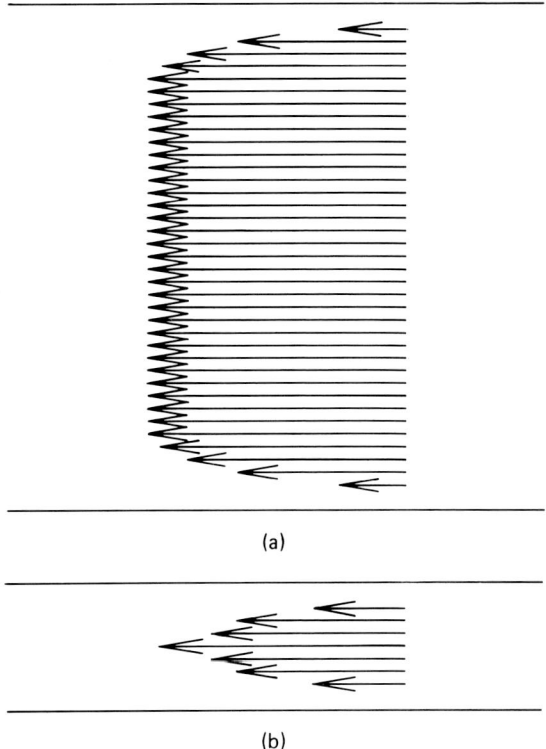

Fig. 1.4a,b. The flow profile is more uniform in a large-diameter vessel (a) than it is in a small one (b).

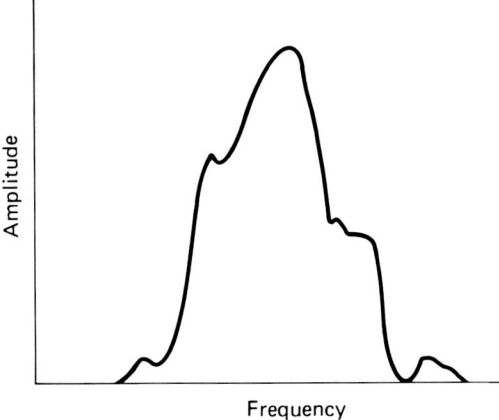

Fig. 1.5. Frequency spectrum plot of the amplitude of each Doppler frequency component present in the returning echoes. Many frequencies are present because of the distribution of flow speed (Fig. 1.4) encountered by the pulse in the gate region. (From Kremkau F: Diagnostic Ultrasound: Principles, Instrumentation, and Exercises. Orlando, Grune & Stratton, 1984. Reprinted with permission.)

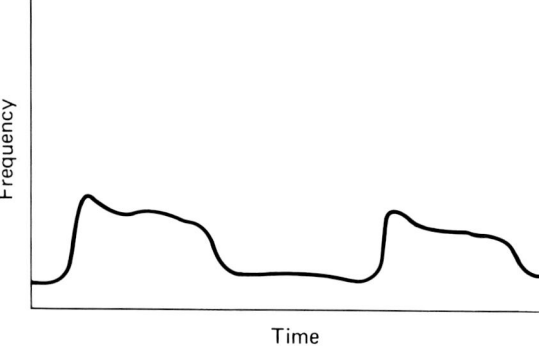

Fig. 1.6. Display of Doppler spectrum as a function of time (cardiac cycle). (From Kremkau F: Diagnostic Ultrasound: Principles, Instrumentation, and Exercises. Orlando, Grune & Stratton, 1984. Reprinted with permission.)

are a combination of many frequencies and do not appear as a pure tone. These frequencies may be presented visually on a spectral display of frequency versus amplitude as shown in Figure 1.5. For venous flow this presentation would remain fairly constant with time. However, for arterial flow, which is pulsatile, the flow increases during systole and decreases during diastole. Therefore, the presentation in Figure 1.5 would continually be oscillating right (during systole) and left (during diastole), that is, as flow increases (systole), Doppler shift increases, and as it decreases (diastole), Doppler shift decreases. The character of this flow variation over cardiac cycle is useful information and can be presented as a function of time as shown in Figure 1.6. Here the Doppler shift frequencies are presented on the vertical axis with time on the horizontal. The amplitude or strength of each frequency component at any instant of time is presented in gray scale or color so that this third item of information can be presented on the two-dimensional display.

In a pulsed-Doppler system, each Doppler shift frequency is built in the instrument from samples of it that are obtained from the pulses interacting with the moving blood cell. This is therefore a sampling system from which the Doppler shift frequency must be derived. In any sampling system if the sampling rate is too low, an incorrect frequency will result (Fig. 1.7). This phenomenon is known as aliasing, and it occurs if the pulse repetition frequency is less than two times the correct Doppler shift frequency. In other words, it will occur if the flow is so great that Doppler shift exceeds half the pulse repetition frequency of the instrument. When this

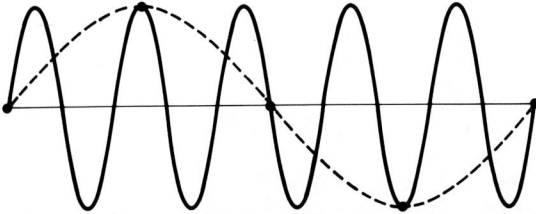

Fig. 1.7. Aliasing occurs when the Doppler shift frequency is undersampled in a pulsed system. Here only one sample (•) occurs each cycle, resulting in derived frequency (*dashed line*) much lower than the true Doppler shift (*solid line*).

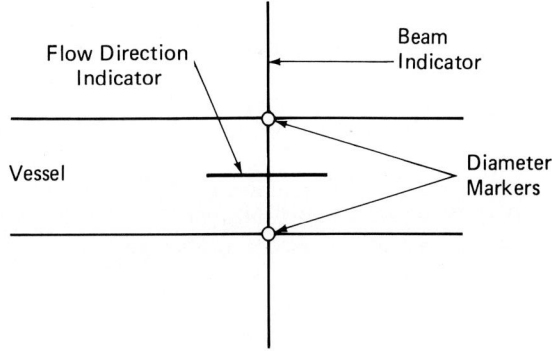

Fig. 1.8. A duplex Doppler instrument display usually has operator-controllable indicators for flow direction and vessel diameter.

occurs the presentation on the spectral display flips over so that positive flow that exceeds the sampling limit appears negative and negative flow that exceeds the sampling limit appears positive (9). To avoid this one might think that the pulse repetition frequency could simply be increased so that it would always be at least double the highest Doppler shift frequency encountered. Unfortunately, at high pulse repetition frequencies, the range ambiguity artifact is encountered (10). This occurs when a subsequent pulse is transmitted before all the echoes have been received from a previous pulse. To avoid aliasing, pulse repetition frequency should be increased. To avoid range ambiguity artifact, pulse repetition should be decreased. High flow rates in superficial vessels can usually be handled satisfactorily with high pulse repetition frequencies. Low flow rates in deep vessels can be handled satisfactorily with low pulse repetition frequencies. The conflict arises when one encounters high flow rates at depth. In this case aliasing can only be avoided by going to continuous wave Doppler. However, continuous wave Doppler has no depth selectivity capability.

The presentation of flow data as a function of time can be as shown in Figure 1.6, in which the vertical axis represents Doppler shift. Alternatively, the vertical axis can represent reflector speed (cm/s) or volume flow (next paragraph). This requires an accurate incorporation of angle into the calculation. Instruments provide means for the operator to enter assumed direction of flow (Fig. 1.8) using the presentation of vessel walls on the anatomic image. Flow is normally assumed parallel to the vessel walls.

Volume flow (mL/s) can be calculated from mean speed multiplied by vessel cross-sectional area. To do this correctly, the various Doppler shifts representing the cells moving at various speeds must be averaged properly, the angle properly accounted for to convert mean Doppler shift to mean speed, and area correctly determined from a vessel diameter measurement aided by the operator (Fig. 1.8) and assuming circular cross-section. Obviously, several things could go wrong in this process, yielding faulty results.

Summary

Duplex sonography combines real-time imaging with pulsed Doppler. This permits flow information to be obtained from known anatomic locations. Flow information is derived from the Doppler shifts produced by blood cell (reflector) motion. It is presented audibly and visually. The visual presentation of the flow data as a function of time aids the audible analysis of the Doppler information and allows assessment of normal and abnormal flow conditions.

References

1. Kremkau F: Diagnostic Ultrasound: Principles, Instrumentation, and Exercises. Orlando, Grune & Stratton, 1984.
2. Powis R, Powis W: A Thinker's Guide to Ultrasonic Imaging. Baltimore, Urban & Schwarzenberg, 1984.
3. Hykes D, Hedrick W, Starchman D: Ultrasound Physics and Instrumentation. New York, Churchill Livingstone, 1985.

4. Hussey M: Basic Physics and Technology of Medical Diagnostic Ultrasound. New York, Elsevier, 1985.
5. McDicken W: Diagnostic Ultrasonics: Principles and Use of Instruments. New York, Wiley & Sons, 1981.
6. Hill C: Physical Principles of Medical Ultrasonics. Chichester, Ellis Horwood, 1986.
7. Atkinson P, Woodcock J: Doppler Ultrasound and Its Use in Clinical Measurement. New York, Academic Press, 1982.
8. Wells P: Biomedical Ultrasonics. New York, Academic Press, 1977.
9. Bom K, de Boo J, Rijsterborgh H: On the aliasing problem in pulsed doppler cardiac studies. J Clin Ultrasound 12:559, 1984.
10. Goldstein A: Range ambiguities in real-time ultrasound. J Clin Ultrasound 9:83, 1981.

2
Duplex Sonography of the Cerebrovascular System

EDWARD G. GRANT

Atherosclerosis is undoubtedly the single most important affliction of the industrialized world. Coronary artery disease is the most frequent cause of death and disability in the United States, and the effect of cerebrovascular atherosclerosis is probably almost as great. The most serious manifestation of cerebrovascular atherosclerosis is stroke. Ranking as the third most common cause of death in the United States, stroke is also the cause for the disability of an additional 1 to 2 million people (1–3). Stroke has long been associated with hemiparesis, aphasia, and even death. Other classic manifestations of cerebrovascular atherosclerosis include transient ischemic attacks (TIAs) and amaurosis fugax. The former is typified by a totally reversible focal neurologic defect originating in an appropriate portion of the brain and the latter is the result of ischemia, or more typically, embolic phenomena in the retinal artery. The importance of TIAs and amaurosis fugax lies less in the effect of the immediate episode than in the ominous heralding of impending stroke. While certain risk factors such as family history, hypertension, obesity, or diabetes mellitus single out a portion of the population who are predisposed to atherosclerotic disease (4), the occurrence of a TIA increases the patient's likelihood of having a stroke within 5 years by threefold (2).

Although atherosclerosis may affect the intracranial vessels directly, it is far more commonly encountered in the extracranial portions of the arteries that supply the brain. Depending on the exact makeup of the population (5), the origins of as many as 88% of all cases of amaurosis fugax or TIAs can be traced to one very important juncture, the carotid bifurcation (6). At present, this concept is so firmly ingrained that it is difficult to imagine that only recently has the association between atherosclerosis at the carotid bifurcation and stroke been appreciated. Chiari (7), in 1904, and Hunt (8), in 1914, suggested that carotid disease might be linked to pathologic events in the brain. This theory, however, went largely unheeded until almost half a century later when Fisher (9) began to investigate the apparent lack of middle cerebral artery thrombosis in stroke patients. He noted that "no source of embolism could be found in the conventional location, the pulmonary veins, the left auricle, the left ventricle, or the ascending aorta" (10). In a series of classic reports (9–12) he demonstrated the now well-known association between carotid bifurcation disease and cerebrovascular accidents. The work of Fisher slowly began to change the accepted concepts surrounding cerebrovascular disease.

The carotid bifurcation became the true focus of attention in the 1950s (13–15) when the surgical community realized that atherosclerotic lesions could be removed from this site, resulting in improvement or total cessation of TIAs or amaurosis fugax. Although surgical techniques were improved (2) and intense research lead to a better understanding of the etiology of carotid disease, its diagnosis has remained somewhat more elusive. In some cases clinical history alone may single out patients with significant carotid disease. The strong correlation between classic TIA symptoms or amaurosis fugax and carotid atherosclerosis is well established (5,6). Other clinical manifestations of bifurcation disease, however, may be

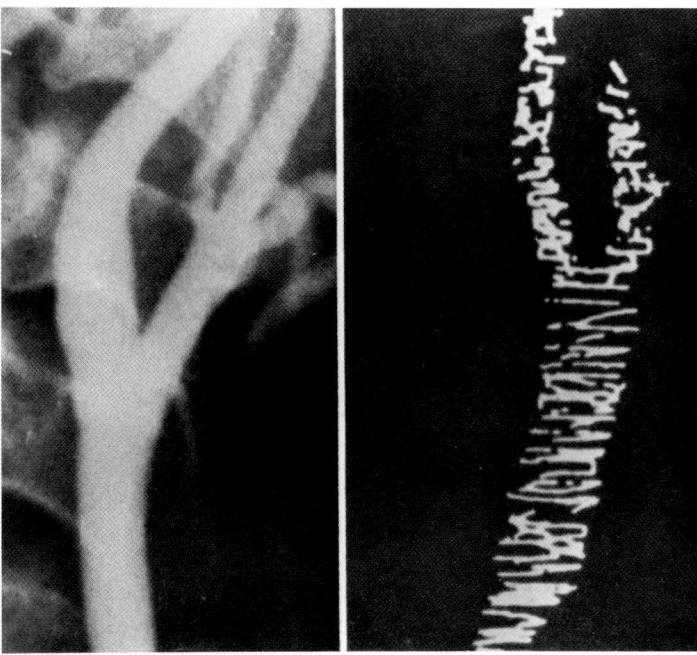

Fig. 2.1. "Doppler angiography" — Movement of mechanized Doppler probe over neck produced lines in areas of returning signal resulting in anatomic image comparable to arteriogram on left. Although relatively sophisticated, pitfalls in interpretation were numerous and accuracy not sufficient to result in widespread application. From Block S, et al: Reliability of Doppler Scanning of the Carotid Bifurcation Angiographic Correlation. Radiology 132:687, 1979. Reprinted with permission.

less easily defined, such as atypical TIAs, symptoms more commonly associated with vertebrobasilar atherosclerosis, and, of course, the cervical bruit. Although arteriography remains the "gold standard" for the detection of carotid atherosclerosis and is imperative before undertaking endarterectomy, it is nonetheless a highly invasive procedure. The risks of modern arteriography are relatively small (16,17), but older patients with significant atherosclerosis have the highest rate of complication (18). Carotid arteriography is not to be recommended without a high suspicion of identifying a significant and hopefully correctable lesion. History and physical examination are simply not sufficiently exact when it comes to the identification of carotid disease. In an effort to decrease the number of negative arteriograms, a host of "noninvasive" examinations have been developed over the years.

Noninvasive evaluations of the extracranial carotid arteries have typically been divided into two categories, direct and indirect. Direct examinations are aimed specifically at the carotid bifurcation. Indirect techniques imply bifurcation disease by identifying abnormal physiology elsewhere, usually in one of the collateral pathways around the eye. Direct noninvasive techniques offer the advantage of specifically localizing the offending lesion to the carotid bifurcation. Unfortunately, they may be ineffective in identifying disease elsewhere, such as at the carotid siphon or within the brain itself. Indirect carotid examinations, on the other hand, rely on abnormal flow to the brain and ideally, would identify all flow-limiting lesions regardless of location. The most widely used indirect examinations include oculoplethysmography (OPG) and periorbital Doppler. Aside from the inability to localize lesions, indirect methods are troubled by the inability to accurately identify bilateral disease and to imply luminal narrowing which does not markedly restrict carotid flow (19,20).

Among both direct and indirect noninvasive techniques, the most extensive research has probably been into the use of Doppler technology. A multitude of often complex adaptions have been devised. Even the possibilities of "Doppler angiography" (Fig. 2.1) were explored (21). Of the many seemingly sophisticated Doppler examinations available, most failed to correctly identify a sufficient percent of lesions to have brought about widespread use. One effort to improve the diagnostic capabilities of Doppler coupled it to real-time ultrasound imaging resulting in what Barber et al (22) termed duplex scanning. Only very slowly did duplex scanning begin to evolve into a viable noninvasive modality with which to evaluate the carotid bifurcation. Originally, the addition of real-time technology to Doppler was envisioned as a method of improving Doppler localization. The beam could be directed, and flow samples could be obtained from one *known* point within the carotid system. The real-time moiety was considered more of a road map than a synergistic diagnostic tool. As real-time technology improved, however, it became apparent that it had anatomic imaging capabilities that were complementary to the physiologic information provided by Doppler. Investigation into the possibilities of real-time evaluation of carotid disease continues. Its role, however, seems to be expanding as more information becomes available about plaque morphology and the natural evolution of carotid atherosclerosis.

Both Doppler and real-time contribute significantly to the diagnostic success of duplex sonography. In the carotid arteries, however, this coupling is particularly effective because each of the two components of the duplex system helps to overcome the deficiencies of its counterpart. The Doppler portion of duplex is particularly accurate in identifying hemodynamically significant, stenotic lesions (23–29). The real-time examination, on the other hand, seems to lose accuracy as the stenoses become tighter (30). Conversely, at least in our hands, nonrate-limiting lesions (those narrowing the lumen less than 50%) are frequently very difficult to quantify using Doppler alone; in this area, modern high-resolution real-time technology seems to work best (25). Further work is needed to fully exploit the potentials of Duplex ultrasound in the carotids. The Doppler component seems quite well established in its ability to detect hemodynamically significant disease. Criteria are available using various types of Duplex equipment, and, overall, experienced users seem capable of identifying 90% or more of rate-limiting stenoses (23–29). The role of the real-time component, beyond acting as a road map for the Doppler, is presently less well defined. As true high-resolution real-time technology has only been available for a brief time, it seems logical that this component may play a greater role in the future. Real-time sonographic evaluation of the carotids provides information that is available through no other means aside from examining the surgical or autopsy specimen. In some regards it even surpasses arteriography, which has no way of depicting events beyond the vessel lumen. The significance of plaque composition, intraplaque hemorrhage, minimal vessel wall thickening, or plaque morphology are poorly understood to date. In the future, plaque evaluation may tell of impending vascular events, but such information will only be available after years of follow-up study.

Technical Aspects of Cerebrovascular Duplex Scanning

Innumerable methods of scanning the extracranial cerebral arteries undoubtedly exist. Because Duplex sonography is a real-time examination, the possibilities are almost limitless. Even the method of archiving the examination can vary considerably. In some institutions, the examination is videotaped; the entire real-time sequence is stored for later use. Although we occasionally videotape real-time examinations (or in some cases, wish we had), we tend to rely heavily on a series of hardcopy images. In an effort to achieve some form of standardization, real-time images and corresponding Doppler spectra are usually taken from specific places within the right and left carotid system, including the proximal, mid-, and distal common carotid artery; the carotid bulb; and the internal and external carotid arteries. Because of the extreme importance of the internal carotid arteries, multiple hardcopy images of this vessel are usually preserved, depending on the length of the internal carotid artery (ICA) that can be examined. In selected patients, evaluation of the proximal vertebral and subclavian arteries is included in the examination as well.

Before proceeding, the reader must become acquainted with the two major Doppler flow patterns encountered in the neck and throughout the body. Doppler spectral analysis is merely a reflection of red blood cell velocity, and the speed at which blood flows is influenced by numerous factors. Most important among these factors is, obviously, cardiac output. Normally, a rapid rise in red cell velocity occurs throughout the body with each systolic contraction; this forward velocity then decreases or ceases altogether as diastole progresses. If arterial blood flow were entirely dependent on the action of the heart, red cell velocity would be the same in all parts of the body at any given point in the cardiac cycle. Needless to say, the heart does have a dramatic effect on arterial blood flow. The Doppler waveforms, for example, of patients with aortic regurgitation are very unusual. Almost as important as the heart, however, is the effect of the distal arteriolar runoff. Two distinctly different flow patterns are encountered throughout the body as a result of the resistance in the distal vasculature. Low resistance vascular beds are generally those of blood-hungry organs such as the brain, liver, or kidneys. These organs require large quantities of blood, and the arteries supplying them primarily act as conduits. The internal carotid and hepatic and renal arteries are all typical examples. Although differences exist, flow in all of these low-resistance vessels follows a *diphasic* or low-resistance pattern—a relatively slow rise with systole and a gradual decrease as diastole progresses. The unique feature of the normal diphasic waveform is the fact that flow never reaches zero; even at end diastole, forward flow continues. The Doppler spectrum never returns to base line (Fig. 2.2 A).

The Doppler signature of high-resistance vessels is somewhat more complex. These vessels supply the vascular beds of the muscular structures of the body. The aorta and subclavian and ilio-femoral artery systems are typical examples. Likewise, the external carotid artery supplies the muscular structures of the face and exhibits a typical high-resistance Doppler signature. Flow in these arteries is always under considerable pressure; the blood flow has a much "snappier" quality than its low-resistance counterpart. Blood velocity rises sharply during systole and falls rapidly with cessation of the cardiac contraction. The normal high-resistance system is also quite elastic; the high arterial end pressure sets up a rebound phenomenon that is its signature. Blood flow actually reverses for a short time after systole. During the remainder of the cardiac cycle no foreward flow occurs and the Doppler signal, therefore, remains on the baseline. This high-resistance flow pattern of the muscular arteries throughout the body results in a triphasic waveform (Fig. 2.2 B).

The two typical modes of blood flow just described are extremely important in all types of Doppler examinations. To some degree they may be used to identify almost any vessel of the body. This distinction is, however, of the utmost importance in the carotid system. Using Doppler alone, the experienced operator should be capable of definitively distinguishing the ICA from the external carotid artery (ECA). Surprisingly, the real-time differentiation of these two vessels can be very difficult or even impossible. Careful evaluation of the Doppler signature of the vessels at the carotid bifurcation is essential if they are to be correctly identified.

We begin a carotid duplex examination by evaluating the most proximal portion of the right common carotid artery (CCA) that can be seen. Practically speaking, we usually locate the mid- to lower portion of the common carotid in an easily accessible part of the neck and move the scan head proximally until it is blocked by the clavicle. Evaluation of the proximal CCA is facilitated by using a wide-angled sector scanner. This type of scan head should enable the operator to identify the CCA-subclavian junction in almost every patient. Because the subclavian artery is sectioned transversely when the scan plane is oriented through the long axis of the CCA, the subclavian artery frequently appears like a bulbous tip at the bottom of the CCA (Fig. 2.3 A–D). The CCA-subclavian junction, therefore, has a relatively distinctive real-time appearance. In addition, the Doppler spectra of the two vessels should be quite different almost right from their origins. The subclavian is a typical muscular artery and should have a sharp triphasic waveform. The CCA, on the other hand, delivers most of its blood to the brain and has diphasic flow in normal patients. The difference in the waveforms of these two vessels should be immediately apparent. The proximal CCA, however, often continues to reflect its origin from the aorta-innominate artery and may produce triphasic waveforms with a moderate amount of turbulence. Real-time images and Doppler spectra should be carefully evaluated at the carotid subclavian junction because significant stenoses may occasionally occur at this point (Fig. 2.4 A–C).

The examination of the CCA is usually relatively simple. The CCA typically bows anteriorly in the lower neck then follows a more or less

Fig. 2.2A,B. Normal Doppler spectra—Diphasic, internal, or common carotid waveform (**A**) shows relatively slow systolic rise, a prominent dicrotic notch, and forward flow throughout diastole. The area beneath the curve is called the "sonic window" or envelope. With normal laminar flow the sonic window should be clear as all red blood cells are traveling at the same speed. Triphasic waveform from subclavian or external carotid has rapid systolic rise and prominent flow reversal phase. Forward flow is absent during diastole.

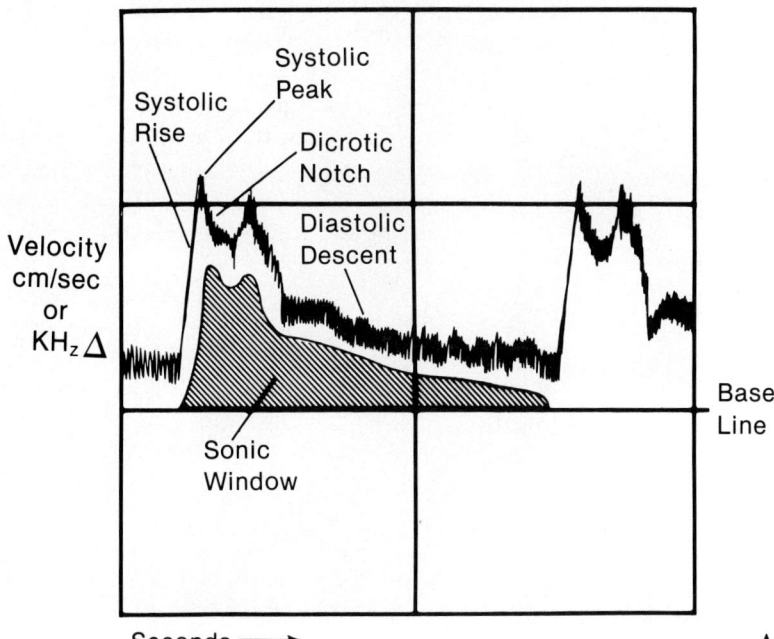

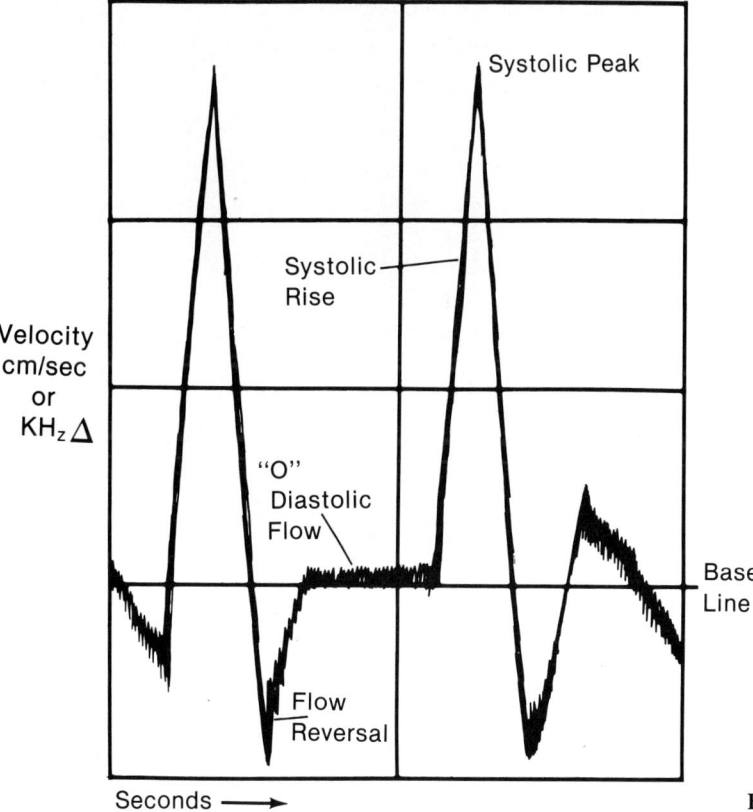

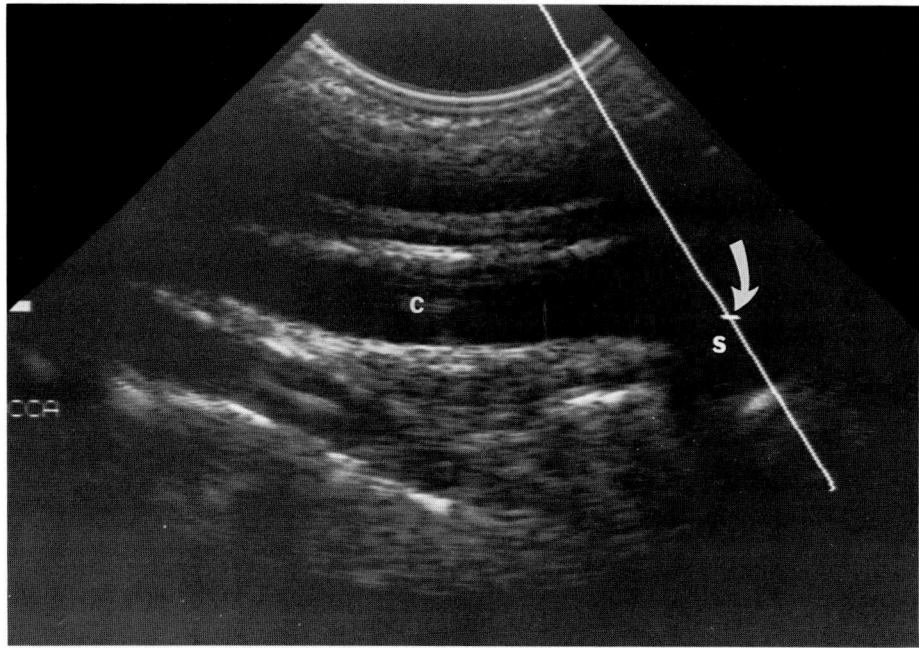

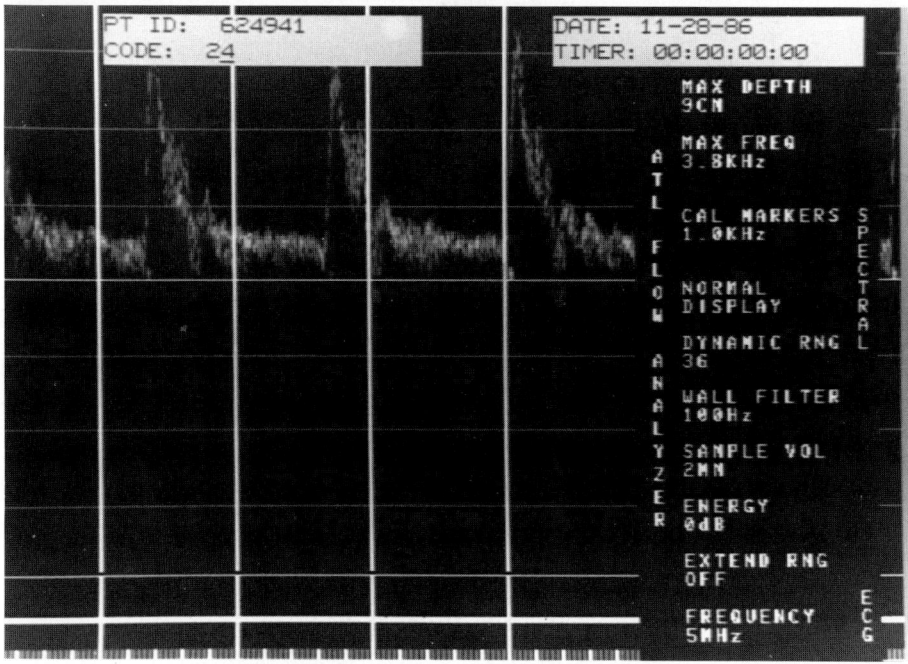

Fig. 2.3A–D. Common carotid artery-subclavian junction—**A**. Bulbous enlargement at the base of the common carotid artery (C) represents the subclavian artery (S) sectioned transversely. Cursor (*curved arrow*) in subclavian artery produces triphasic waveform (**B**). **C**. Same patient, cursor (*curved arrow*) now in CCA (C); note appearance of diphasic signal (**D**). Mild spectral broadening is present in diastole; flow turbulence is often present in the proximal common carotid artery.

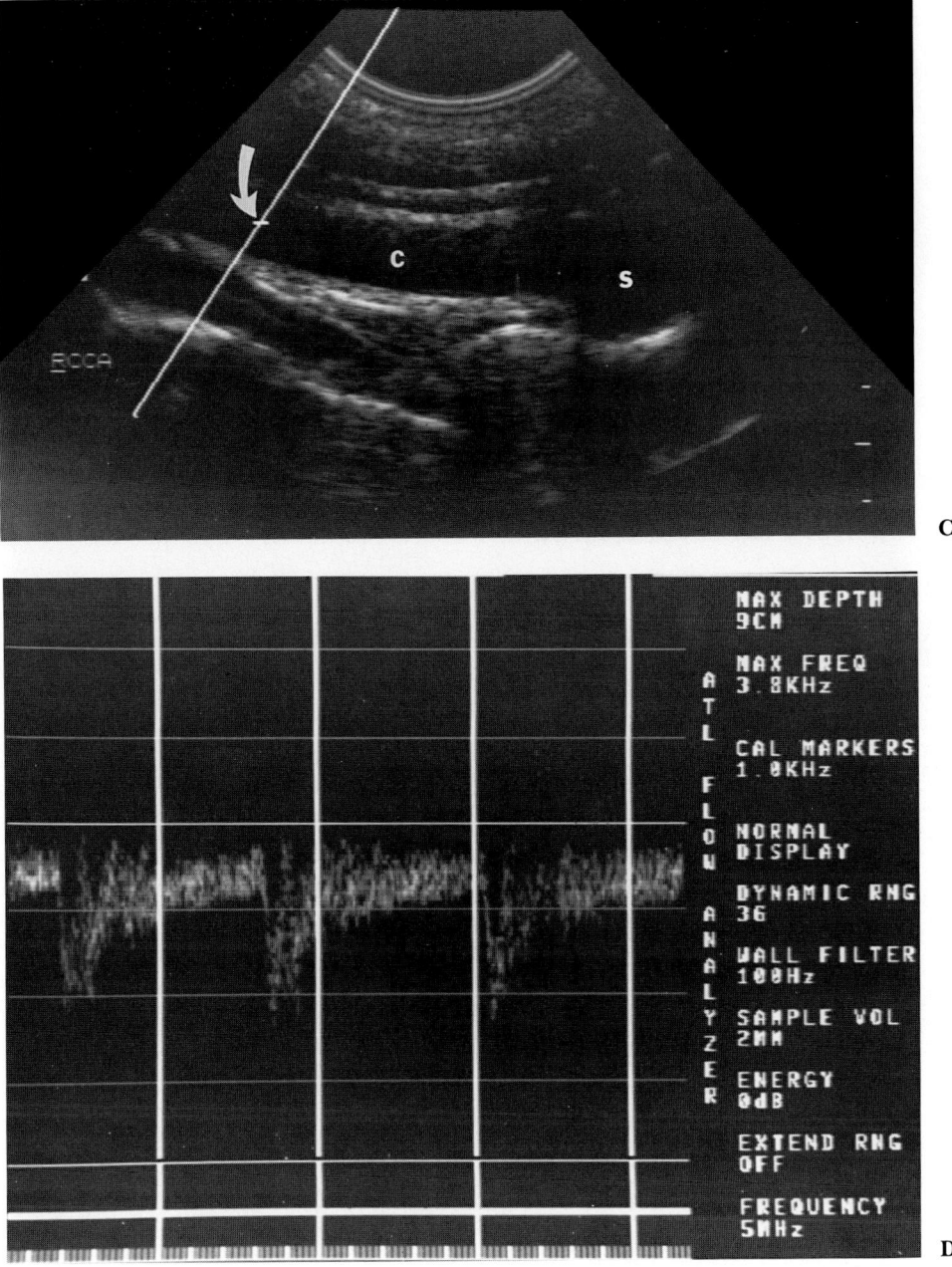

Fig. 2.3.

straight course to the carotid bulb. Although, in an occasional patient, the CCA may be very tortuous. The carotid bulb is usually imaged as a widening of the CCA. The bulb should be clearly identified and in addition to being scrutinized for evidence of intrinsic atherosclerotic disease, it should be used as an essential anatomic landmark.

The evaluation of the common carotid artery can be adequately performed in a brief period of time; the vessel is large and easily visualized. It normally lies lateral to the thyroid and deep to the jugular vein and sternocleidomastoid muscle (Fig. 2.5 A,B). The common carotid artery is not frequently involved with hemodynamically significant atherosclerotic lesions.

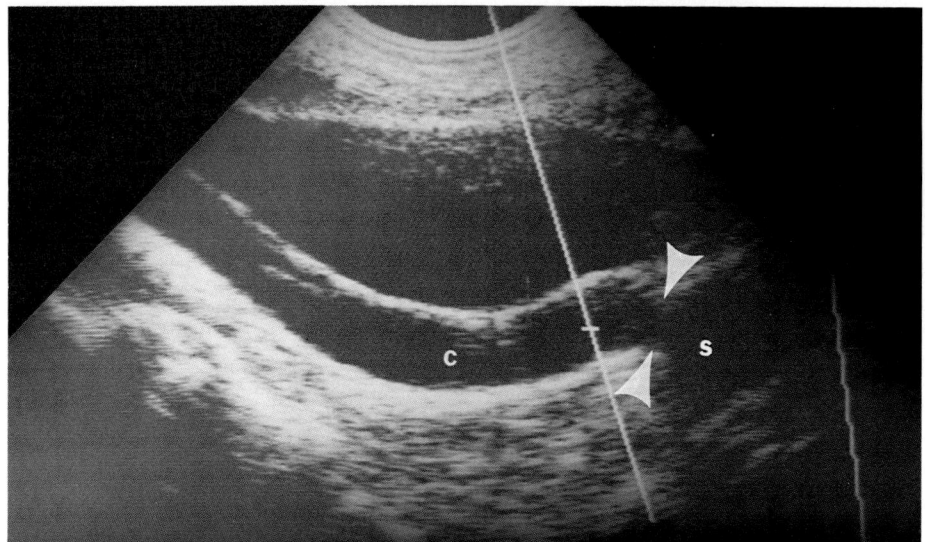
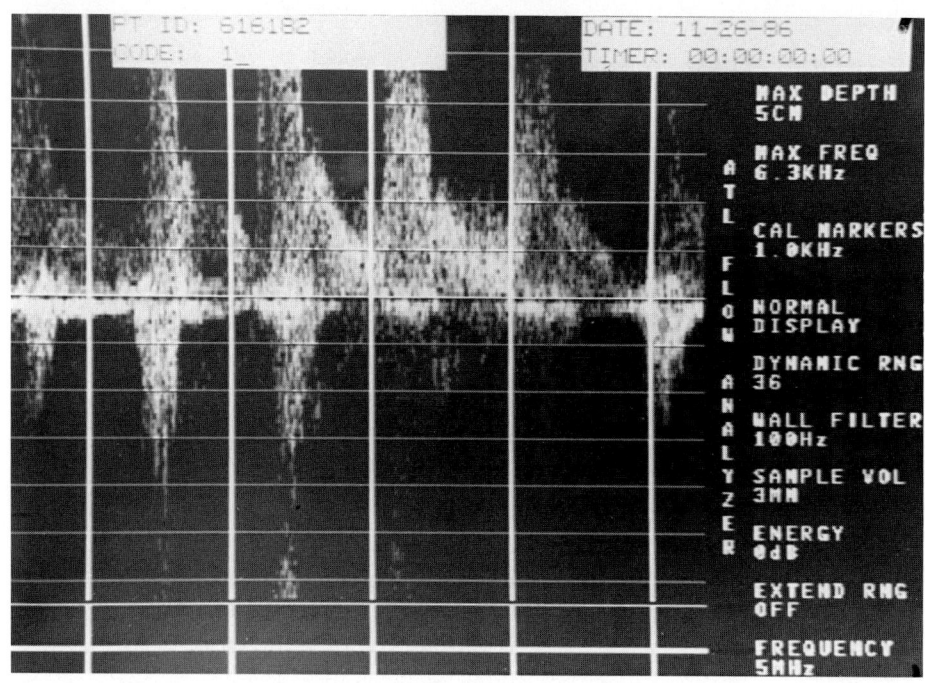

Fig. 2.4A,B. Common carotid artery-subclavian stenosis — real-time image (**A**) suggests narrowing (*arrowheads*) at junction of CCA (C) and subclavian artery (S). Doppler spectra (**B**) are markedly abnormal.

Typically, scattered plaque or long, smooth, fibrofatty deposits will be found. Occasionally, plaque will be encountered that narrows the lumen more than 50% by real-time inspection, whereas the Doppler spectra remain normal. Possibly because of the large size of the common carotid artery, however, moderate stenoses, seem to produce relatively less Doppler abnormality in the CCA or bulb than they do in the ICA. The operator must be aware of this phenomenon and occasionally check lumen size with transverse image (Fig. 2.6 *A–E*).

In most patients, even those with severe atherosclerosis, the scanner may be rapidly moved up the neck. Doppler samples may be obtained as one advances, or the cursor may

Fig. 2.5A,B. Normal common carotid artery—Magnified transverse real-time image (**A**) of right CCA. Blocking sound beam in center of neck is shadow caused by air in trachea (T). Between trachea and common carotid artery (C) lies the homogeneously gray thyroid (Tr). Lateral to the carotid is the jugular vein (J). Anterior portion of sternocleidomastoid muscle (S) separates vessels from transducer. Arrow points to longus colli muscle. Longitudinal section of CCA (**B**) shows a 4-cm portion of artery in one image. Entire vessel lies at relatively constant angle with transducer. Doppler cursor may, therefore, be moved along the CCA quickly (*arrow*).

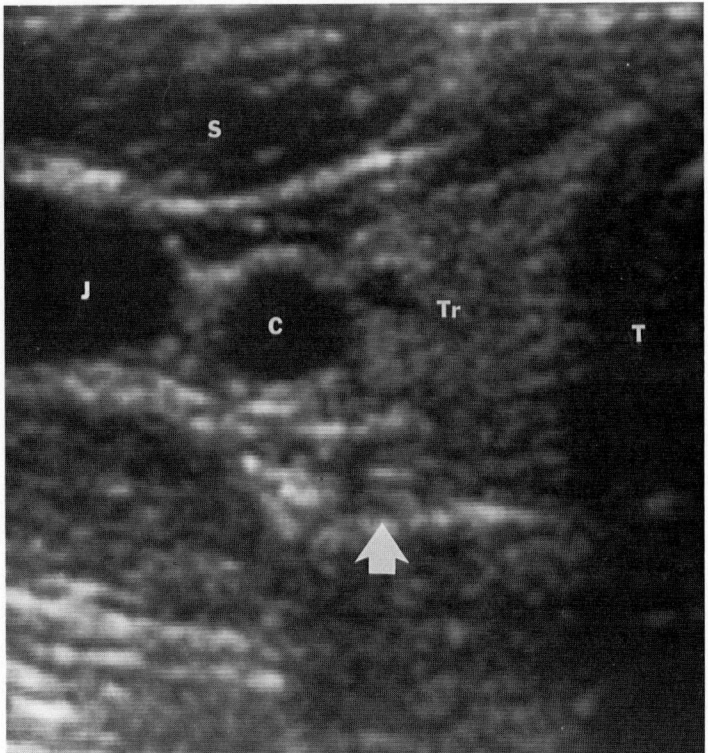

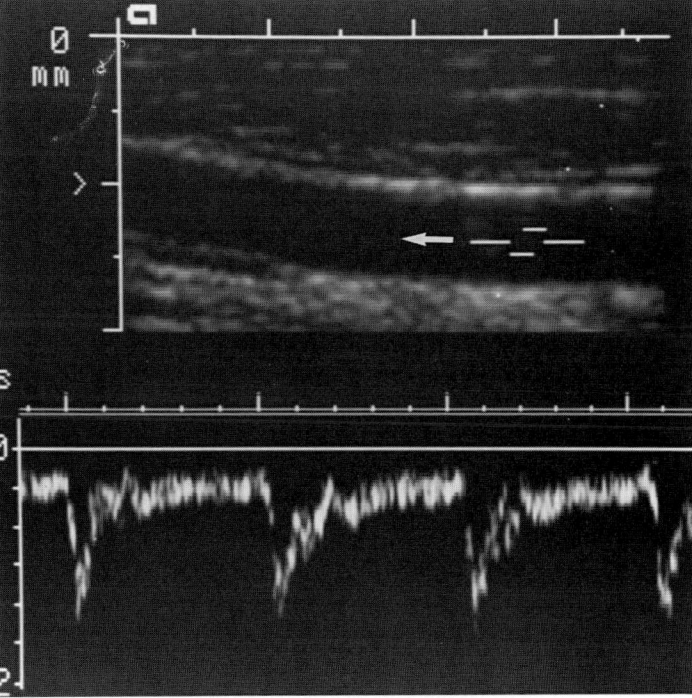

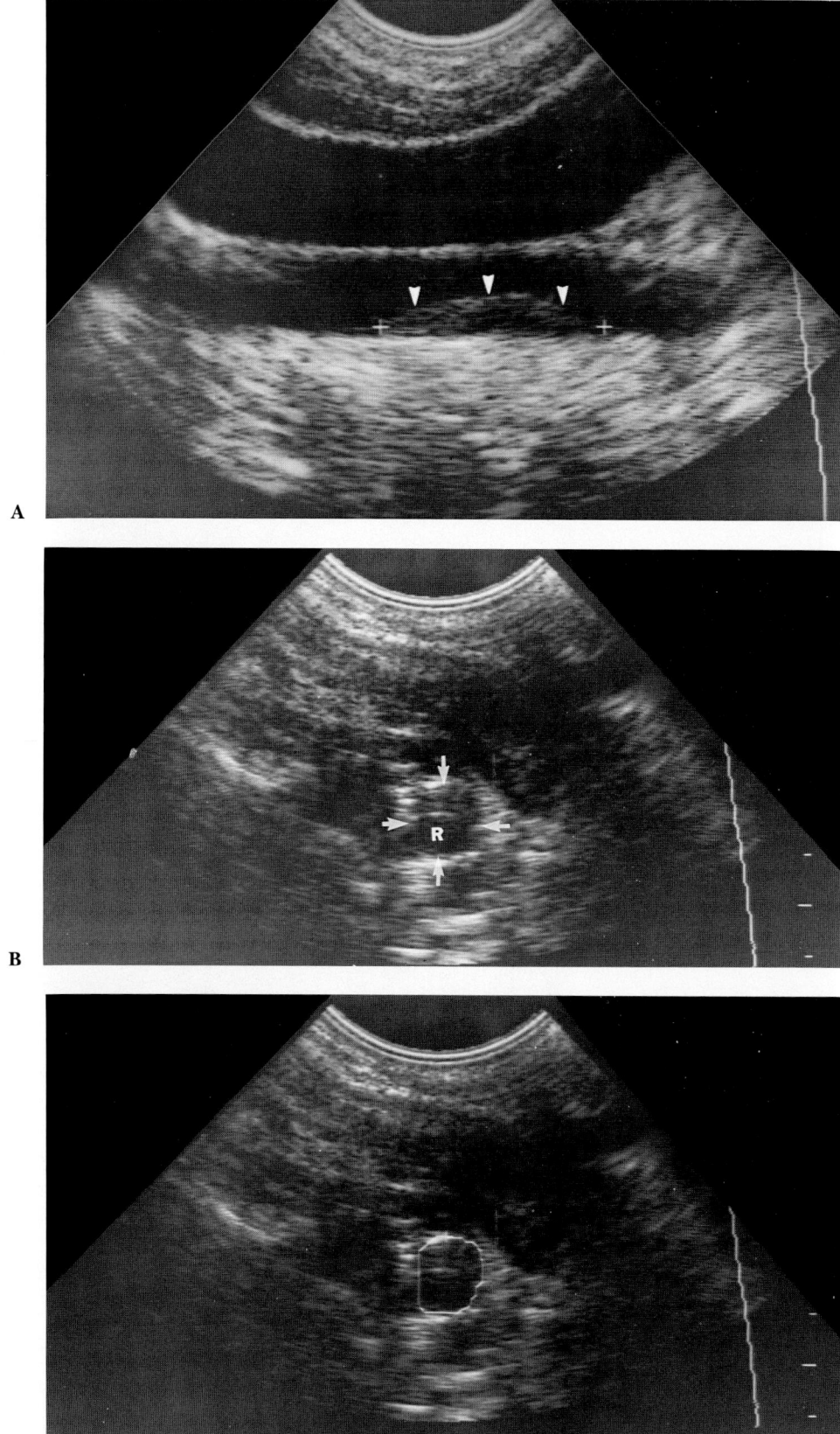

Fig. 2.6.

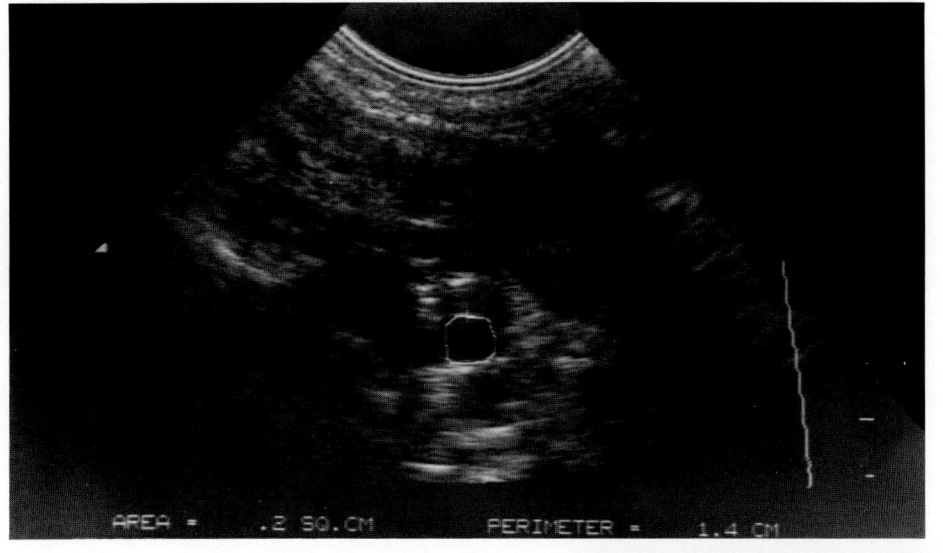

Fig. 2.6. A–E. Moderate narrowing of CCA—Longitudinal image (**A**) depicts long, smooth fibrofatty plaque (*arrowheads*) in CCA. Transverse image (**B**) gives more adequate impression of degree of luminal narrowing. R = residual lumen, arrows outline vessel. Area plots of outer vessel (**C**) and residual lumen (**D**) are often of value in assessing the degree of narrowing. Longitudinal image was taken while scanning from behind sternocleidomastoid. Transverse images were made from anterior neck. Arteriogram confirms long, smooth area of luminal compromise (*black arrows*).

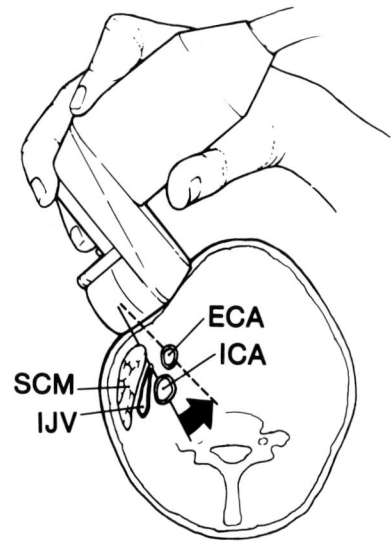 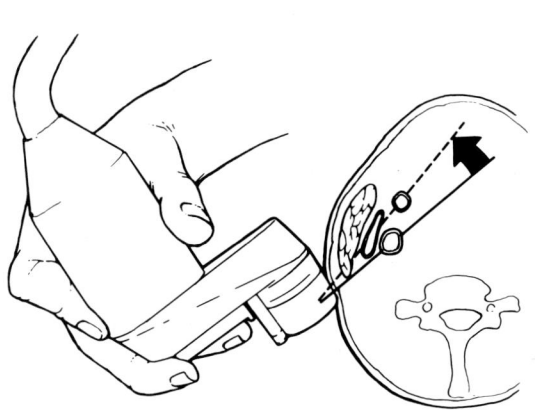

Fig. 2.7A,B. Orientation of transducer—Scanning may be performed from either anterior (**A**) or posterior (**B**) to sternocleidomastoid muscle (SCM). With minimal transducer pressure, the internal jugular vein (IJV) is often flattened and not visible. Slight changes in transducer angulation will usually bring the ICA or ECA separately into the scan plane. From Grant EG: Duplex ultrasonography: Its expanding role in noninvasive vascular diagnosis. Med Clin North America 23:563, W.B. Saunders, 1985. Reprinted with permission.

be positioned in the most proximal part of the CCA visible and moved distally through the scanning field. The latter is particularly easy with longer, linear array transducers (see Fig. 2.4*B*). Depending on the position of the bifurcation, the carotid bulb should be encountered rapidly. It is at this point that the major work begins.

The carotid bulb should be evident as a mild widening of the common carotid artery. Scanning distal to the bulb in a small minority of patients, both the ICA and the ECA will come into view in the same section (see Fig. 2.8 *D*). In the majority of patients, however, first one vessel then the other will be identified as the operator fans the ultrasound beam from medial to lateral (Fig. 2.7 *A, B*). For reasons not entirely clear, scanning at the bifurcation is almost always better accomplished from a posterior orientation than from an anterior (Fig. 2.8 *A, B*). In general, we conduct routine scanning from the back of the neck, behind the sternocleidomastoid. This is even done in the CCA although it is less essential. At the bifurcation, it is very unusual to be able to scan to good advantage with the transducer anterior to the sternocleidomastoid. Because most scanning is done from a posterior orientation, the ICA will be typically located closer to the scan head and, therefore, above the ECA in most of our images. I might add that in

Fig. 2.8A–D. Normal carotid bifurcations—Transverse image (**A**) shows that ICA (I) and ECA (E) lie beside each other. Longitudinal sections (**B** and **C**) show a larger vessel, which bows somewhat anteriorly (**B**). Diphasic Doppler spectra identify this vessel as the ICA. Scanning more medially, a second vessel is identified (**C**). This vessel courses more posteriorly. Posterior vessel is almost as large as its counterpart and has mild widening at the base simulating ampullary region usually associated with ICA. Triphasic Doppler spectra confirm that this vessel is the ECA. Ideal bifurcation (**D**) shows both ICA (I) and ECA (E) arising from CCA (C). Note normal ampullary widening (A) at origin of ICA (see p. 20).

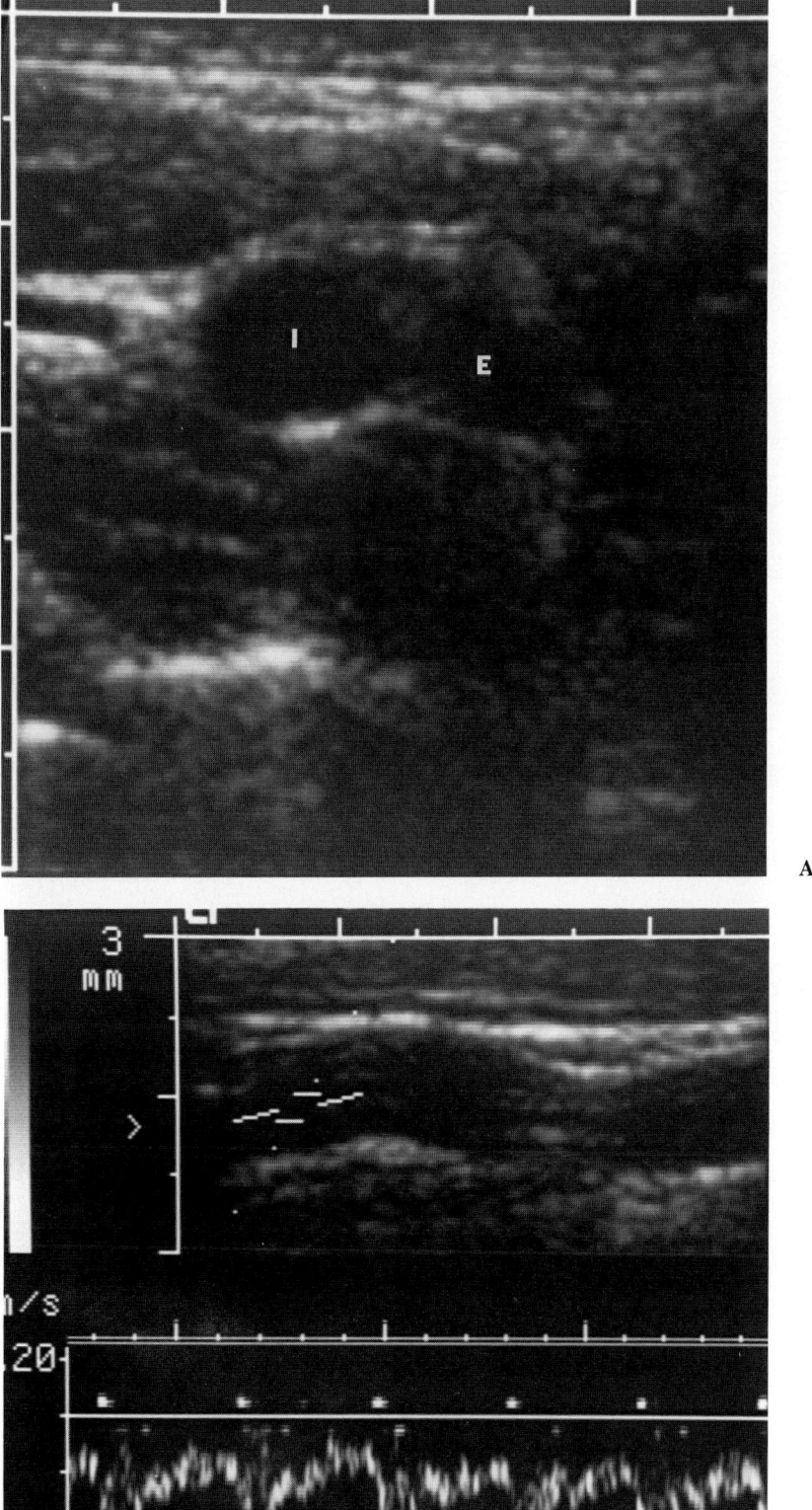

Fig. 2.8.

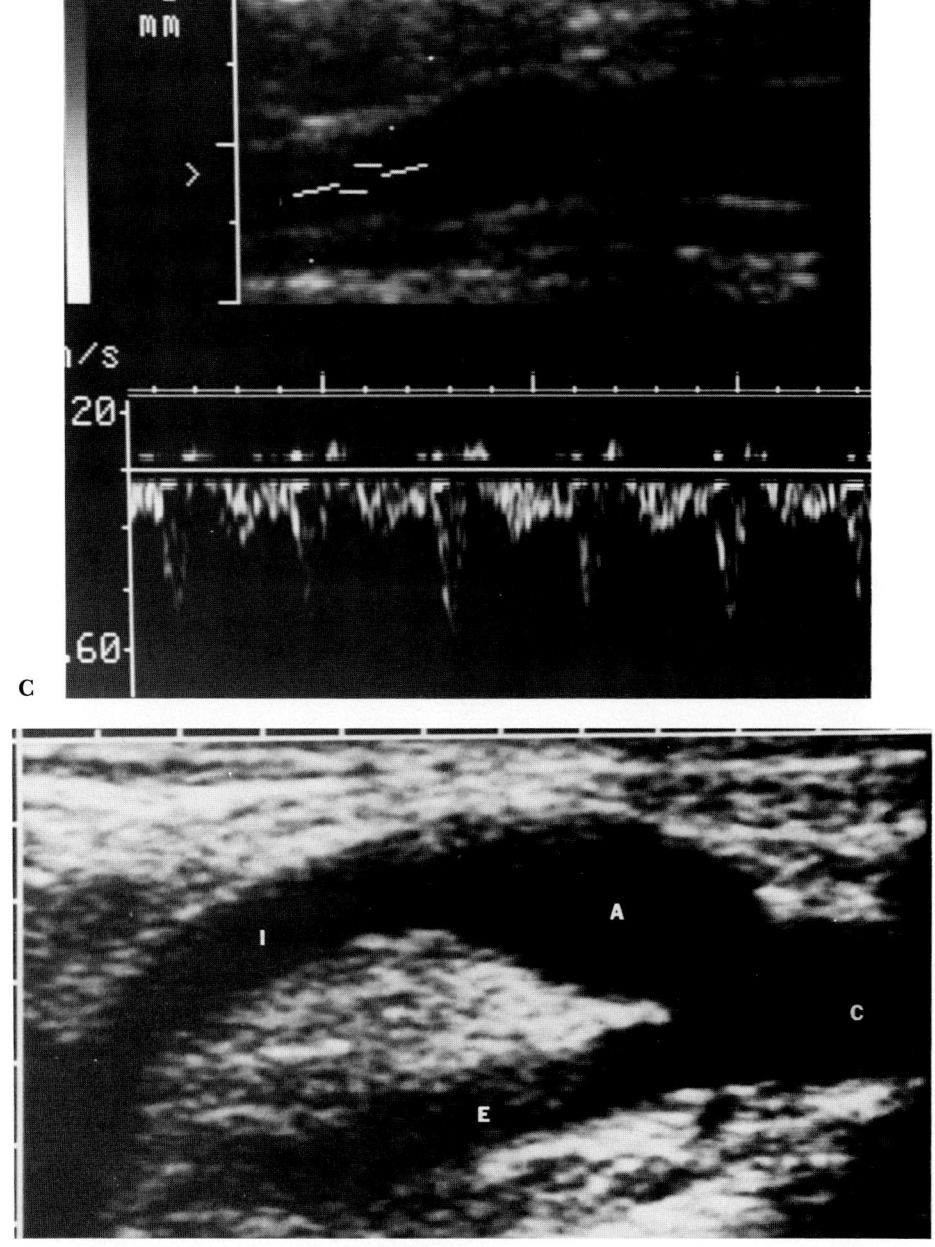

Fig. 2.8.

an occasional patient, placing the transducer on the anterior neck will lay the bifurcation out beautifully after much unsuccessful scanning from behind. Whichever scanning position opens up the bifurcation, it is obviously the correct one. Our marked preference for the posterior position may also be directly linked to the shape of the transducer with which we have the most experience. Other manufacturers' scan heads, in fact, may favor the anterior approach. In some patients it may be impossible to identify two separate vessels in the longitudinal orientation. Assuming they are both present, a transverse view may yield a better idea of their orientation; one may then return to a more optimum longitudinal scanning angle (Fig. 2.9 A–C).

Assuming that two separate vessels are identified, the most technically difficult task in carotid scanning follows, the differentiation of the ICA from the external. Nature has not been kind in this regard; the clear-cut differentiation of internal from external vessel may be very difficult. Anatomically, in about 95% of patients, the ECA will lie superficial to the internal. In the majority of patients the proximal ICA will also have an ampullary region of normal mild dilitation just beyond its origin. The ICA will also usually be larger than the external. Unfortunately, in 5% of patients the anterior-posterior orientation of the ICA and ECA will be reversed (29), and this anatomic reversal is not always bilateral. In addition, the latter two features of the ICA are also not constant. Occasionally, the ECA will be the larger of the two vessels, and the ampullary dilitation of the ICA may be very subtle. The anatomic or real-time differentiation, therefore, of the internal and external carotid arteries is not reliable. The ability to anatomically distinguish between these two vessels becomes even more difficult when atherosclerosis is present. The vessels may become ectatic, leave the bulb at odd orientations, wrap around each other, and even double back upon themselves in a series of "S curves." The only totally reliable real-time sign is the clear identification of the superficial thyroid artery (Fig. 2.10 A, B). This vessel is the first branch of the ECA; the ICA has no branches at all in the neck. One must be certain the supposed superficial thyroid artery is actually a vascular structure and not a thin muscle bundle. If any question exists, Doppler should demonstrate relatively low-resistance flow in the opposite direction from the ECA. In practice, on the basis of the "unreliable" anatomic information just discussed, the sonographer rapidly decides which vessel is being insonated. By visual inspection alone one can usually get a correct impression. This impression must then be confirmed by evaluating the Doppler signal.

After definite identification of the ICA, its origin must then be meticulously evaluated for anatomic abnormalities with real-time and for physiologic flow alterations using Doppler. The abnormalities encountered with each of the two components of the examination will be discussed under the appropriate headings. The sonographer should follow the ICA as far distally as possible until the vessel is lost behind the mandible. In some patients a considerable amount of the ICA will be visible, in others only the immediate origin of the vessel will be accessible. Very rarely, the bifurcation may not be visible at all. In our experience this situation is actually so unusual that one must be suspicious of some form of pathology if the bifurcation cannot be identified. The field of view of the sector scanner sometimes facilitates imaging of areas covered by bone. It is not unusual for experienced sonographers to be capable of following the Doppler signal beyond the point where the real-time image is lost. Although this is very useful, it must be done with circumspect as the angle between the probe and the vessel is unknown, and spurious Doppler signals may occasionally be obtained (Fig. 2.10 A–C).

After following the ICA as far distally as possible, attention may then be returned to the bulb and the ECA. Which vessel is actually examined first is of no importance. Again, identification of the ECA may be made with certainty if the superficial thyroid artery is identified. This small artery will not be found in many patients; it seems to be particularly difficult to find when it is most needed, such as when the ICA and ECA are reversed in anatomic orientation or in cases of severe atherosclerosis. Atherosclerosis of the external carotid is less common than of the internal; it is also of little clinical significance. In an effort to shorten scan time, only the origin of the external carotid needs to be evaluated. Stenoses of the ECA should, however, not

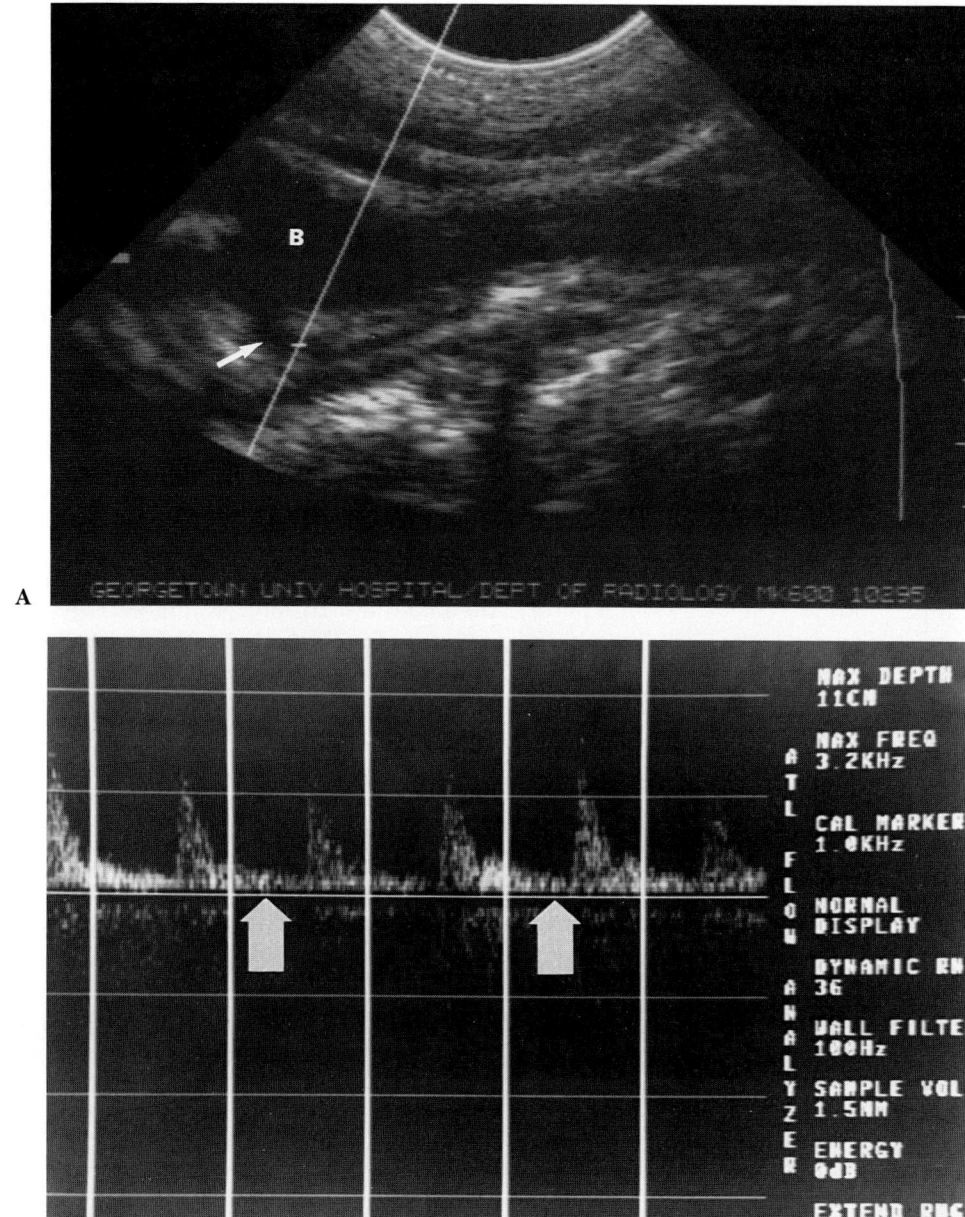

Fig. 2.9A–C. Superior thyroidal artery — Real-time image (**A**) shows carotid bifurcation (**B**). Anterior vessel is confirmed as ECA by presence of superior thyroidal artery (*arrows*). Doppler spectra (**B**) are typical. Trace is above baseline (*white arrows*) indicating flow is toward cursor, opposite of ECA. Subtraction arteriogram (**C**) of carotid bifurcation shows superior thyroidal artery (*arrowheads*) to good advantage.

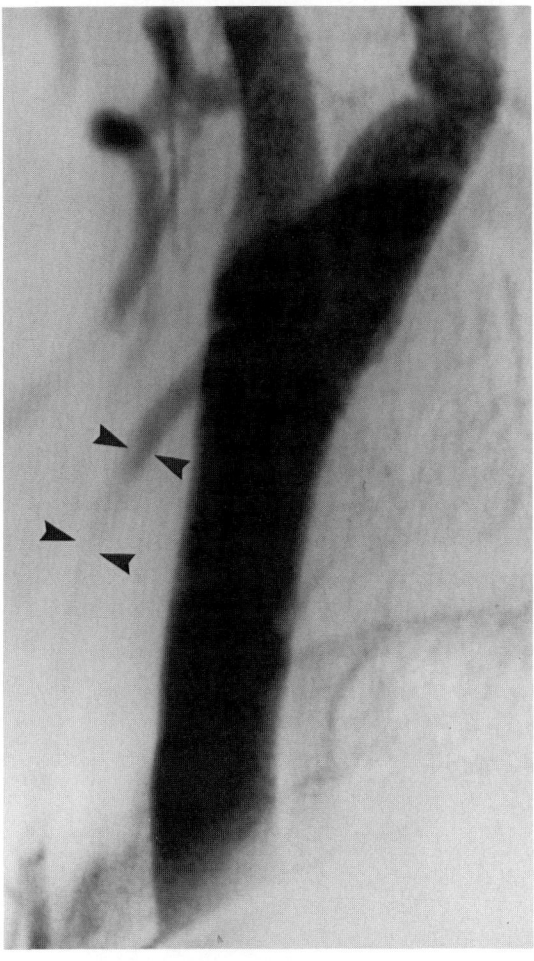

E

Fig. 2.9.

be overlooked. An ECA stenosis may account for a worrisome cervical bruit when the ICA is normal. With the evaluation of the right carotid system complete, the transducer is brought across the neck to the left carotid. In general, this portion of the examination is quite similar to the right, except that the left CCA arises directly from the aorta.

Before ending the examination, an attempt at visualizing at least the origins of the vertebral arteries should be made. The vertebral arteries are subject to considerable congenital variation; in some cases one or the other may be entirely absent. When present, however, the vertebral arteries, should be visible in the majority of patients (32). Scan technique for these vessels is relatively simple. The transducer is placed on the anterior part of the neck and the proximal common carotid artery identified. In most instances, slight lateral angulation of the ultrasound beam will bring the vertebral artery into view (Fig. 2.11 A–D). An alternative method for locating the right vertebral artery is to follow the CCA proximally to the subclavian and scan laterally until a vessel branches superiorly. Caution must be urged, however, because the costocervical and thyrocervical arteries also arise from the subclavian and may present confusion. More frequently another large vessel, the subclavian vein, will mimic the vertebral. Doppler evaluation will easily determine the nature of the vessel in question. Distinction between the arteries, however, may be more difficult. One should follow the vessel distally; no other artery passes through the transverse foramina of the cervical vertebrae except the vertebral. This anatomic peculiarity produces a vessel that is striped by clear-cut periodic shadowing (Fig. 2.12).

The vertebral artery supplies a large amount of blood to the brain. It, therefore, exhibits a low-resistance flow pattern. Because the vessel is small, flow tends to be somewhat turbulent and the clear sonic window expected in the normal carotid system is usually filled in. The origins of the vertebral arteries are the second most commonly stenosed regions of the cerebral vessels (33). Therefore, evaluation at this juncture may be important. More distally, stenoses are rare, and careful evaluation of flow direction to eliminate the possibility of subclavian steal should complete the cerebrovascular examination.

Cerebrovascular Duplex Sonography: Real-Time Imaging

Real-time imaging is by far the more familiar component of duplex scanning. When applied to carotid occlusive disease, however, this otherwise successful technology has proven less than impressive. In theory, the carotid artery seems an ideal candidate for real-time sonography. The carotid is a large, fluid-filled structure located almost directly beneath the skin, thereby lending itself to easy high-resolution scanning. Numerous authors have investigated

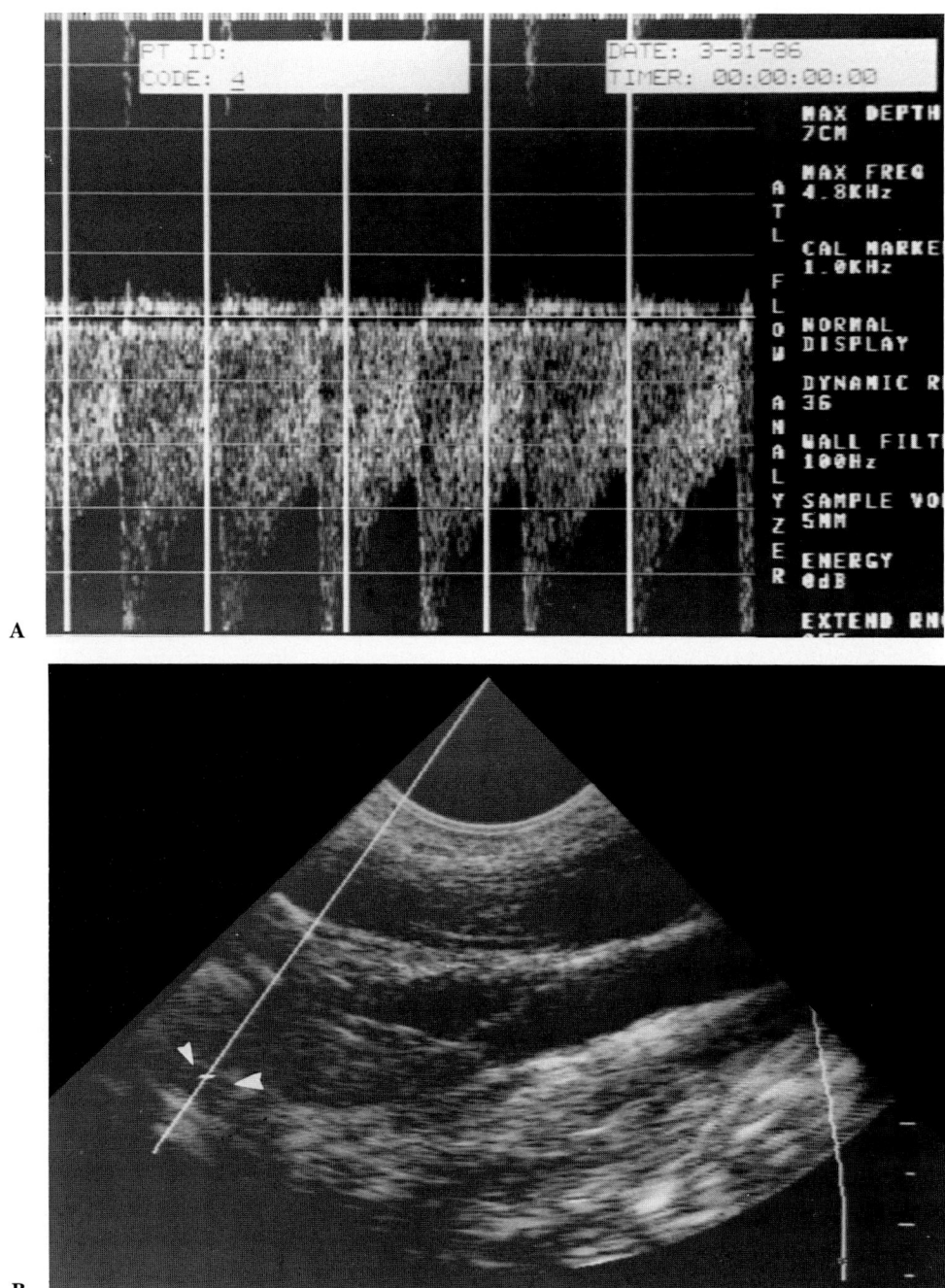

Fig. 2.10A–D. Misleading Doppler spectra — 42-year-old physician with migraine-like symptoms and blackout. Normal Doppler patterns are found throughout both carotid systems except in area shown in **A** (*arrowheads*). Markedly abnormal Doppler spectra (**B**) are encountered. Arteriogram (**C,D**) shows unusual folding or kink (*arrows*) in corresponding region. Doppler trace was obtained from area where angle and vessel course were unknown. Sharp angles in vessels often produce marked alterations in flow; such alterations are, however, not usually believed to be clinically significant.

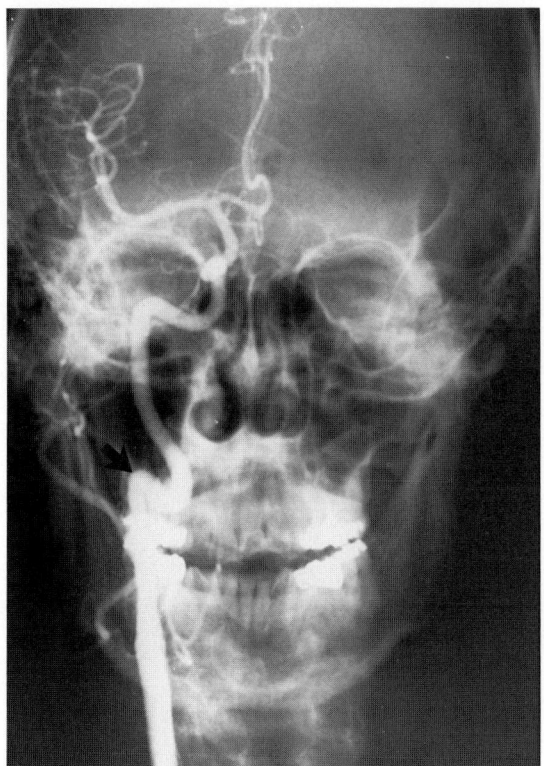
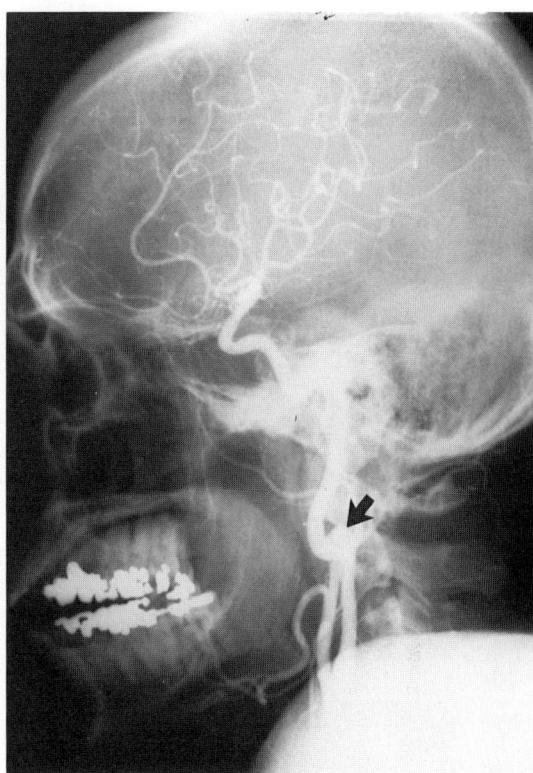

C D

Fig. 2.10.

these possibilities; as early as 1975 Anderson et al (34) tried conventional B-mode ultrasound. He concluded, however, that the technology "was not quite appropriate." Following such leads, Cooperberg et al (35), in 1979, applied high-resolution real-time scanning to the carotid artery and produced what appeared to represent rather promising results. Unfortunately, later studies by a series of authors failed to find real-time evaluation alone an adequate method of diagnosing carotid stenoses (30,36–38).

The reasons for these disappointing results are many and the study by Comerota et al (30) of more than 1,000 patients goes right to the heart of the matter. Simply stated, as the severity of the occlusion increases, the quality of the real-time scan decreases. Unfortunately, scan quality is directly proportional to diagnostic accuracy. Several different physical principles work against successful real-time evaluation of the carotids. Most problematic is the inherent acoustic impedance of many atherosclerotic lesions. Ironically, problems occur at both ends of the acoustic spectrum. On one hand, plaque may be composed of material that closely resembles the soft tissues of the neck. As echogenic plaque fills the vessel, it becomes indistinguishable from its surroundings. The artery is simply not seen as a discrete structure on the ultrasound examination. On the other hand, "soft plaque" often has acoustic properties similar to flowing blood; some plaques or thrombi are almost anechoic. The latter problem is most apparent in vessels that appear sonographically normal yet are totally occluded. The difficulty of distinguishing between normal and total occlusion is referred to in almost every real-time study (30,36–38). The inability to differentiate a normal vessel from a totally occluded one is, needless to say, rather disconcerting. The acoustic properties of blood and plaque may, however, work to our benefit in situations in which much flowing blood is present in an artery. Flowing anechoic blood provides an excellent contrast to plaque. Real-time ultra-

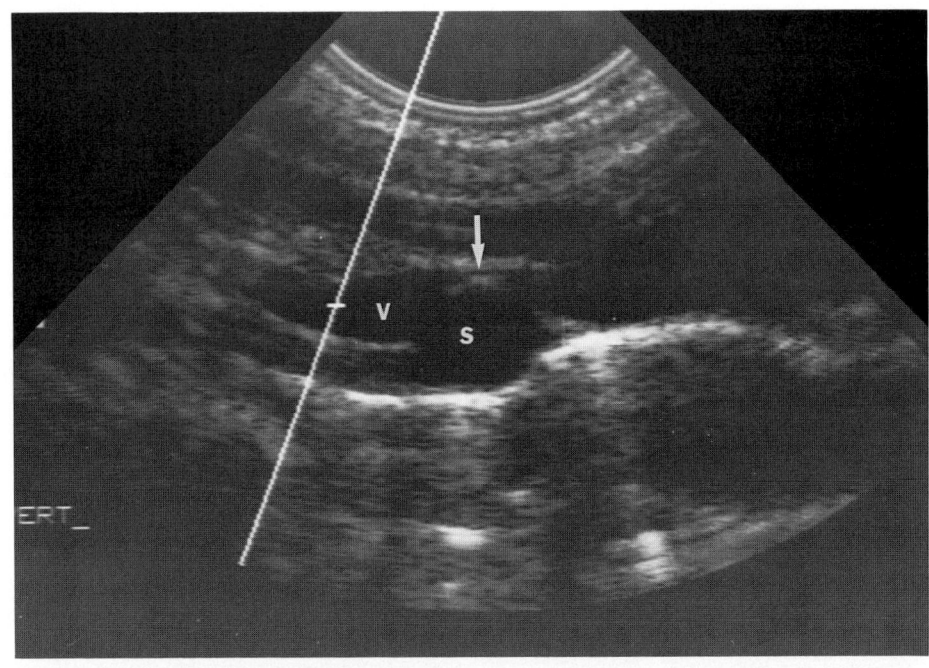

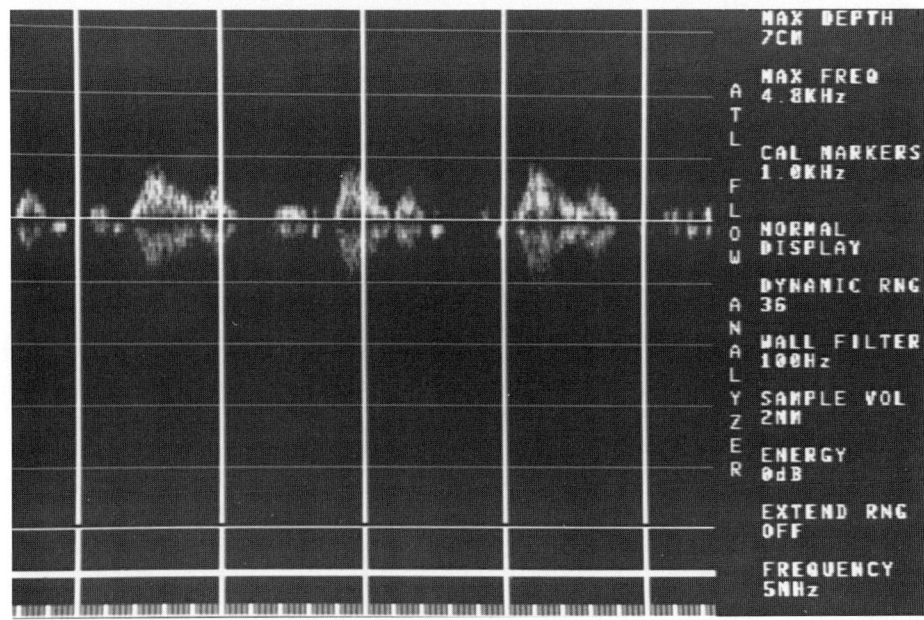

Fig. 2.11A–D. Vertebral artery-vein — **A**. Longitudinal images obtained slightly lateral to CCA section subclavian artery (S) transversely. Two vessels appear to arise from it. The larger and more anterior of the two (V) is a vein. Note "choppy" venous flow characteristics and positive deflection of waveform indicating flow toward transducer (**B**). Vein is compressed into a narrow waist (*arrow*) as it passes over subclavian artery. **C, D.** Lower vessel (A) is vertebral artery. Doppler characteristics are typical. Note relatively low systolic amplitude, negative diphasic waveform, and spectral broadening. Spectral broadening is a normal feature of smaller vessels.

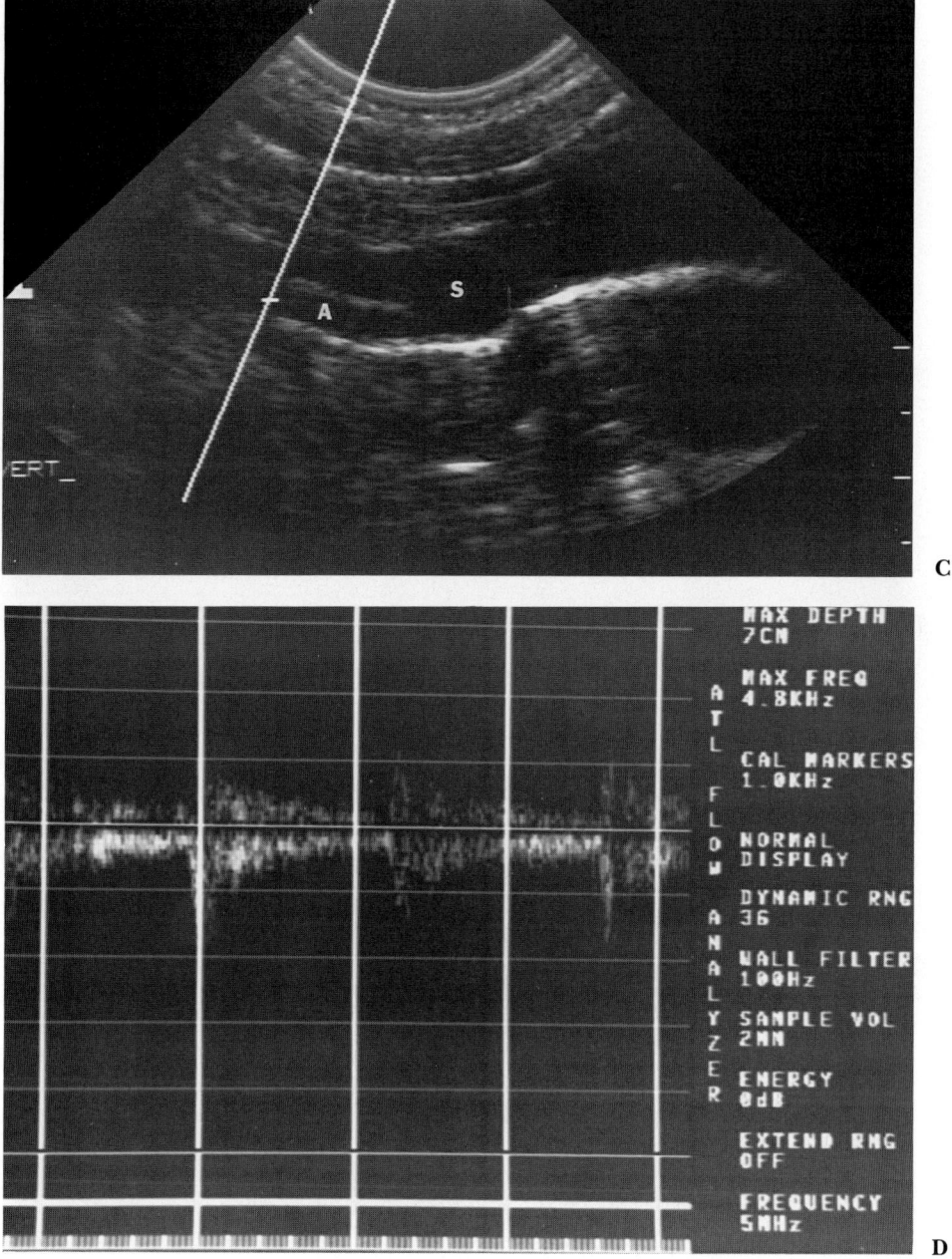

Fig. 2.11.

sound seems, therefore, best suited for the evaluation of nonrate-limiting lesions and not for diagnosing stenoses (25). Luckily, Doppler performs most optimally in situations involving hemodynamically significant disease.

When examined using high-resolution real-time technology, atherosclerosis exhibits a number of rather specific features. Benign, flat fibrofatty plaques are common in asymptomatic older patients. Such plaques often appear as smooth echogenic lines paralleling the intimal surface (Fig. 2.13 A, B). Fibrofatty plaques are typically 4 mm or more in thickness and may contain hypoechoic areas postulated to represent lipid deposits (39). Examples of fibrofatty plaque are often best demonstrated in the

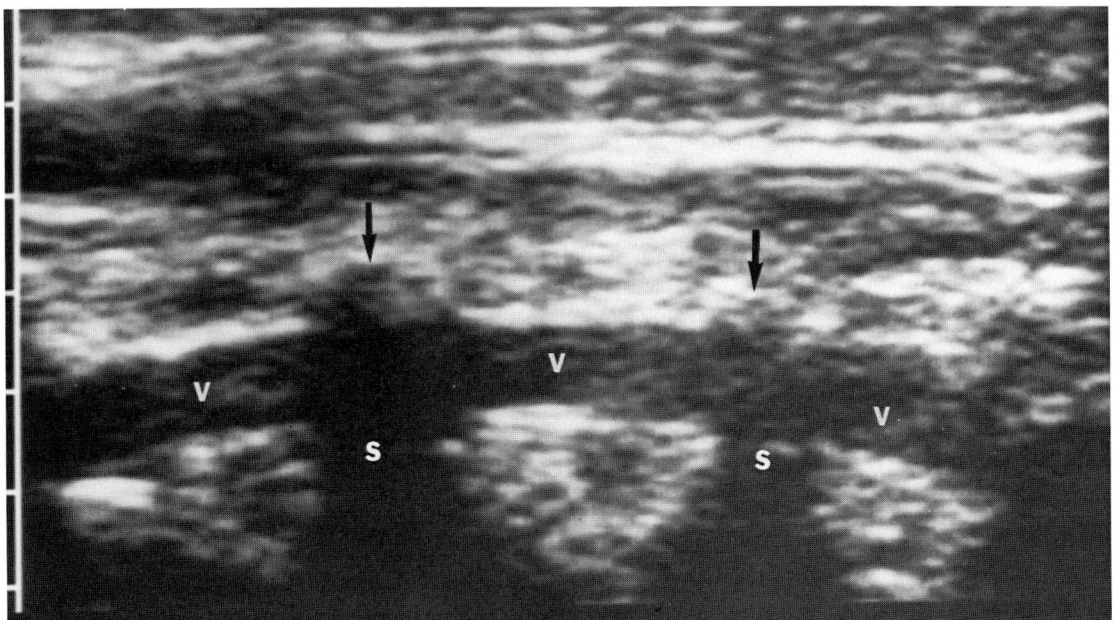

Fig. 2.12. Vertebral artery—If followed distally, the vertebral artery (V) passes through the transverse foramina of the cervical spine (see Fig. 2.30). Bone (*arrows*) causes sharp periodic acoustic shadowing (S) and confirms vessel to be the vertebral artery.

CCA (also see Fig. 2.6). Calcific plaque is also common. Calcific plaque seems to have little bearing on outcome and is frequently found in asymptomatic patients (40,41). Dense, calcific plaque may, however, cause enough shadowing to lead to uncertainty about the status of the portion of the carotid within the shadow. Angling the Doppler cursor steeply up or down into the real-time shadow may yield information about flow dynamics. Approaching the lesion from the opposite side of the neck may also help overcome this problem.

Plaque ulceration also has been scrutinized with real-time sonography. Ulcerated plaque has long been the arteriographic hallmark of operable nonrate-limiting carotid disease. The actual significance of many carotid "ulcerations," however, remains unclear. When seen by real-time examination, ulcerations demonstrate the expected excavation or niche within a plaque (Fig. 2.14 A–C). Unfortunately, cross-sectional imaging has inherent difficulty with ulcerations: If the lesion is not caught in exactly the right plane, it may not appear as an ulcer. Distinguishing between ulceration and multiple and adjacent plaques also may present considerable difficulty (Fig. 2.15 A–C). Finally, it is well known that the angiogram (the usual "gold standard" to which duplex is compared) does not recognize a significant number of ulcerations, some of which are well-visualized with high-resolution sonography (37,42,43).

Recently, a number of impressive studies (40,41) have implicated intraplaque hemorrhage as a possible cause for many ischemic cerebral events. The theory is an attractive one. Arteries have an inherent blood supply, the vasa vasorum. Ischemia of the vasa vasorum may actually lead to infarction of an existing atherosclerotic plaque: Hemorrhage into an infarcted plaque "may erupt through the intima like a volcano" (39,44) and send any number of emboli on their devastating way to the end arteries of the brain. Intraplaque hemorrhage may also acutely increase the size of an atheroma and actually lead to the rapid development of a rate-limiting lesion. Some would even postulate that many ulcerative lesions actually represent the pocket of a previous intraplaque hemorrhage (39,44,45). The work of Imparato et al (46,47) indicates that intraplaque hemorrhage is the single most significant lesion in stroke-related symptoms.

The real-time finding most associated with intraplaque hemorrhage appears to be inhomogeneity of an atheroma. A homogeneous pat-

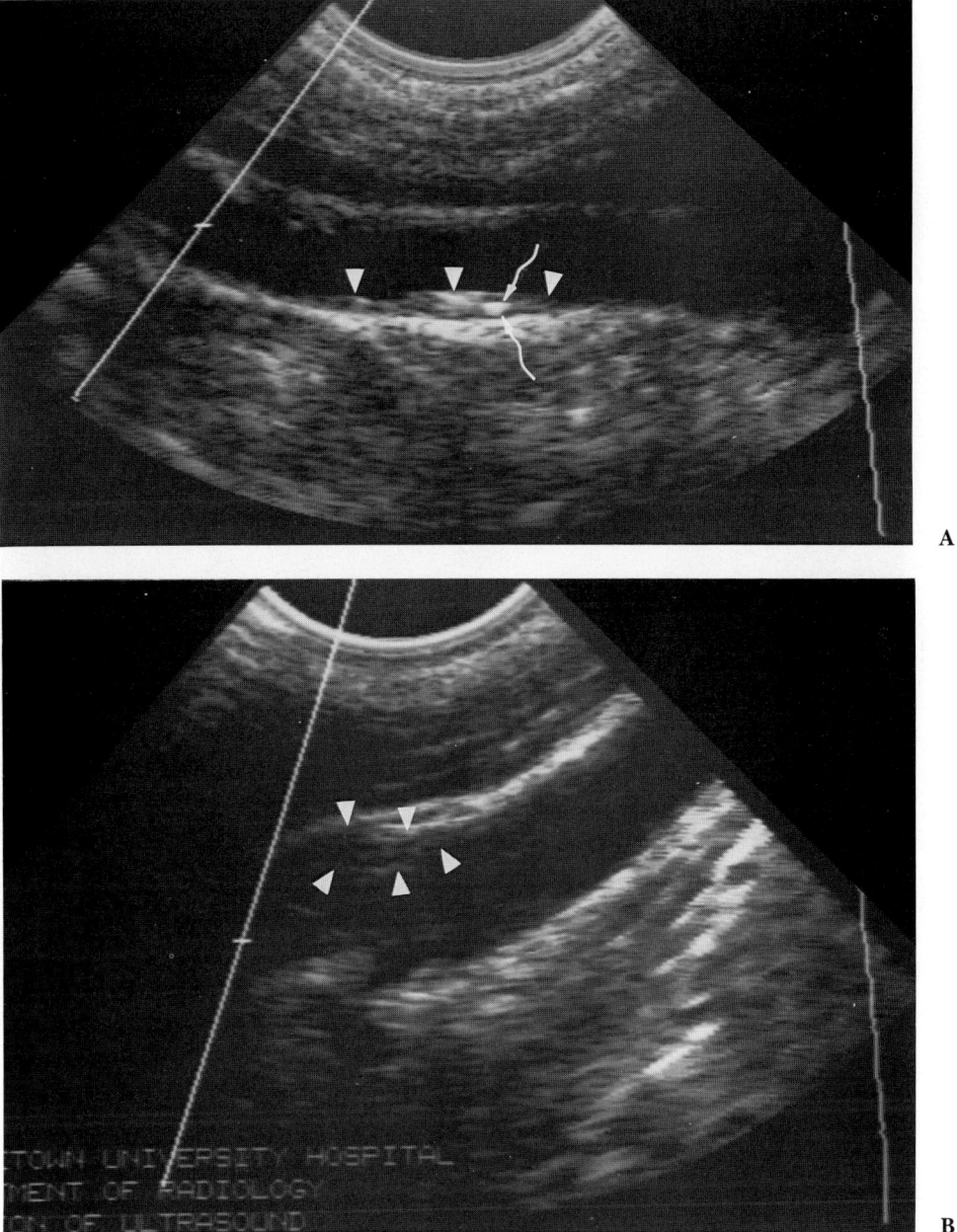

Fig. 2.13A, B. Fibrofatty plaque—**A.** Smooth, echogenic plaque (*arrowheads*) parallels surface of CCA. Note small internal calcification (*curved arrows*). **B.** Shows homogeneous fibrofatty plaque in ampullary region of proximal ICA (*arrowheads*).

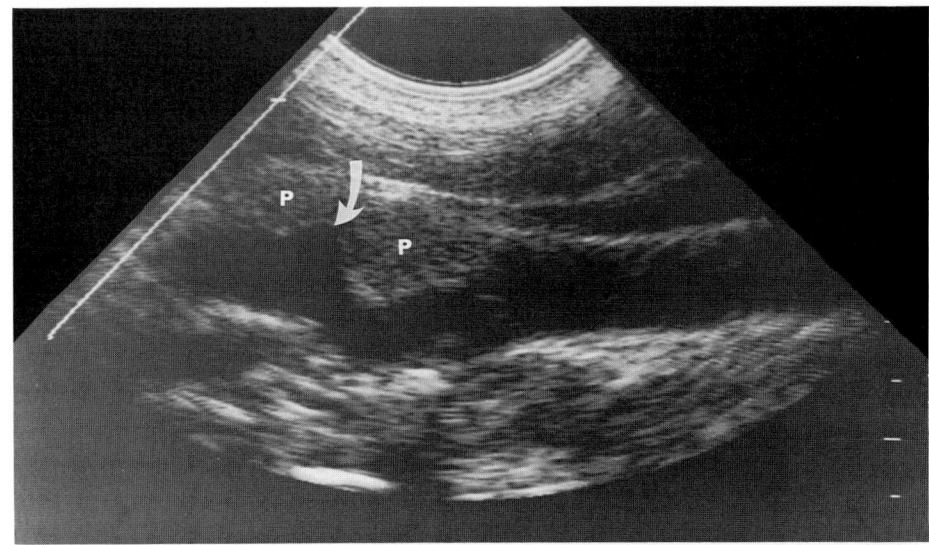

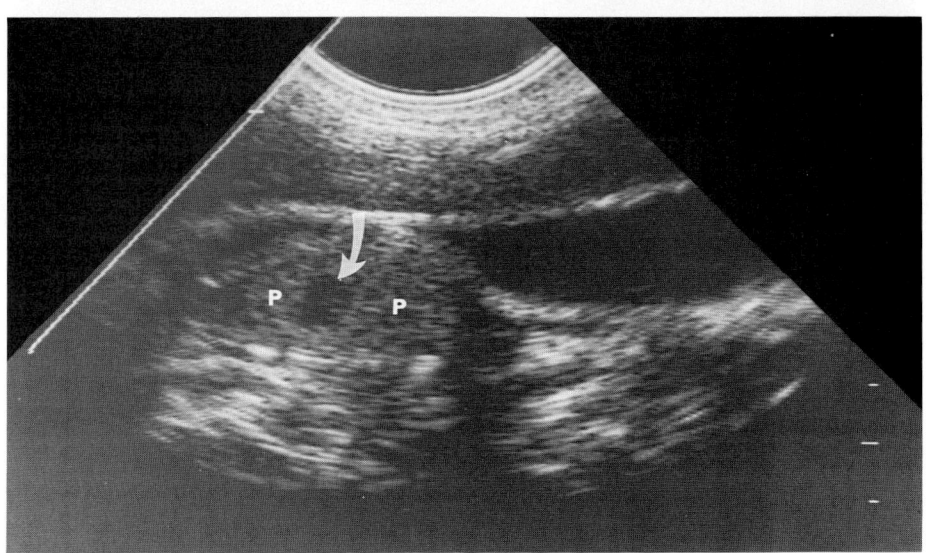

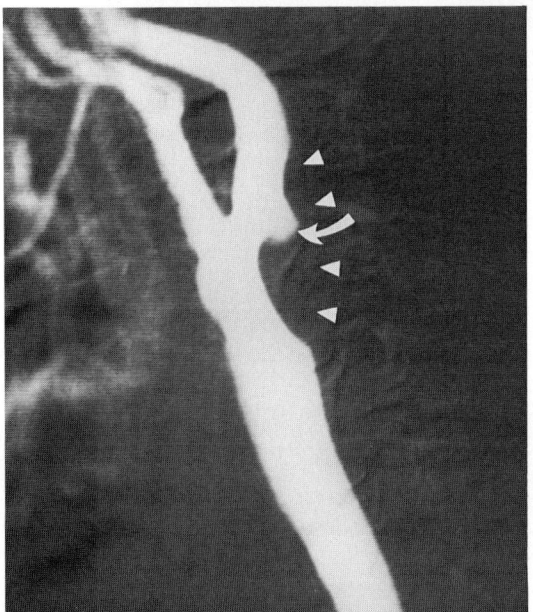

Fig. 2.14A–C. A. Giant ulcer—64-year-old woman presented with multiple episodes of amaurosis fugax. Extensive soft plaque (P) identified in ipsilateral carotid bulb and proximal ICA. Large ulceration (*curved arrow*) is present in plaque. **B.** An unusual section across the plaque showing the ulcer actually invaginating into it. Arteriogram (**C**) confirms sonographic findings. Arrowheads outline the approximate area of the plaque; curved arrow points to ulcer.

Fig. 2.15A–C. Ulcerated plaque—54-year-old man with poorly defined TIA-like symptoms. **A.** Duplex evaluation of right carotid shows possible ulceration (*curved arrow*) by real-time. **B.** Doppler trace has extensive spectral broadening but only 4 KHzΔ. Each graticule of the x-axis = 2 KHzΔ. Low flow in CCA was suggested by maximum systolic KHzΔ (at a similar angle) of less than 1. Fourfold increase in flow velocity indicates a hemodynamically significant lesion. Arteriogram (**C**) confirms presence of ulcer (*curved arrow*) and a marked stenosis. *(See p. 32.)*

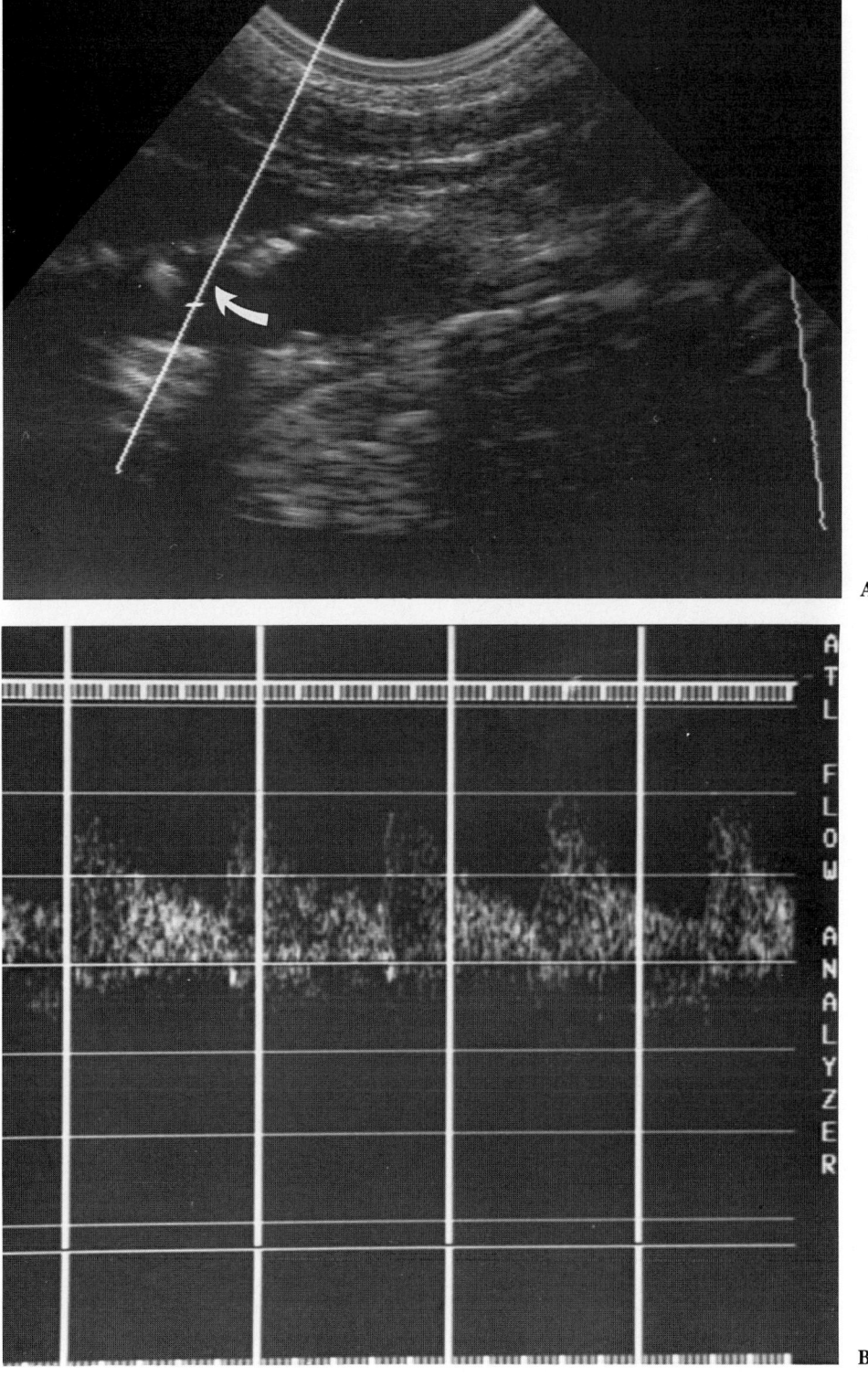

Fig. 2.15.

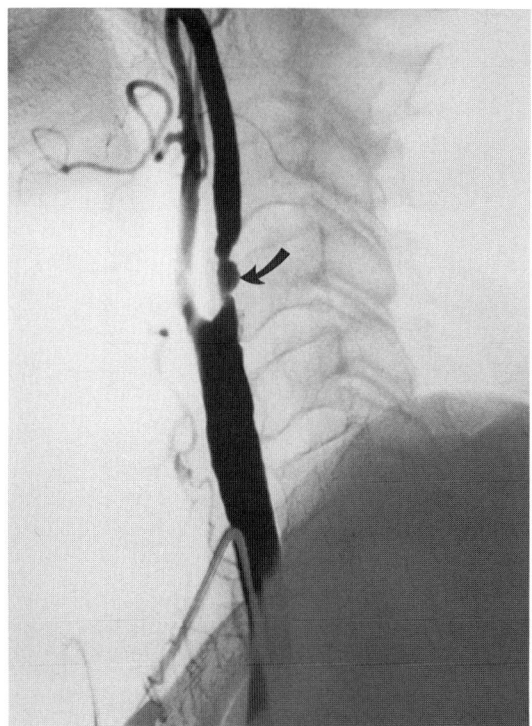

C

Fig. 2.15.

tern with uniform high or medium level echoes seems to indicate the presence of relatively benign, dense fibrocollagenous material as shown in Figure 2.13 A, B. In the series by Reilly et al (41) intraplaque hemorrhage did not occur in association with homogeneous plaque. Interestingly, no cases of ulceration were ever identified in association with this pattern. Conversely, Reilly's work (41) and that of Bluth et al (40) found heterogeneous plaque associated with a high percentage of intraplaque hemorrhages and ulcerations at pathology. Heterogeneous plaque frequently consists of a mixture of differing echogenicities. The classic feature, however, is the finding of anechoic regions, which may actually represent intraplaque hemorrhage (Fig. 2.16 A–C).

If the recent theories about the significance of intraplaque hemorrhage hold true, real-time imaging of the carotids may actually prove of considerably more value than previously thought. Real-time technology is the only effective means of diagnosing extraluminal events. Arteriography is useless beyond the intact intima and indirect testing can only identify lesions that significantly impede flow.

The foregoing discussion on the use of real-time ultrasound shows that, indeed, it may prove far more useful than merely providing a road map for better Doppler localization. The astute sonographer will use the real-time component to its fullest advantage. With further research we may eventually have a tool that identifies those patients who have the highest risk for future cerebral damage from carotid bifurcation disease.

Cerebrovascular Duplex Sonography: Doppler

The potential of Doppler to quantify blood flow has been well known for many years. Unfortunately, numerous drawbacks inherent in older Doppler technology have detracted significantly from its success. Although the human ear is quite sensitive to the range of Doppler shifts produced by moving blood cells, auditory cues are quite difficult to quantify precisely. Other drawbacks of conventional Doppler, including the inability to localize the source of the signal and summation of signals from multiple sources decreased the accuracy of the Doppler examination significantly. In spite of this, for many years, conventional Doppler represented one of medicine's best methods by which to noninvasively evaluate blood flow.

In an attempt to eliminate some of the shortcomings of the Doppler examination, investigators coupled it to a real-time image to better localize the source of the signal. The addition of pulse-gating actually allowed the operator to select one specific point along the Doppler beam for evaluation. These improvements allowed considerable technical advantages over conventional Doppler systems. The problem of quantification of the signal was finally overcome by various computer manipulations resulting in spectral analysis. These manipulations transform auditory information into a quantifiable, graphic image.

Nonquantitative Doppler presently seems to suffice in many areas of the body. Exact quantification of blood flow and, therefore, stenosis, may be less important, for example, than flow direction or identification of inappropriate vascular resistance. In many areas this may change with increasing research, but at the outset, pre-

Fig. 2.16A–C. Heterogeneous plaque-intraplaque hemorrhage—Heterogeneous plaque (*arrowheads*) at origin of ICA (**A**). Note central hypoechoic areas (*arrow*). Transverse (**B**) and longitudinal (**C**) images reveal crescentic plaque having extensive anechoic area (*arrowheads*) within. Such anechoic areas frequently indicate intraplaque hemorrhages.

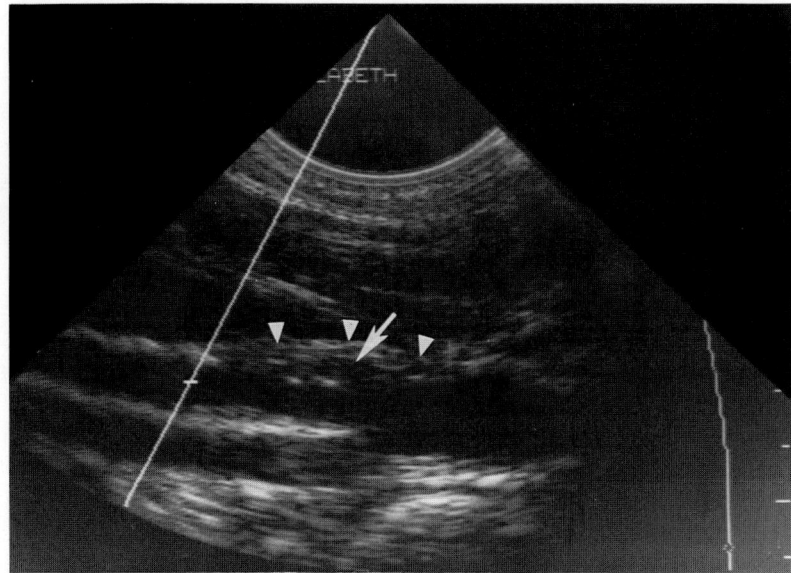

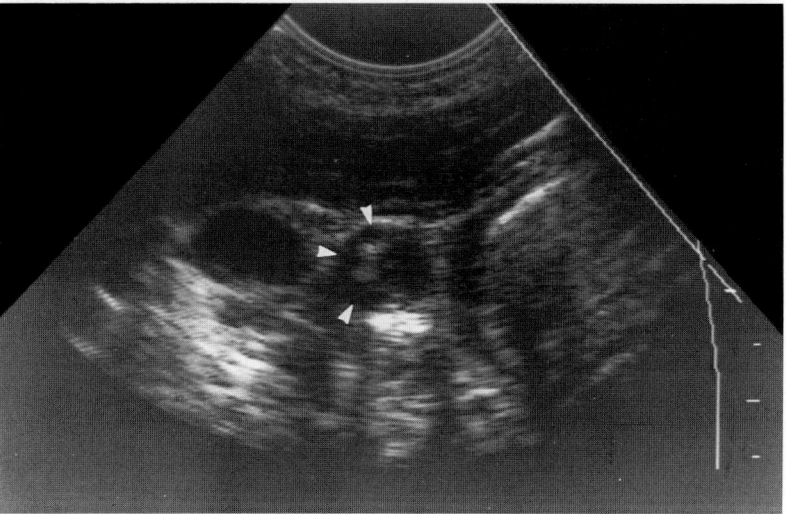

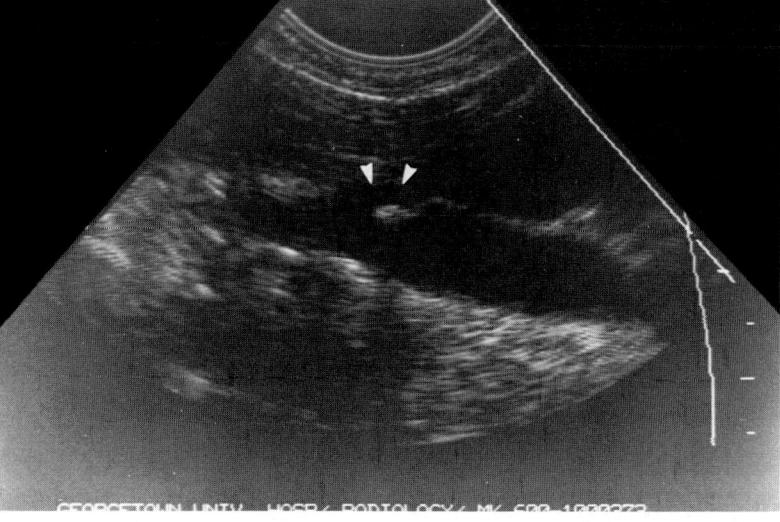

cise quantification of carotid blood flow was required if any noninvasive test was to be successful. Historically, precise and reproducible Doppler measurements have been quite elusive. With the proliferation of duplex technology around 1980, however, the Doppler criteria for internal carotid stenoses fell into place during a remarkably brief period. In rapid succession, authors published impressive data using the duplex scanner to identify rate-limiting stenoses of the carotid (23–29). It was primarily the Doppler component of duplex that produced the impressive diagnostic results that led to its popularity. In fact, as stenoses become tighter and exert an increasing effect on flow dynamics, the job of the Doppler becomes easier. Despite increasing resolution and the use of the real-time component, Doppler continues to yield most of the significant diagnostic information desired from a duplex examination.

Doppler criteria for diagnosing internal carotid artery stenoses vary considerably depending on the equipment used, the method of evaluation and one's own philosophy about the interpretation of Doppler data. At best, Doppler results are an estimation of blood flow velocity based on the effect of a frequently ragged and tortuous plaque (Fig. 2.17 A, B). Unlike flow dynamics studied in the laboratory, Doppler spectra produced by a diseased artery are not directly dependent on one variable. Cardiac output, systemic blood pressure, and the length, shape, and position of the stenosis, to name a few, all enter into the equation when attempting to estimate the severity of carotid disease. For this reason, basing one's impression on a single set of criteria will lead to a loss of diagnostic accuracy. For example, given similar degrees of stenosis, the flow velocity will be quite different in a patient with low cardiac output compared with one with severe hypertension. One should also be aware of the limitations of the usual "gold standard" to which duplex is compared. Arteriography is typically performed in only two planes and is well known to be relatively reader dependent (1,39,48). Both duplex and arteriography have shortcomings. It is comforting to find, however, that although some variations in interpretation are frequent, major discrepancies are relatively uncommon.

Numerous authors have explored the possibilities of duplex Doppler and philosophies vary. Some would claim that Doppler is useful in diagnosing the entire spectrum of carotid occlusive disease from minimal narrowing to high-grade stenoses. Subtle Doppler abnormalities, particularly spectral broadening during certain parts of the cardiac cycle (27), have been said to imply minimal (less than 50%) vessel narrowing. Our own experience with lesions less than 50% occlusive, however, has indicated that Doppler is not particularly reliable in this range (25). Other groups have also noted that Doppler criteria are far less accurate in lesions that are not hemodynamically significant (less than 50%) (27,49,50). Theoretically, a plaque protruding into the vessel lumen and narrowing it by 30% should result in flow turbulence. Although this may be so in theory, turbulence is reflected as spectral broadening and, therefore, subject to considerable operator error. Minor variations in gain setting can easily simulate or erase true spectral broadening (Fig. 2.18 A–C). Although most experienced sonographers can easily make this distinction and accurately identify minor flow turbulence, in general, we have not found Doppler to be reliable in the diagnosis of nonrate-limiting lesions. This seems to be the area where the real-time component of duplex does best. Regardless, nonhemodynamically significant lesions are only important if ulceration or intraplaque hemorrhage is found. Clearly, neither ulceration nor intraplaque hemorrhage are Doppler diagnoses!

In evaluating rate-limiting stenosis, many researchers have found the maximum systolic velocity or KHz shift (KHzΔ) to be the single most important feature of the Doppler data (25,27,28,51,52). Increased peak systolic velocity is present in almost every hemodynamically significant lesion unless some factor extrinsic to the carotid artery is present (see Figs. 2.15 and 2.21). As shown in Table 2.1, for most subjects, the maximum KHzΔ should be less than 3.5 to 4.0. Scan angle is assumed between 45 and 60°, and all of our equipment uses a 5 MHz Doppler transducer. We have relied more heavily on KHzΔ than velocity in our Doppler diagnoses and have found it quite adequate thus far. This probably stems from our learning duplex before the availability of scanners that easily incorporated angle adjustments and gave direct centimeters per second data. Certainly in theory, the use of velocity would seem preferable because the scanning angle is incorporated into

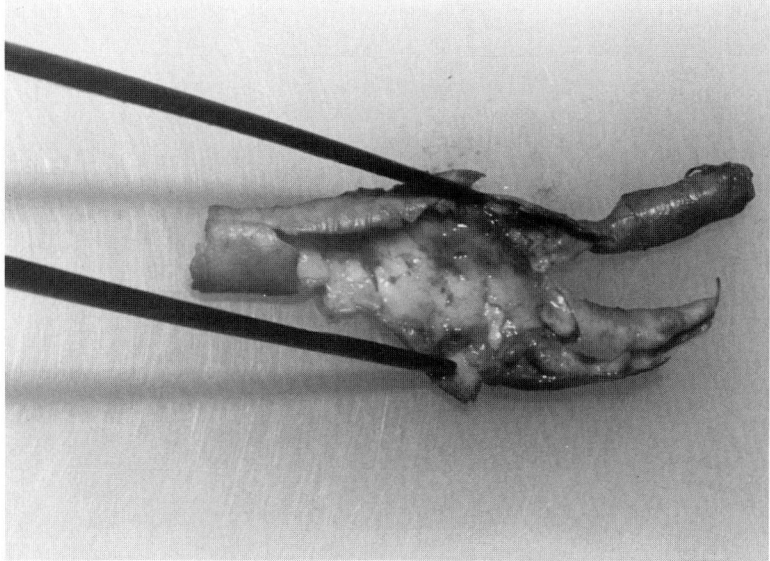

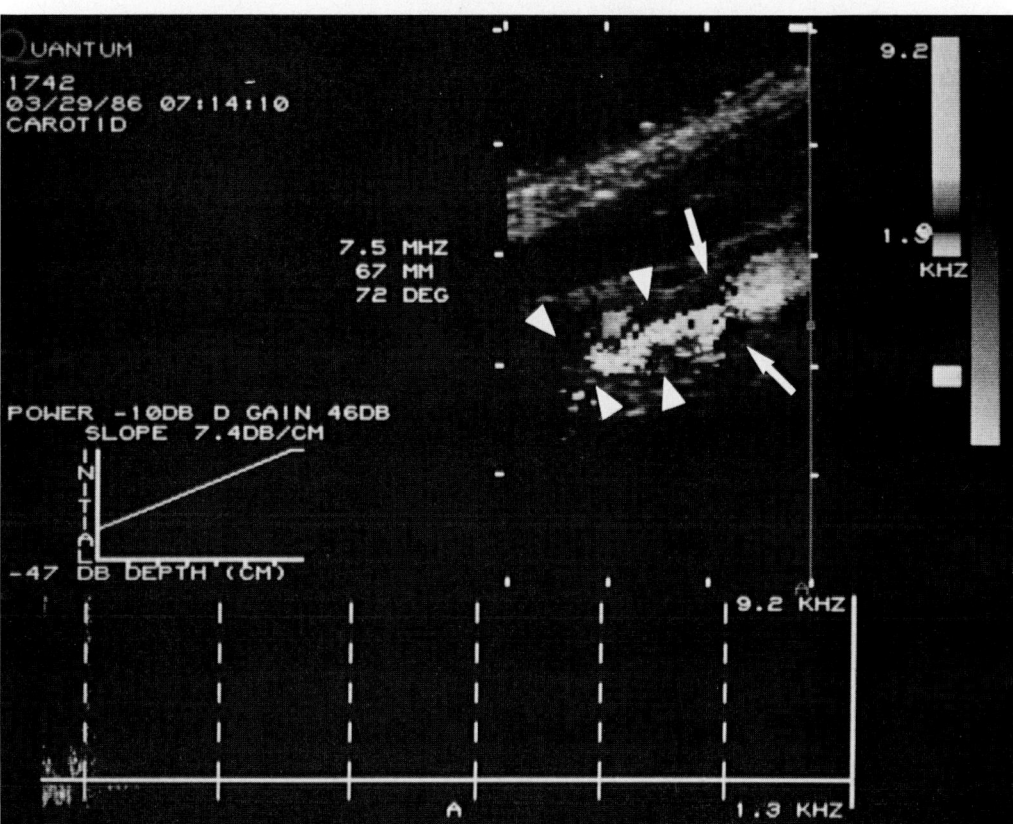

Fig. 2.17A–B. Effect of atherosclerotic plaque on blood flow—**A**. Operative specimen demonstrates vessel narrowing and typical irregularity of plaque surface. Courtesy of Dr. Mario Gomes, Department of Surgery, Georgetown University Hospital. **B**. Color flow image depicts effect of vessel narrowing and irregular surface of plaque on flow. Various colors are seen as blood travels through the lesion. Differing colors (*arrowheads*) reflect an increase in flow velocity beyond an area of stenosis (*arrows*) and marked turbulence. Courtesy of Dr. Eugene Strandness, University of Washington Hospital, Seattle, Washington. (For a color reproduction of this figure see frontmatter.)

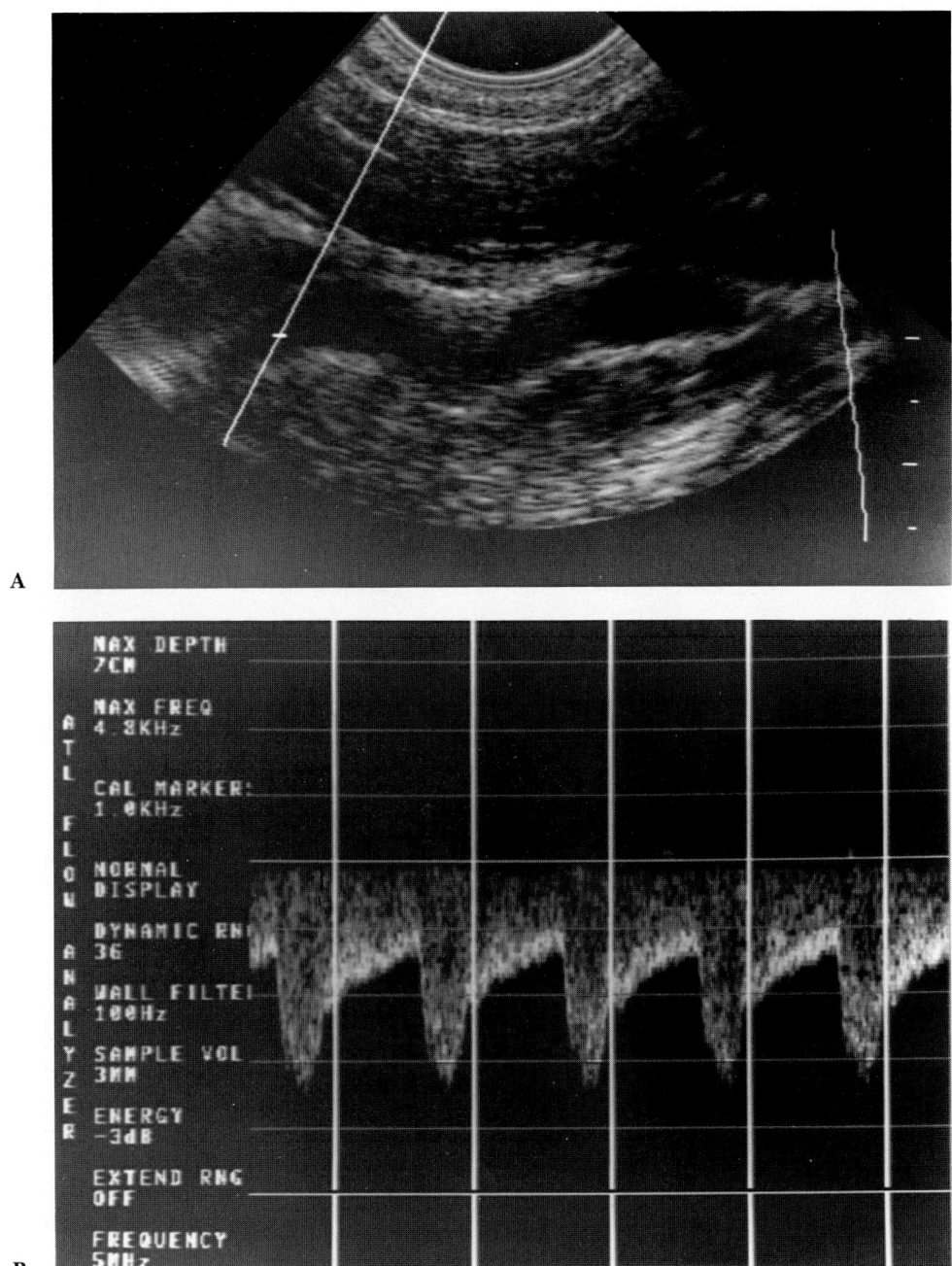

Fig. 2.18A–C. Artifactual spectral broadening—(**B**) might lead one to suspect a moderate degree of luminal narrowing. Properly adjusted Doppler gain shows clean diphasic trace (**C**) of normal ICA. Although spectral broadening may be artifactually induced, excessive high gain settings should leave peak velocity relatively unaffected. Improper angle has the opposite effect; velocity throughout cardiac cycle will be artifactually raised or lowered.

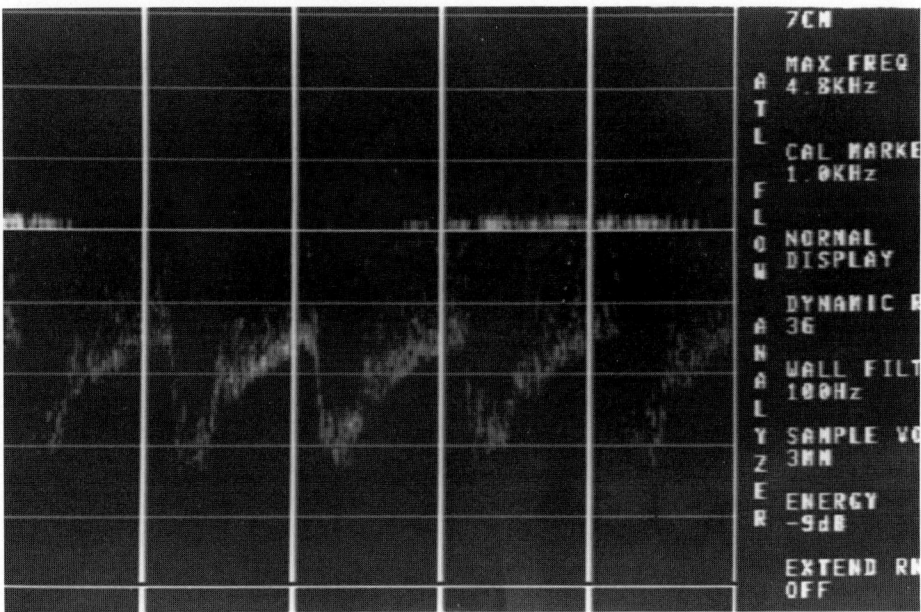

Fig. 2.18.

Table 2.1. DCS Criteria for Stenosis

Percent Stenosis	KHz Shift	Waveform
0–30%	<3.5	Real-time US helpful in differentiating ≤30% stenosis from normal
31–50%	3.5–4	50–67% of window under waveform filled in during systole; real-time US particularly helpful in the occasional case of a smooth stenosis at the carotid bulb, where Doppler criteria may be inadequate
51–90%	>4–8	67% of window usually filled in; waveform recognizable
91–99%	>8	Window filled in; waveform becoming distorted
>95–99%	Variable (can be <4)	Window filled in; waveform markedly distorted
100%	0	No waveform; series of dots seen along the baseline

From Jacobs N, Grant E, Schellinger D, et al: Duplex Carotid Sonography: Criteria for Stenosis, Accuracy and Pitfalls. Radiology 154:385–391, 1985. Reprinted with permission.

the results. The use of velocity eliminates two possible variables: angle and transducer frequency. Velocity may, therefore, be used interchangeably regardless of equipment.

In the normal patient, a clean, thin spectrum of sound should be both visible and audible. The systolic rise should be relatively slow and capped by the dicrotic notch. Diastole should consist of a gradual down slope and, of course, flow should be present throughout the cardiac cycle. Unfortunately, considerable variation is frequent in the waveforms from one patient to the next. A 3 KHzΔ or lower is common in the older, atherosclerotic-prone population who form the vast majority of our patients. Young, apparently healthy subjects may actually generate considerably higher systolic velocities. The added effects of caffeine, tobacco, stress, and other extrinsic factors may occasionally result in peak KHzΔ over 6 in young hospital employees (Fig. 2.19 *A, B*). Such a reading in a 65-year-old with a bruit could easily lead to an arteriogram. Other somewhat unusual flow patterns also may be encountered in young patients with presumed normal vessels. Phillips (53) actually raises the possibility that *absence* of some mild spectral broadening might imply early atherosclerosis. Luckily, such patterns would only be associated with minimal disease. At the carotid bifurcation, spectral broadening may also be encountered in normal patients in certain portions of the vessel lumen (Fig. 2.20 *A–E*). These areas of turbulence are most likely

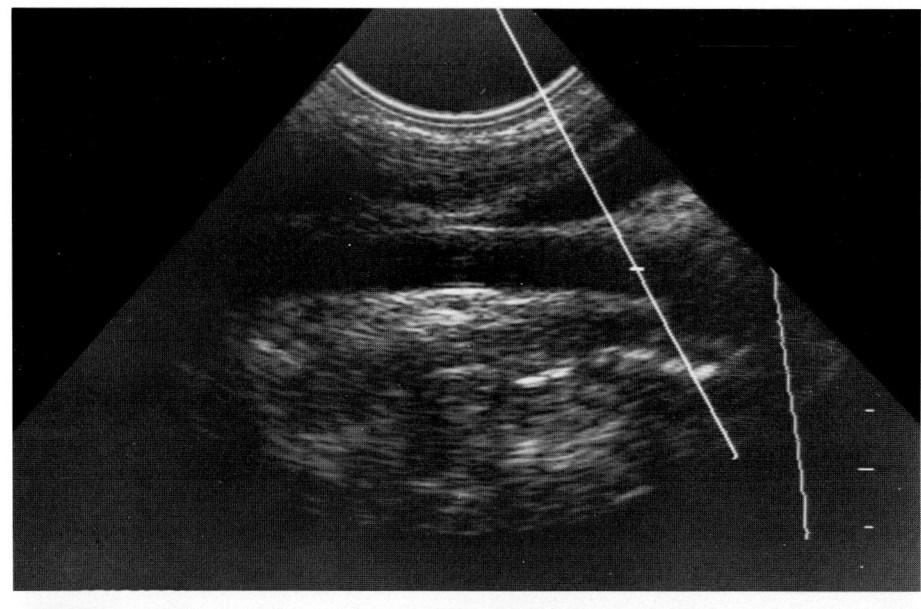

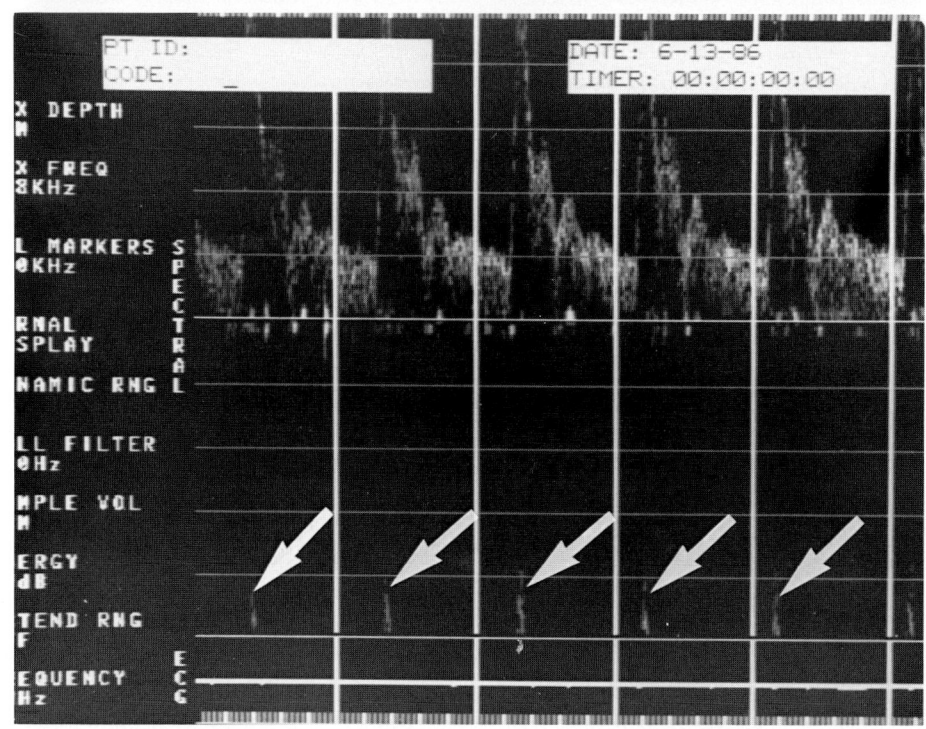

Fig. 2.19A,B. Healthy hospital employee—Presumed normal 24-year-old exhibits a 6 KHzΔ (or greater) throughout both carotid systems. Note aliasing of Doppler signal (*arrows*).

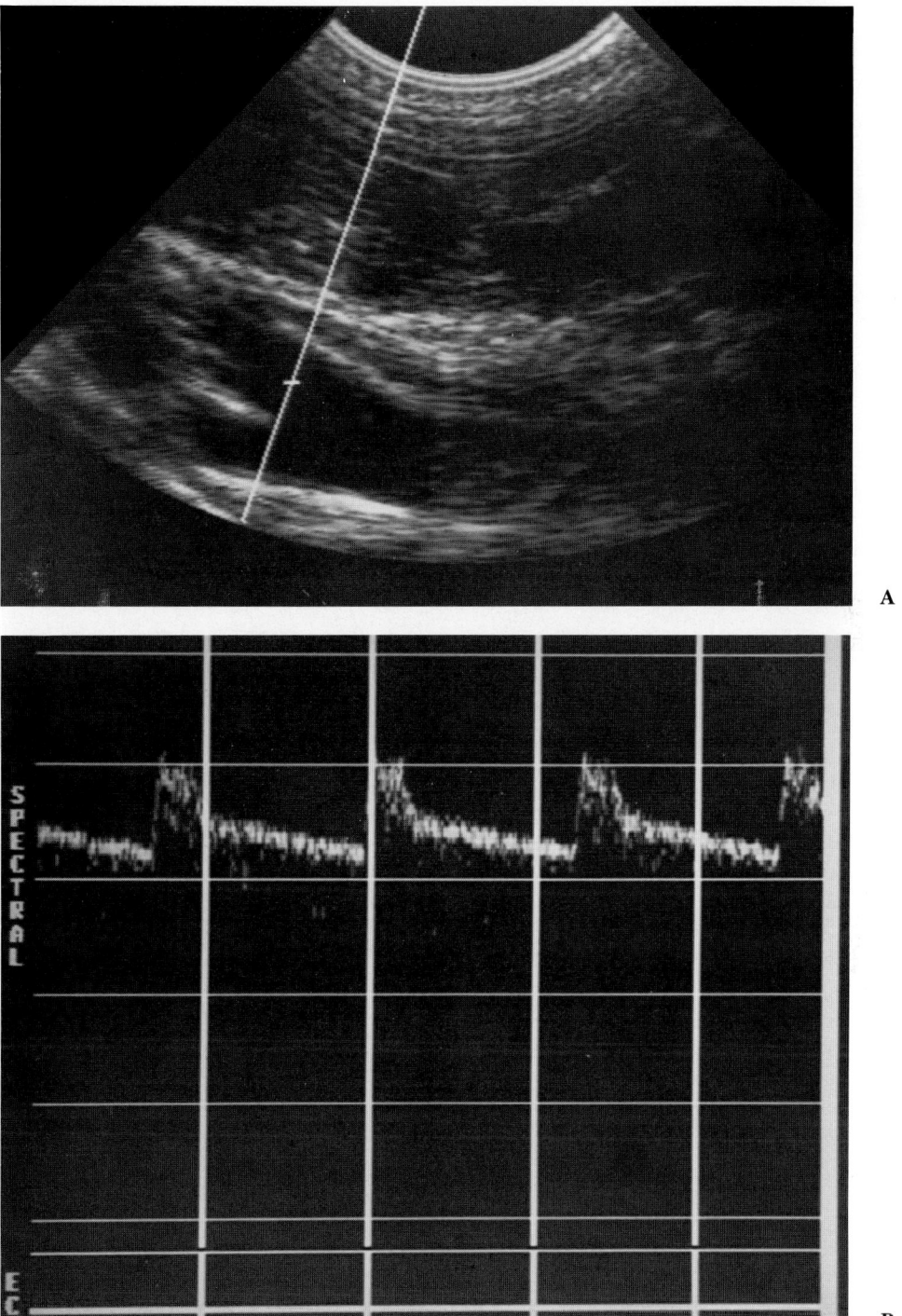

Fig. 2.20A–F. Boundary separation zone—Center stream sample from proximal ICA (**A**) produces typical diphasic waveform (**B**). A normal region of low flow, the "boundary separation zone," (**C**) produces rather bizarre traces that are frequently of low amplitude and may have prominent negative components (**D**). Color flow image (**E**) shows areas of blue (*arrows*), confirming flow reversal in boundary separation zone. (For a color reproduction of this figure see frontmatter.) Courtesy of Quantum Systems, Inc., California. The unusual flow patterns of this area may render it prone to atherosclerotic disease. **F.** Isolated plaque (*arrowheads*) is commonly found in area corresponding to boundary separation zone. *(See next pages.)*

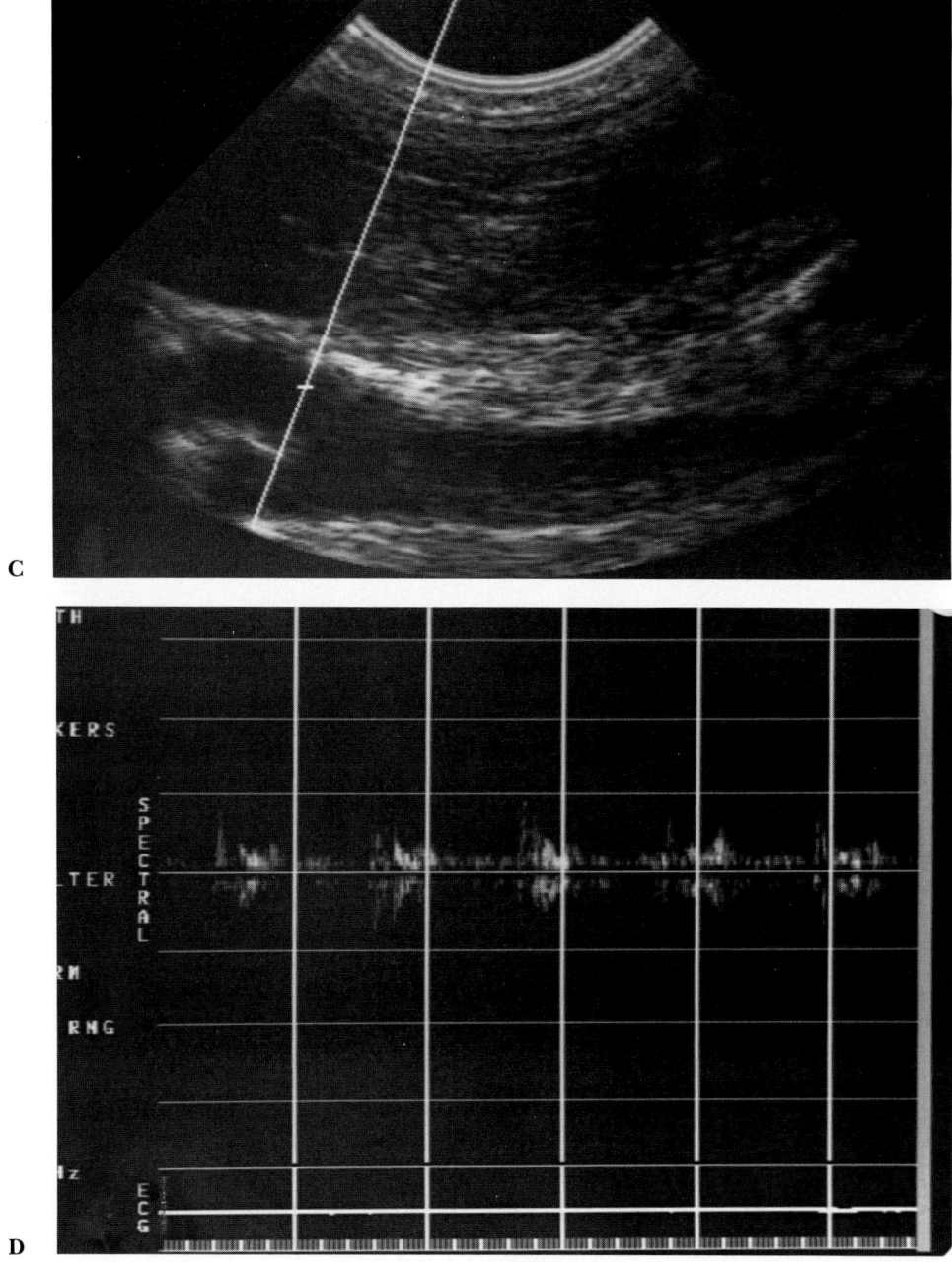

Fig. 2.20.

the result of the complex flow dynamics that occur as the common carotid divides. In addition to bifurcating and interacting with the vessel walls, flow is being directed into two very different conduits, one of which is high resistance and the other of which is low resistance. Some researchers, in fact, have linked the early and common appearance of atherosclerosis in the proximal ICA to the particularly turbulent flow patterns that are found in its proximal ampullary region (53).

Minor bifurcation turbulence and the unusual flow patterns of hospital employees aside, in general, flow velocity is directly proportional to the degree of luminal compromise. With increasing velocity one also fre-

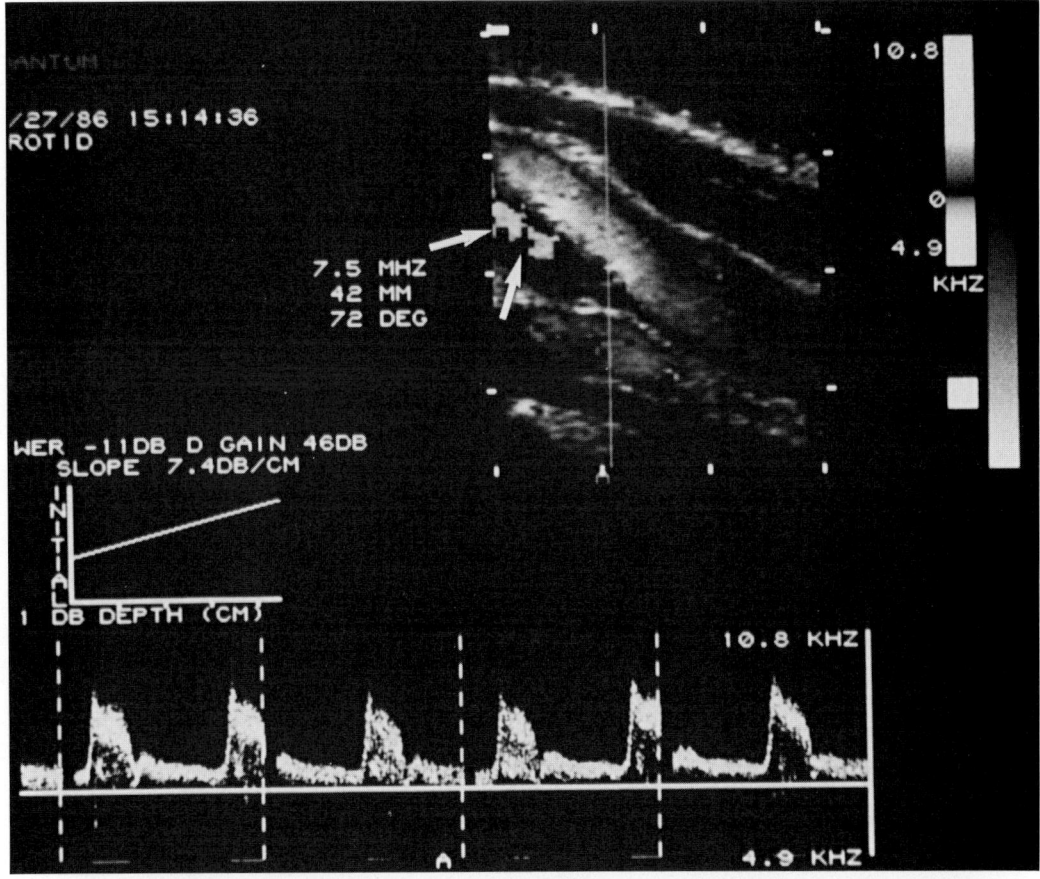

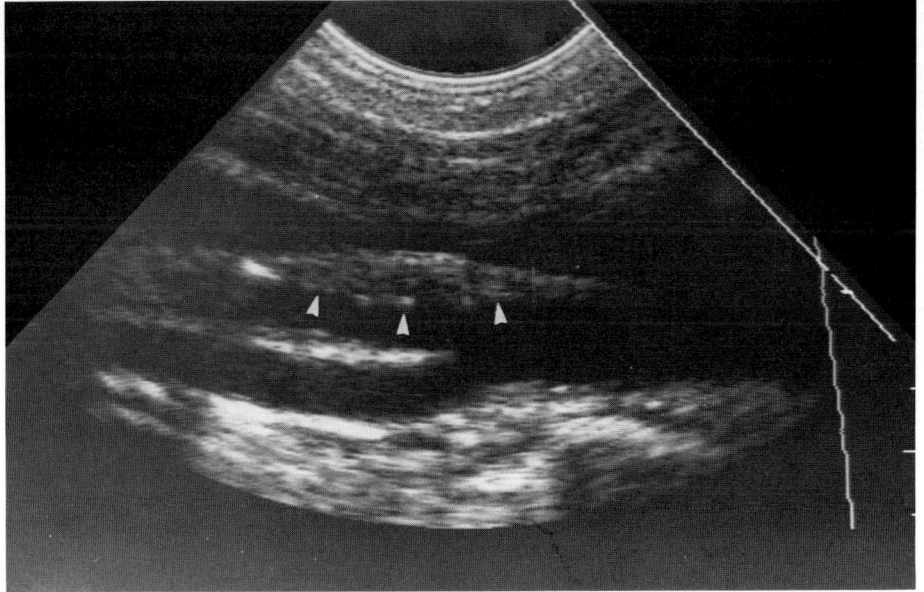

Fig. 2.20.

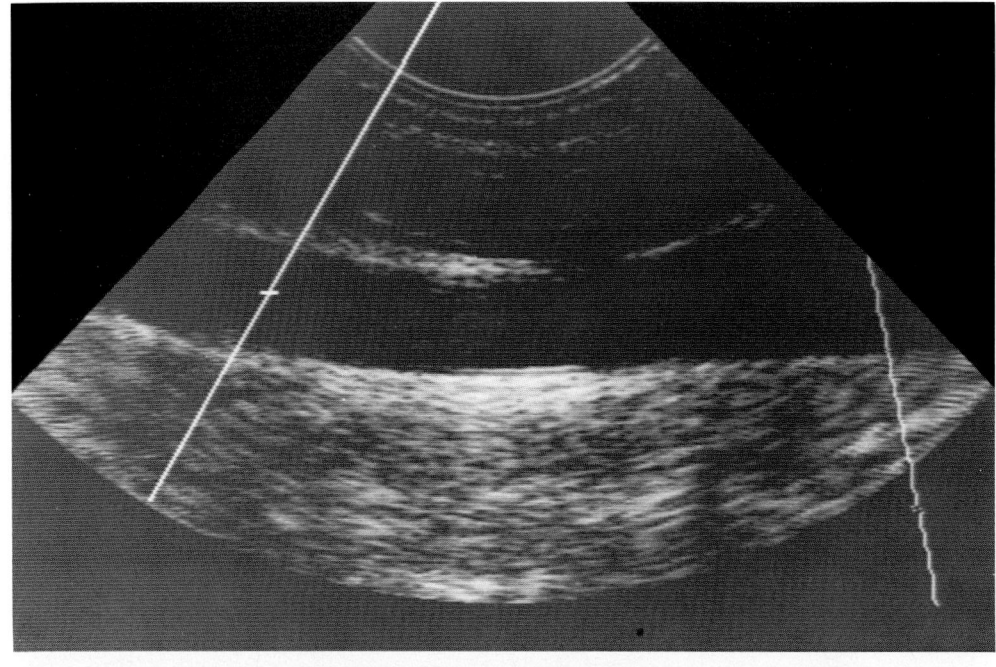

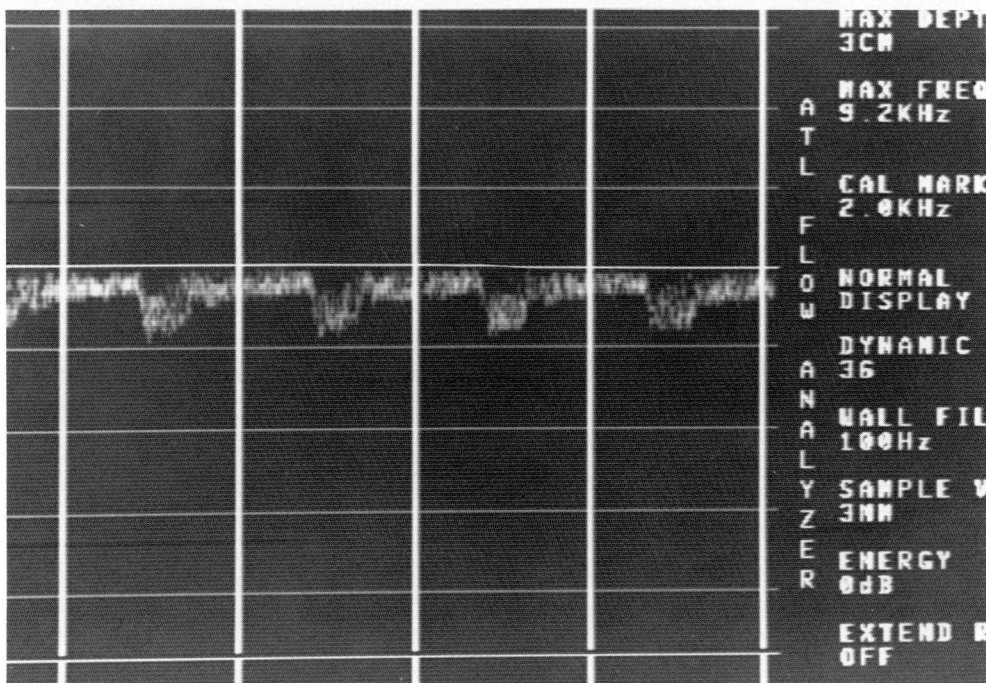

Fig. 2.21A–H. Moderate ICA stenosis (50 to 75%) – Evaluation of distal CCA is normal (**A**, **B**). Beyond ICA origin a localized area of flow abnormality is encountered. Real-time image (**C**) is unremarkable. Doppler evaluation (**D**) shows complete filling in of sonic window (*arrows*). A mild focal velocity increase is present. Each graticule = 2 KHzΔ. Although 4 KHzΔ is within normal range, it does represent a doubling of flow velocity when compared with the CCI. VICA/VCCA is, therefore, diagnostic, whereas peak KHzΔ is misleadingly normal. More distally, ICA flow returns to normal (**E**, **F**). Anteroposterior and lateral views from arteriogram (**G**, **H**) confirm abnormality; lesion (*black arrows*) called 60% stenotic by neuroradiologist. *(See next pages.)*

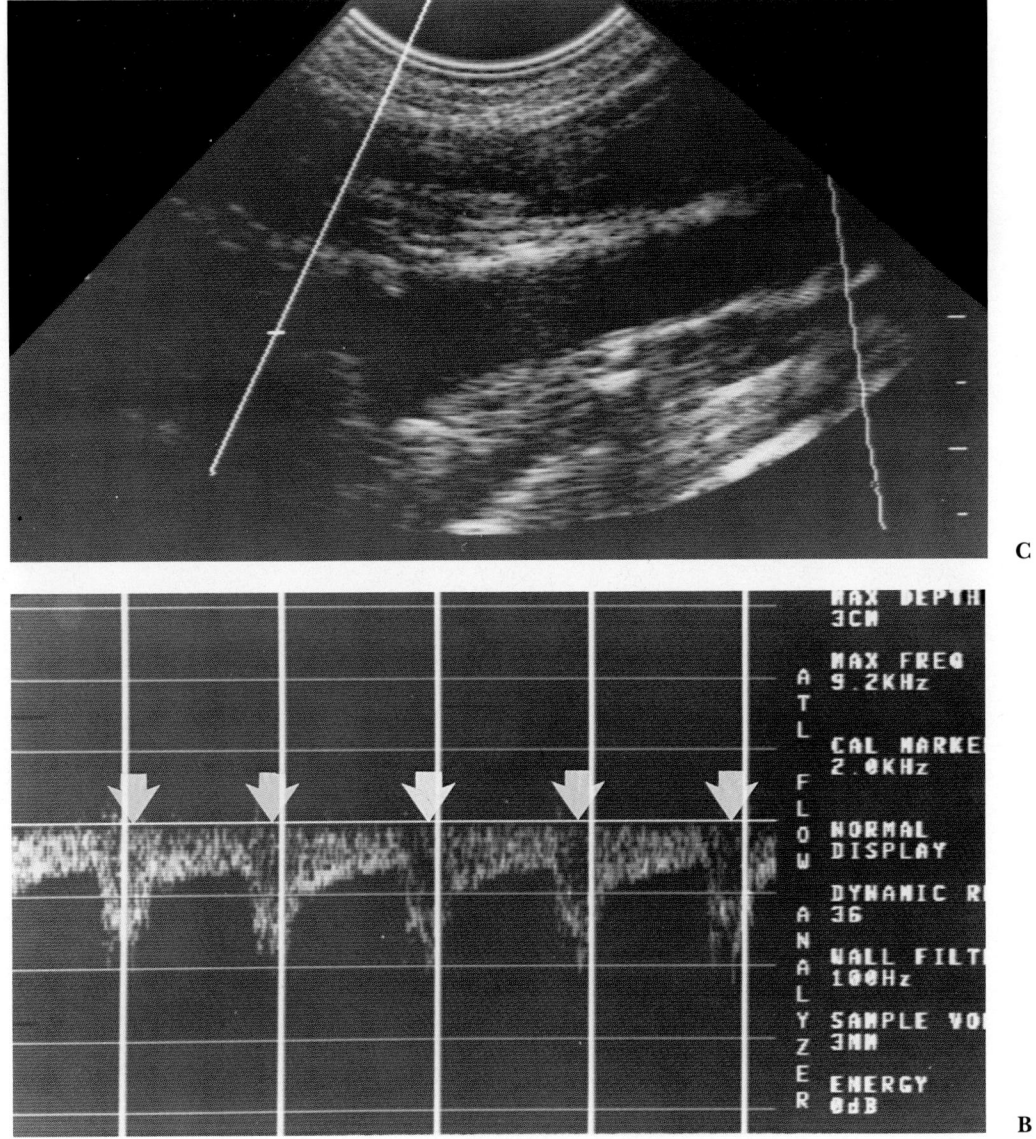

Fig. 2.21.

quently encounters more pronounced spectral broadening. Although this is the rule, we have occasionally encountered patients with abnormally high velocities and relatively clean Doppler traces who had high-grade stenoses. Assuming the increased velocity represents a true localized phenomenon and is not the result of an unusually steep scanning angle, even in the absence of spectral broadening, significant luminal compromise should be suspected. Conversely, true spectral broadening of sufficient magnitude to fill in the sonic window but without a marked velocity increase should also be viewed with suspicion (Fig. 2.21 A–E). In the latter case, however, a lesion greater than 75% would seem extremely unlikely unless the patient had generalized low flow velocity. Low velocity is usually encountered in patients with poor cardiac output. In any atypical situation, the use of multiple Doppler criteria, particularly ratios, may be very important.

As carotid stenoses become tight, high-flow velocities are almost invariably generated. Stenoses that narrow the lumen 75 to 90% are

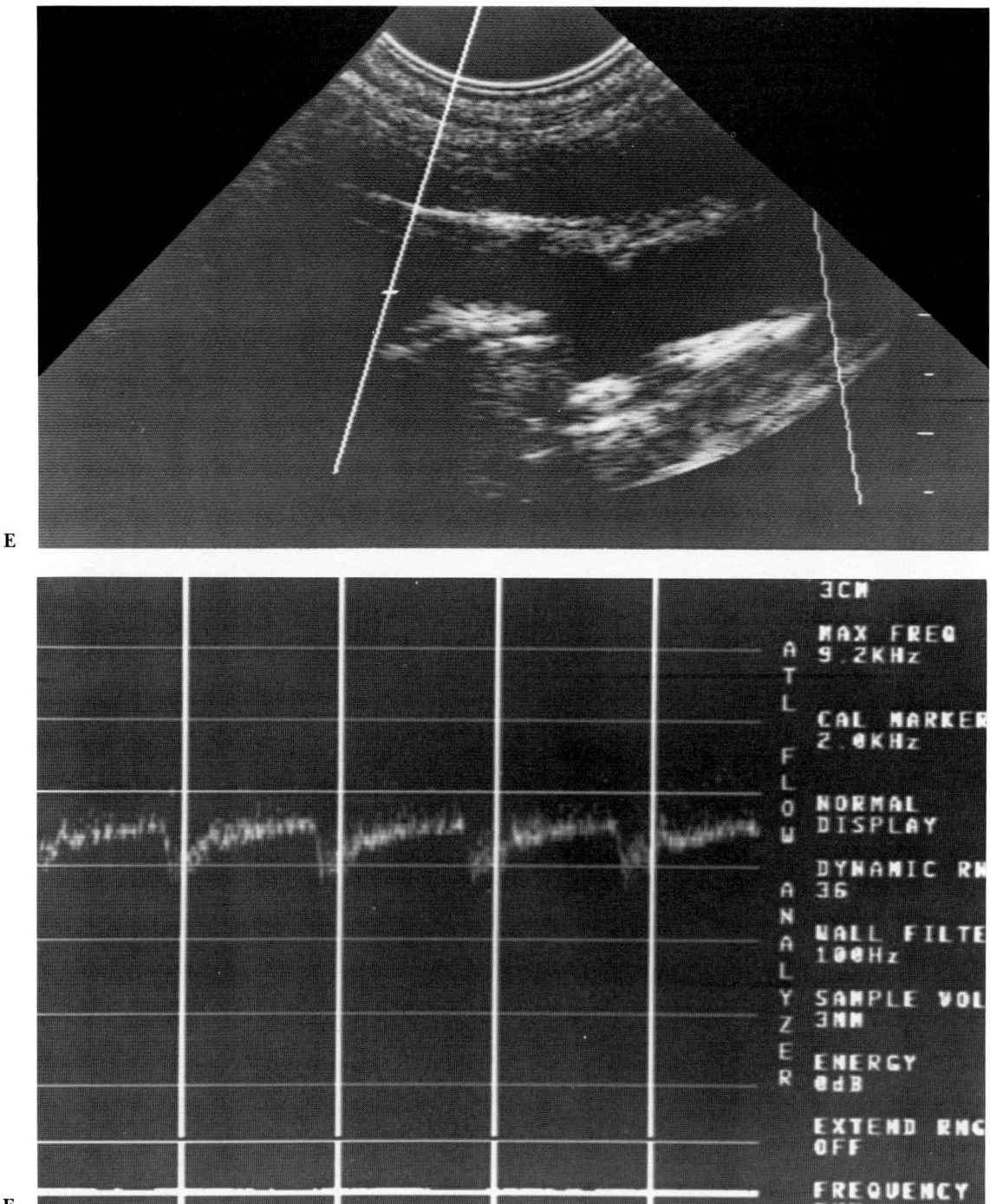

Fig. 2.21.

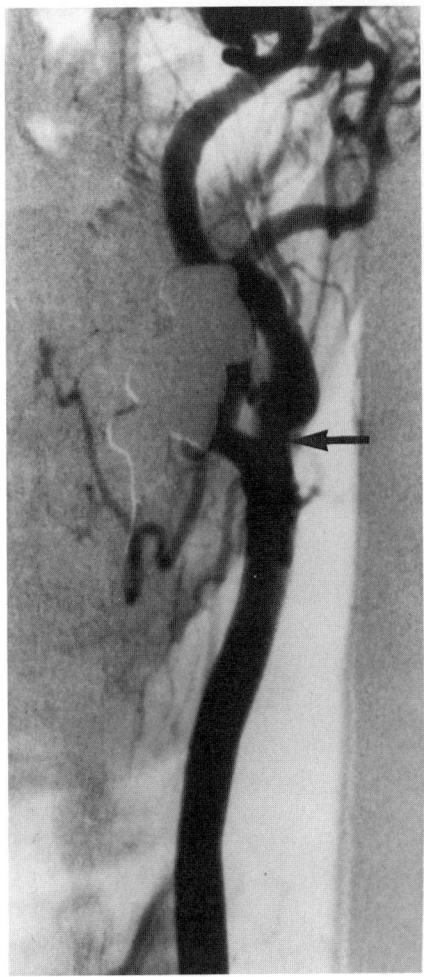
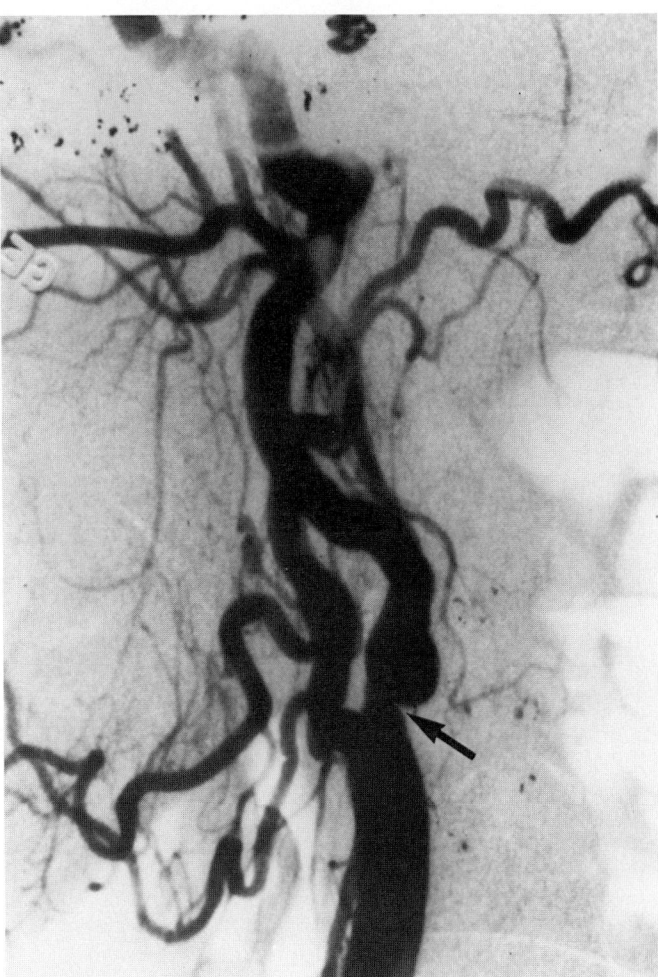

G H

Fig. 2.21.

typically the most obvious lesions for Doppler examination (Fig. 2.22 A–E). Doppler reaches its highest accuracy in this clinically important area. The thin, high-pitched, scratchy sound is often obvious even to the passerby outside of the examining room. In addition to peak systolic velocity, diastolic flow may increase markedly in tight stenoses. Strandness (personal communication), in fact, contends that an increase in diastolic flow velocity beyond 4.5 KHzΔ is actually the mark of stenoses greater than 80%. Although a diastolic KHzΔ of 4.5 or greater almost certainly implies a high-grade (or very importantly, surgically correctable) lesion, it has been my own experience that end diastolic flow of 4.5 KHzΔ or greater is quite unusual. Again, the most typical abnormality encountered is the markedly increased velocity at peak systole.

As the carotid lumen becomes compromised beyond 90%, a different phenomenon begins to emerge. Flow velocity actually begins to decrease through the extremely tight residual lumen (54,55). These lesions may present difficulty in their diagnosis as their maximum flow velocities are frequently well within the normal range. In the majority of cases, however, they will be easily recognized by an extremely distorted waveform (Fig. 2.23 A–E). Although the diagnosis can be made using the spectral display, the ears often recognize it best. Subtotal stenoses simply sound very abnormal. They typically sound much more abnormal than they look. A harsh hissing is often encountered,

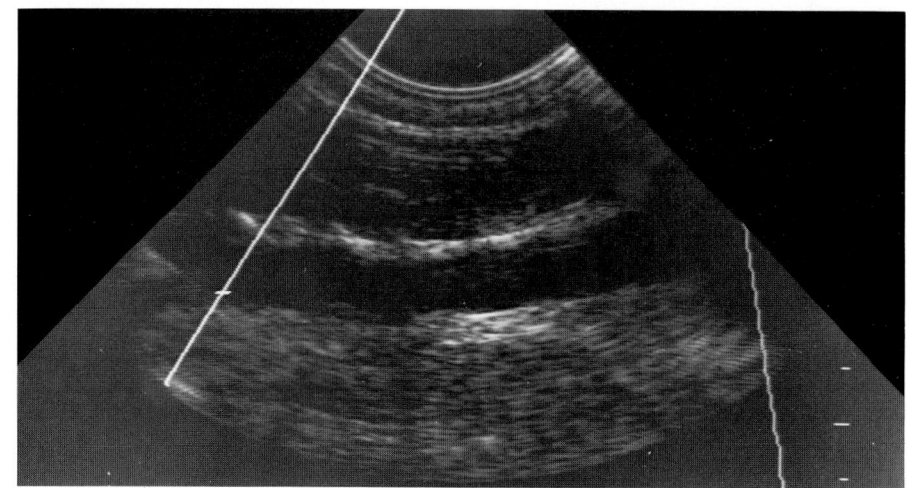

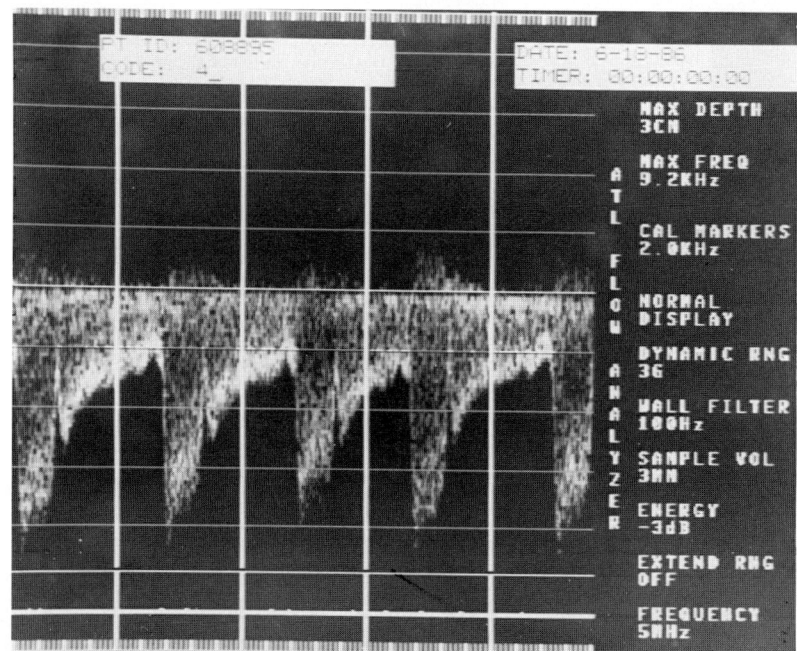

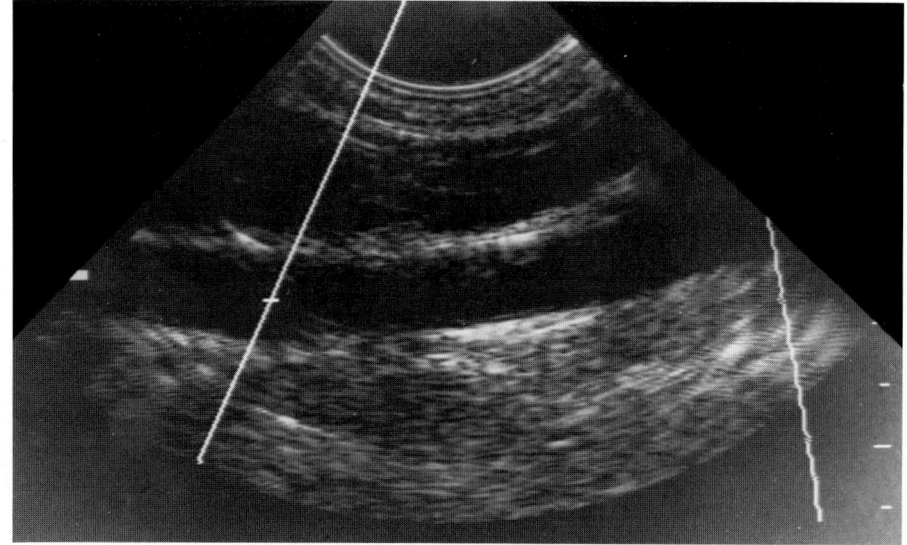

Fig. 2.22.

2. Duplex Sonography of the Cerebrovascular System

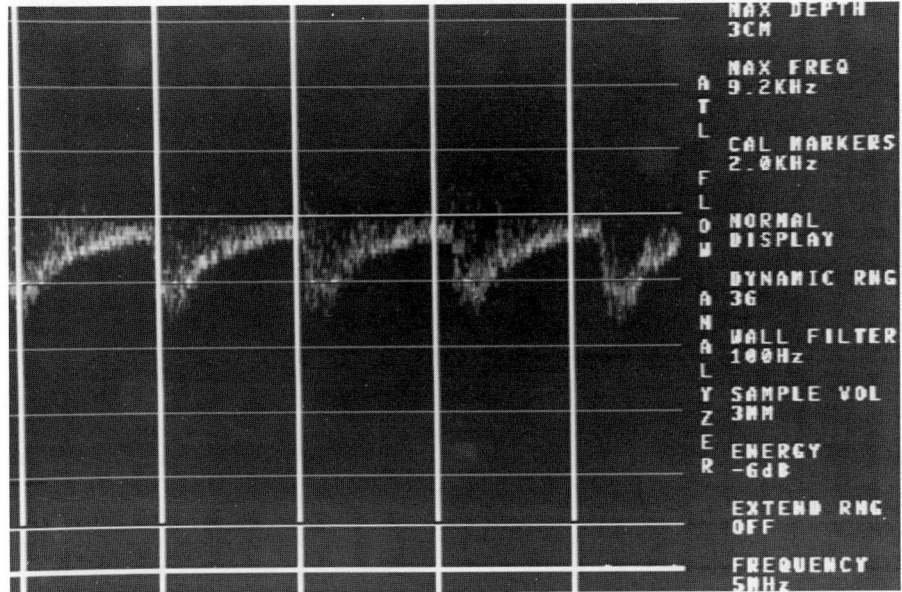

which probably represents the vessel's last desperate attempt at maintaining flow. In this regard, it should be emphasized that subtotal lesions, like atherosclerosis in general (56), are not static. We have encountered a number of patients who returned a short time after a diagnosis of subtotal occlusion was made and no flow was present at all. If intervention is contemplated in patients with high-grade lesions, it should be carried out as soon as possible. Total occlusions are not surgical lesions.

From the foregoing discussion, one would logically presume the diagnosis of total occlusion to be quite simple using duplex. Large, solid, or calcific plaque should fill the origin of the ICA, and the absence of a Doppler trace confirms the diagnosis (Fig. 2.24 A–D). This scenario is, unfortunately, encountered too infrequently. More typically, externalized (high-resistance) flow will be found throughout the CCA, but at the origin of the ICA a normal appearing anechoic lumen will be found. The

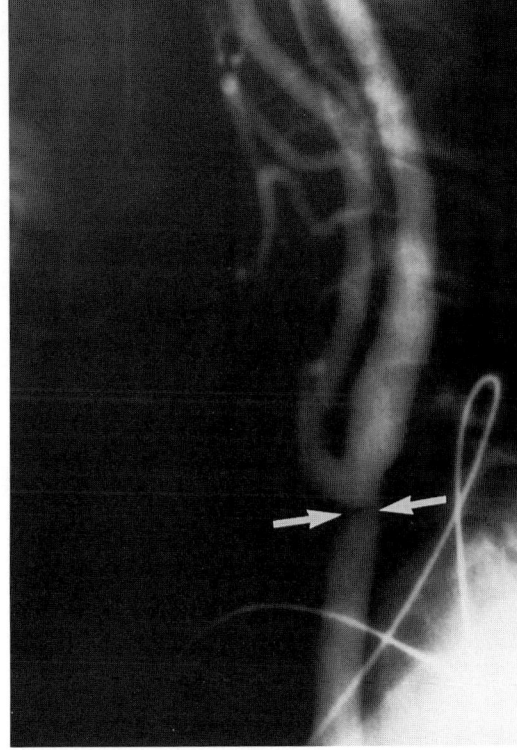

Fig. 2.22A–E. High-grade (75 to 90%) stenosis—59-year-old woman with history of transient left arm weakness. Contralateral bifurcation has a markedly abnormal Doppler pattern (**B**). Peak systolic KHzΔ is greater than 8 (graticules = 2 KHzΔ), and pronounced spectral broadening is present. Note that flow at end diastole does not exceed 2 to 3 KHzΔ. Lesion is actually in carotid bulb. Real-time image is remarkably normal in appearance (**A**). Doppler trace taken distal to lesion (**D**) has reverted to normal, indicating a segmental stenoses. Arteriogram (**E**) confirms ultrasound findings. Note bandlike area of stenosis (*arrows*) in carotid bulb.

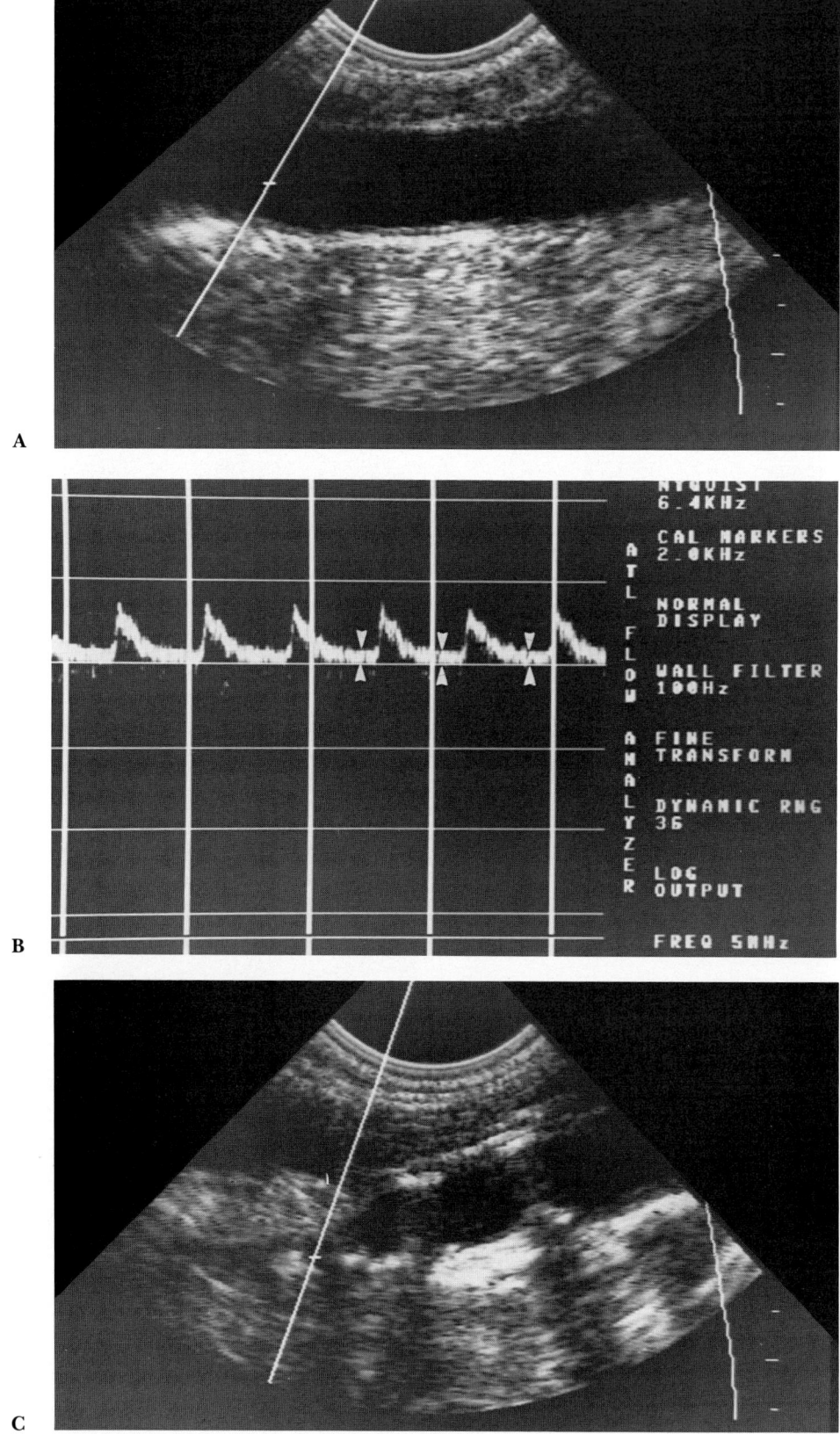

Fig. 2.23.

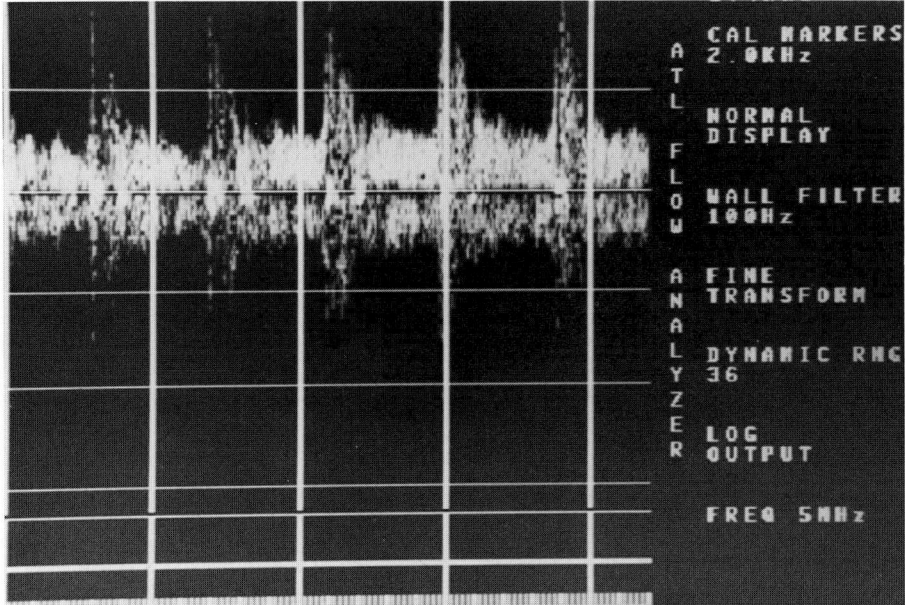

Doppler probe, however, will fail to identify flow after an exhaustive search (Fig. 2.25 A–D). The accurate diagnosis of total ICA occlusion is often, however, not as straightforward as these two cases might imply. In our own early experience (25) and in that of Zweibel and Crummy (57), duplex was actually only capable of diagnosing total occlusions approximately 50% of the time! In fairness, however, I should add that many groups have been quite accurate in diagnosing total occlusions (26–29). The reasons for the apparent difficulty in diagnosing total occlusions are many. In some cases, the occlusion may not actually begin at the carotid bifurcation. A patent ICA stump may be encountered that exhibits a very unusual flow pattern (Fig. 2.26 A–E). This pattern is probably the result of blood merely sloshing back and forth in the lumen and has a peculiar audible "thudding" quality. We have called this "stump flow."

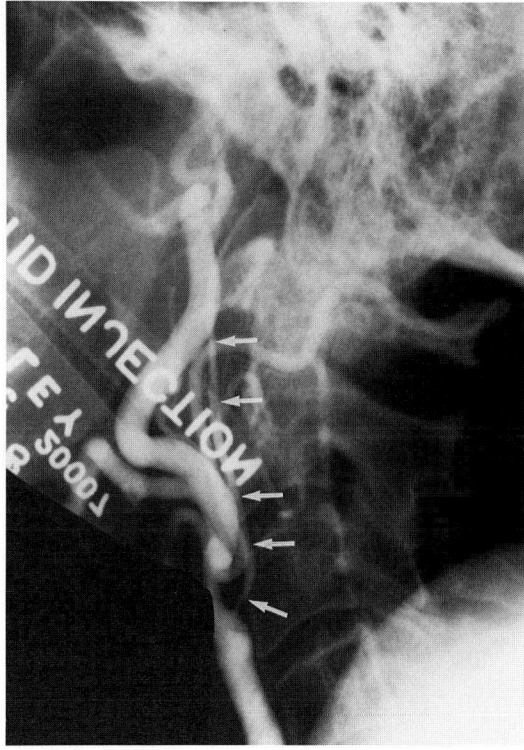

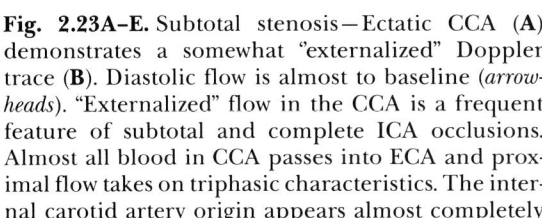

Fig. 2.23A–E. Subtotal stenosis—Ectatic CCA (**A**) demonstrates a somewhat "externalized" Doppler trace (**B**). Diastolic flow is almost to baseline (*arrowheads*). "Externalized" flow in the CCA is a frequent feature of subtotal and complete ICA occlusions. Almost all blood in CCA passes into ECA and proximal flow takes on triphasic characteristics. The internal carotid artery origin appears almost completely blocked by soft and calcific plaque (**C**). Doppler trace is disorganized (**D**). Systolic peak is reduced to a few sharp lines. Note that maximum systolic velocity is within normal range. Audible Doppler signals in this patient were very abnormal. Angiogram confirms sonographic findings of subtotal stenosis; the entire ICA is markedly narrowed (*arrows*) (**E**).

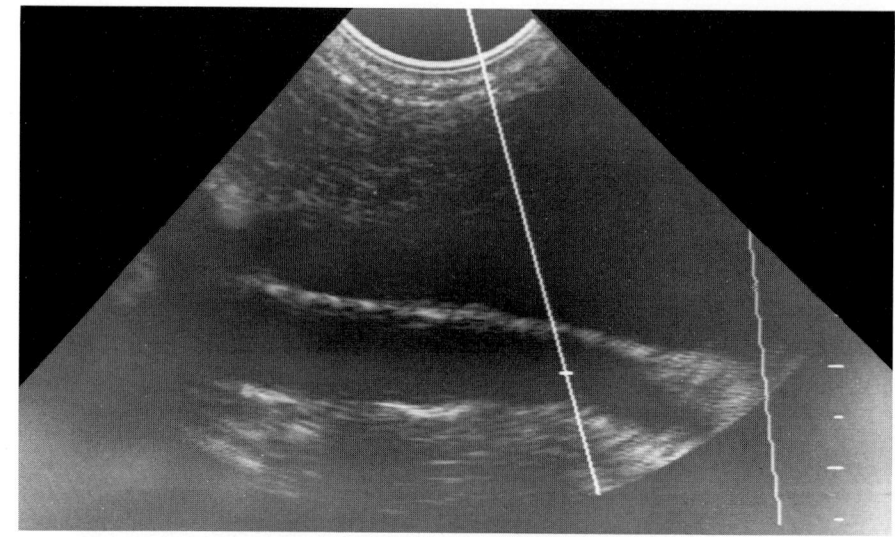

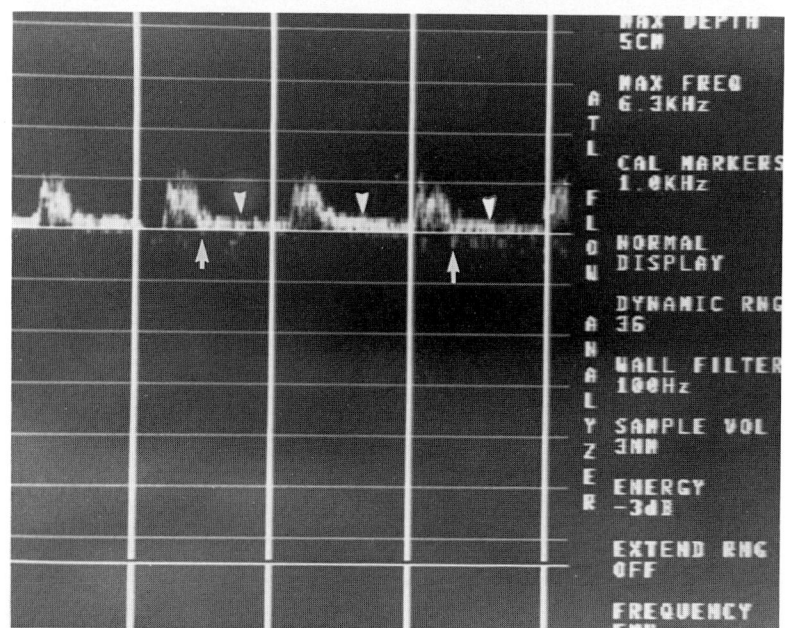

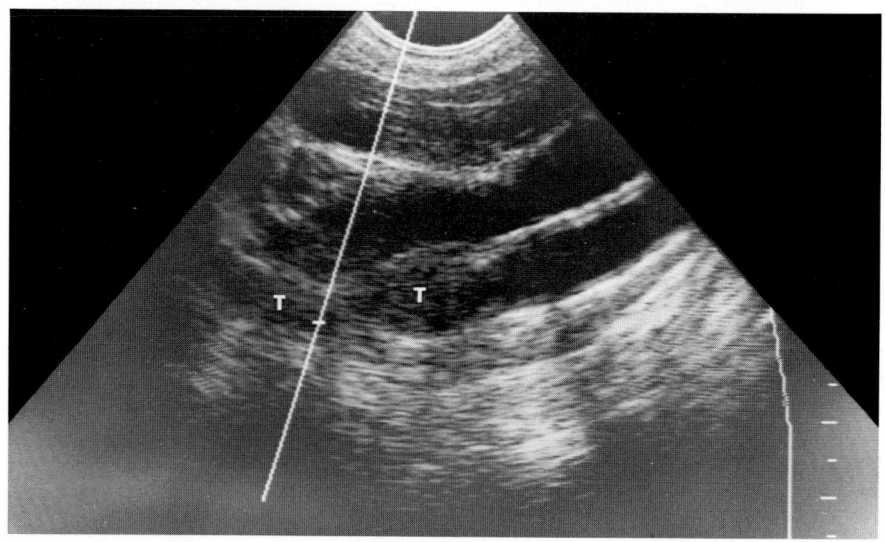

Fig. 2.24.

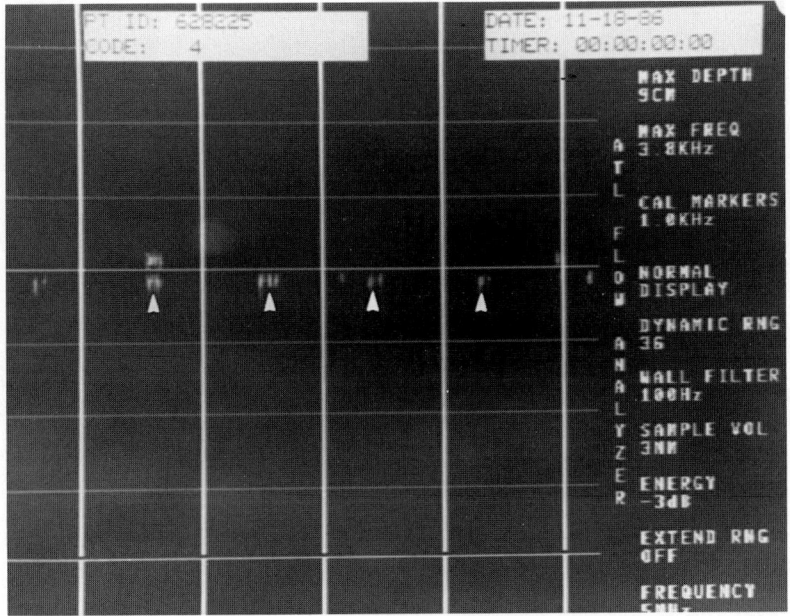

Other difficulties in the diagnosis of high-grade total occlusions may involve mistaking the ECA (or more typically one of its branches) for the ICA. Not infrequently one will encounter flow somewhat distal to the bifurcation in a vessel thought to be a severely diseased ICA, when the ICA origin is actually occluded. In these cases, the Doppler signal most likely arises from a tortuous ECA or one of its branches (Fig. 2.27 A–C). Further complicating the diagnosis of subtotal-total occlusion is the fact that as the ICA narrows, the ECA frequently begins to take on more low-resistance flow characteristics. This is probably the result of the opening of widespread ECA/ICA collaterals.

Particularly confusing ECA flow patterns may be found in patients with totally occluded internal carotid arteries who have undergone external carotid (temporal) artery-middle cerebral artery bypass. In these patients, flow in the ECA may be very internalized and all but impossible

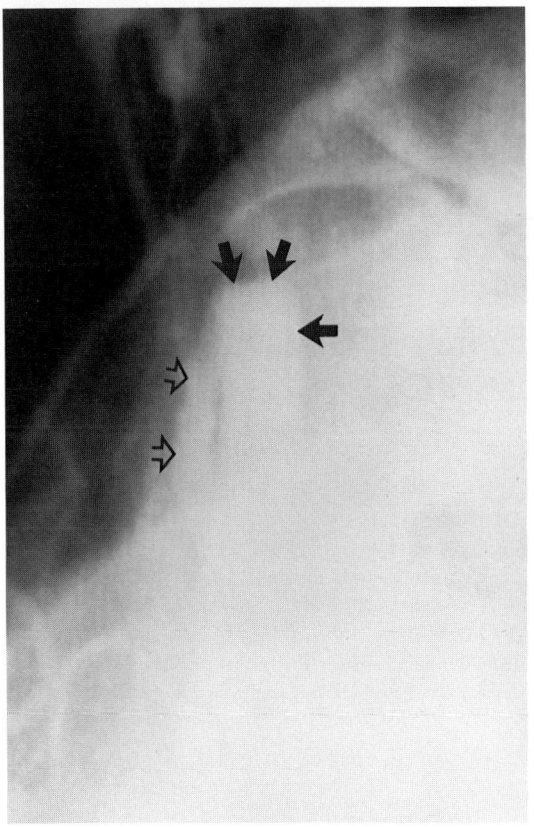

Fig. 2.24A–E. Total ICA occlusion—Mid-CCA appears normal (**A**) but exhibits an externalized waveform (**B**). Note diastolic flow to baseline (*arrowheads*) and occasional flow reversal (*arrows*). Solid thrombus (T) completely occludes bulb and visible portions of ICA (**C**). Doppler trace is absent (**D**). Small pulsations as shown (*arrowheads*) are common in total occlusion. They should not be taken to represent true flow. Arteriogram (**E**) confirms complete occlusion to distal CCA (*arrowheads*). Superior thyroidal artery (*open arrows*) remains patent.

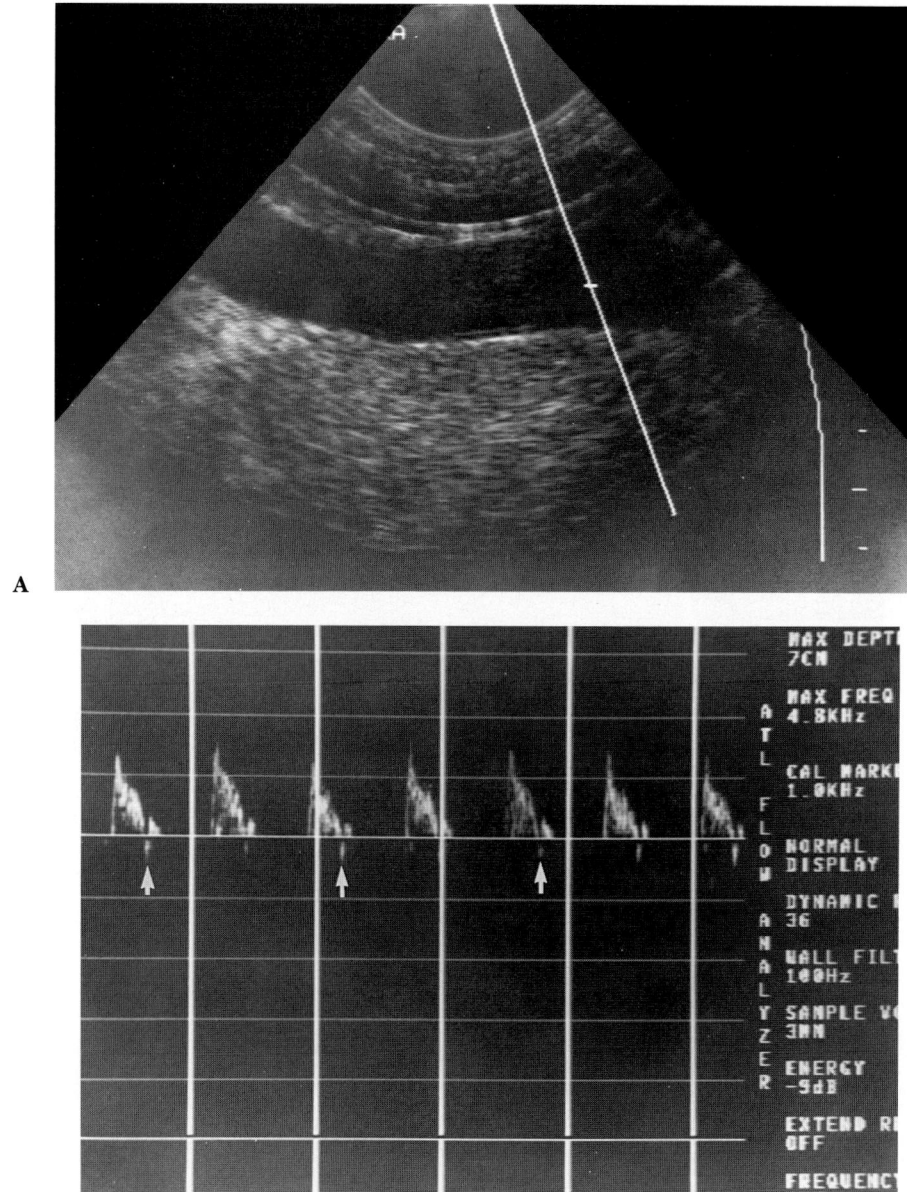

Fig. 2.25A–D. Total ICA occlusion—65-year-old woman immediately postendarterectomy with right-sided weakness and facial droop. Common carotid artery (**B**) waveform is markedly externalized. Flow is completely absent in diastole, and the negative component (*arrows*) is quite pronounced. Proximal ICA (*arrowhead*) is totally anechoic (**C**), but Doppler trace is absent (**D**). Patient was immediately returned to operating room; large thrombus was removed. Patient did well after surgery. Anechoic thrombus is common and often found in association with total occlusion whether postsurgical or not.

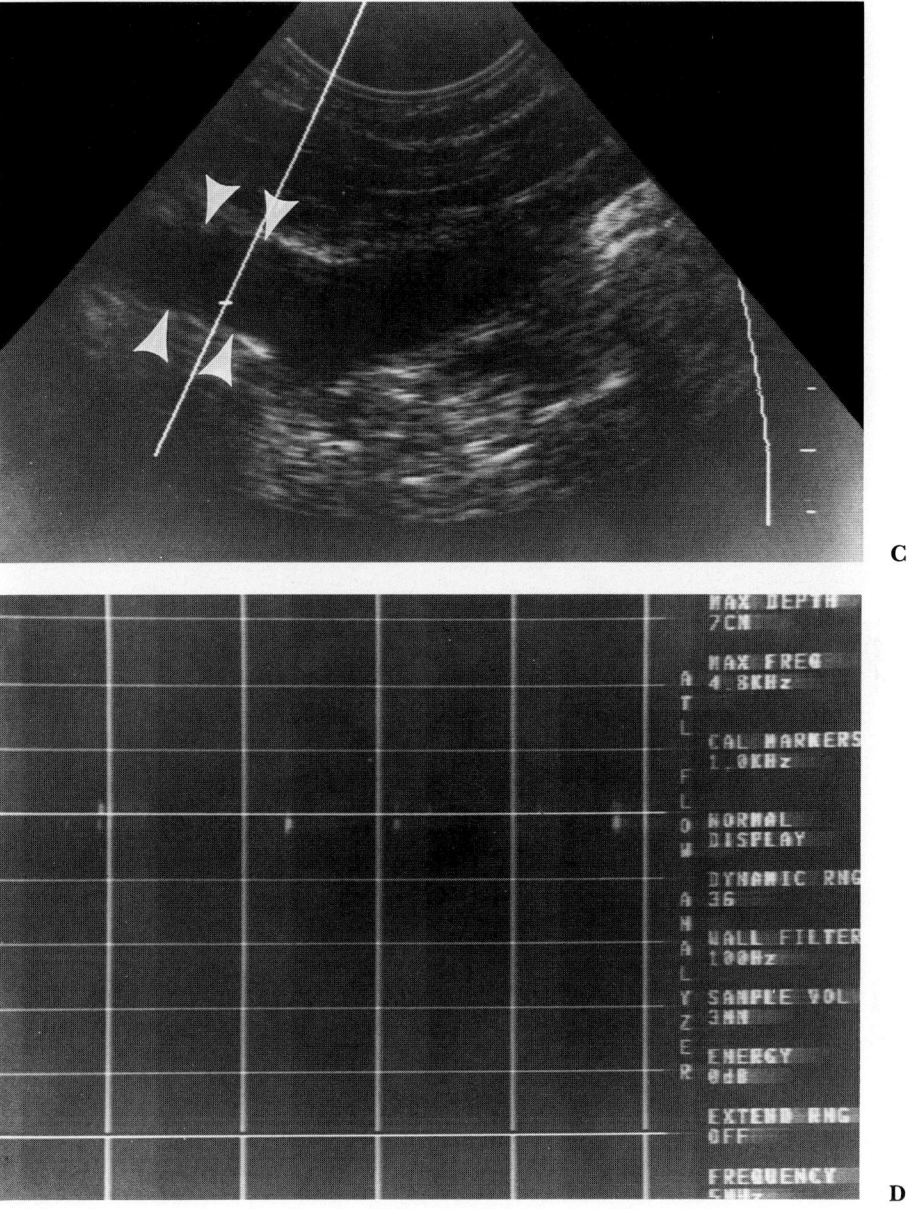

Fig. 2.25.

to identify from its Doppler signature (Fig. 2.28 A–D). As an aid in sometimes better determining if a vessel is truly the ECA, one may continue to scan at its base and simultaneously "milk" back or tap over the area of the patient's temporal artery. This return of blood may briefly dampen flow in the ECA; the ICA, on the other hand, will show no effect from this maneuver.

Another difficulty that may arise in the evaluation of subtotal-total occlusion is the inability to find a small residual lumen. Plaque or thrombus is frequently anechoic at real-time rendering the residual lumen invisible. The Doppler cursor, therefore, must be serendipitously placed in the minute stream of flow. Extensive sampling must be done before the diagnosis of total occlusion is entertained. Temporarily increasing the size of the sample volume may be of assistance in such cases. Conversely, real-time scanning may actually identify a tiny thread of

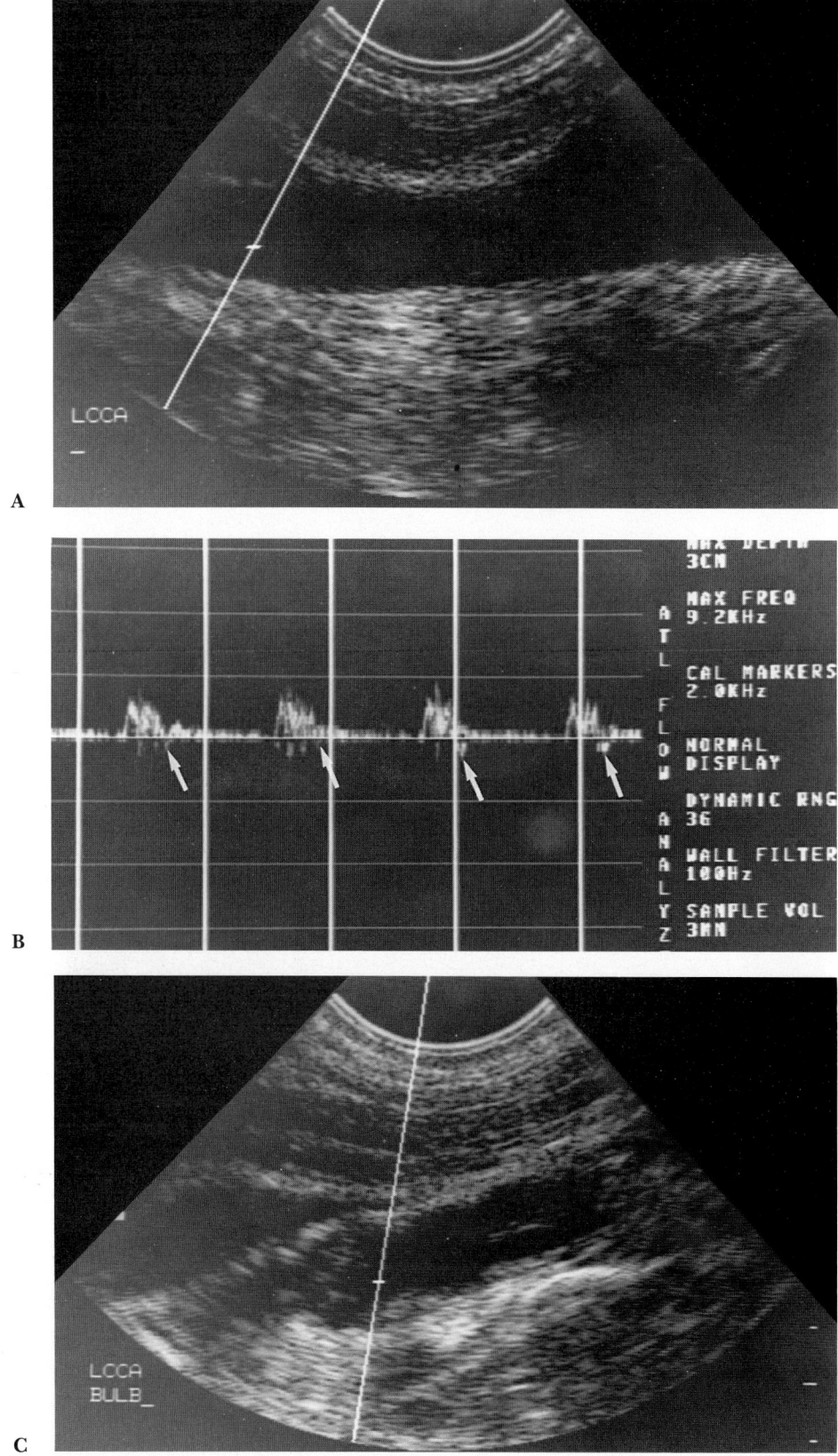

Fig. 2.26.

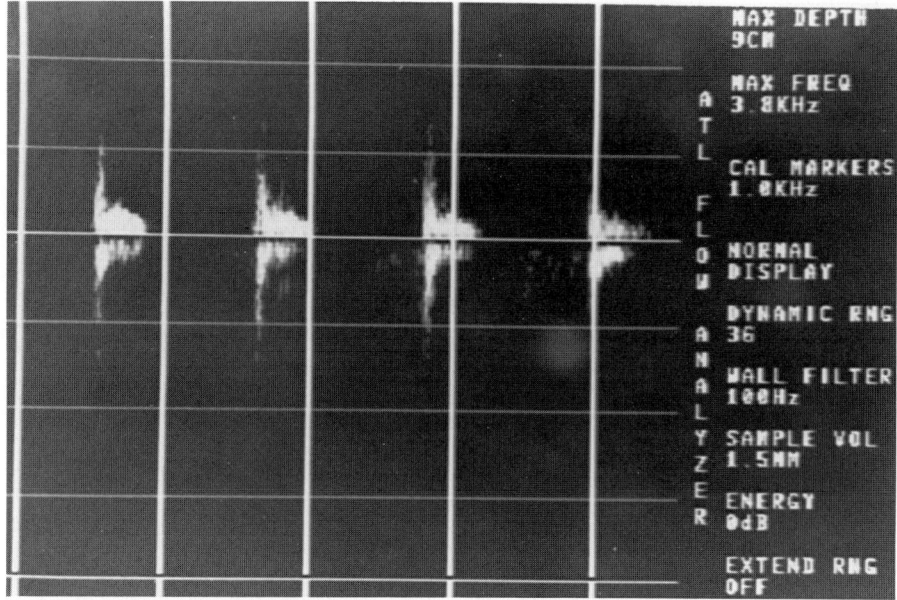

patency in the proximal ICA, and some flow may be confirmed by Doppler, leading to a diagnosis of subtotal occlusion. Occasionally, the end of the lumen may be further distal and unseen by the sonogram. The identification of "stump flow" in a minute lumen may accurately imply such a distal obstruction.

A final difficulty encountered in subtotal-total occlusion is transmitted pulsations. The Doppler cursor may be clearly in the ICA lumen and pulsatile flow identified. One must pay close attention to the direction of flow and the nature of the pulsations. True center stream sampling should be documented by transverse scanning and the sample volume reduced in size as much as possible. Extraneous pulsations should seldom be transmitted to the center of a thrombus. Pulsatile flow from the jugular vein can be excluded by the shape of the waveform and the fact that flow is in the opposite direction from that of the carotid. If any question

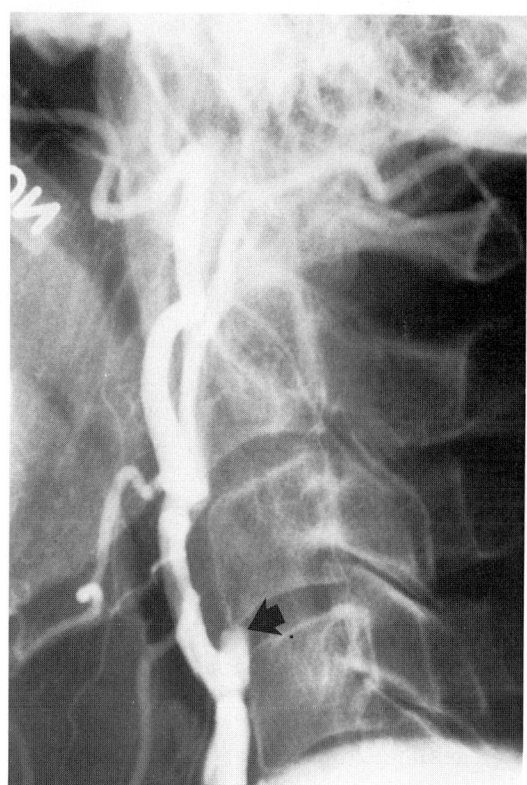

Fig. 2.26A–E. "Stump flow"—Distal CCA (**A,B**) exhibits dampened and markedly externalized flow pattern. Note almost complete absence of diastolic flow and prominent negative components (*arrows*). Small patent stump (around Doppler cursor) of ICA is noted to be surrounded by thrombus by real-time examination (**C**). Doppler spectra (**D**) are quite peculiar, being both above and below baseline with absent diastolic component (**B**). To the listener, stump flow sounds as if something is "thudding" against the Doppler speaker. Angiogram (**E**) shows total ICA occlusion with small patent stump (*arrow*), which corresponds nicely to real-time image.

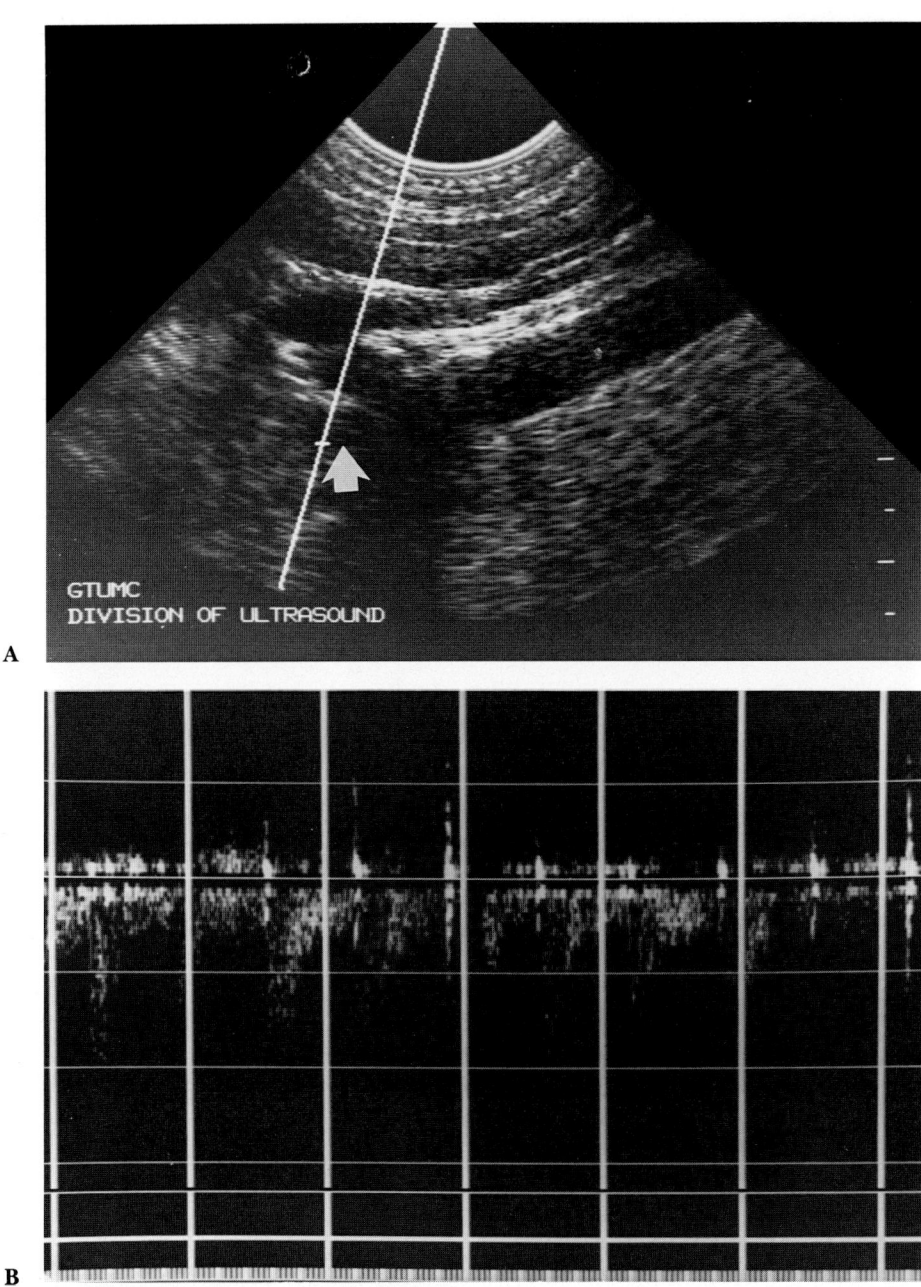

Fig. 2.27A–C. Totally occluded ICA – Flow was demonstrated in a vessel beyond the carotid bulb (**A**). The trace was extremely distorted (**B**) but interpreted as representing a severely diseased ICA. Arteriogram (**C**) shows a number of ECA branches, one of which was presumably responsible for the Doppler signal. The ICA is totally occluded.

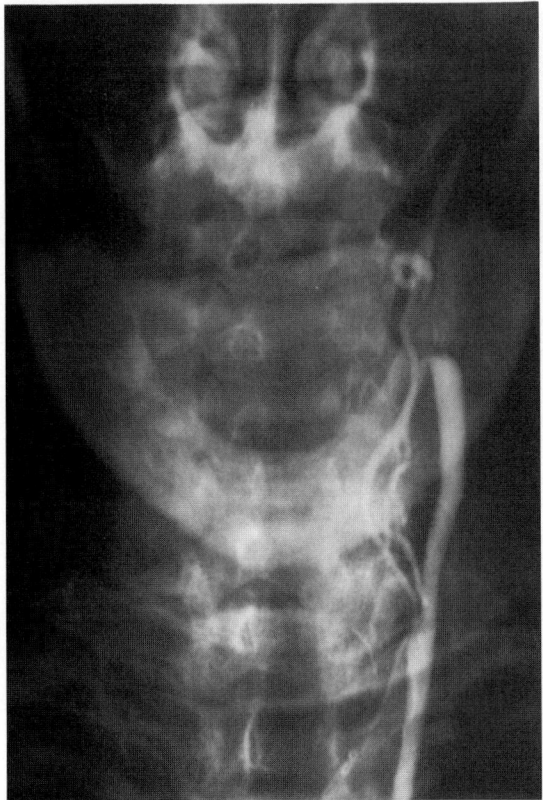

Fig. 2.27.

exists, the vein may be easily compressed manually, thereby briefly eliminating the flow. The venous flow pattern will also be affected by breath holding or the Valsalva maneuver.

When evaluating total occlusions, one should never assume that thrombus always propagates distally into the head. Although distal propagation almost invariably occurs with ICA occlusions, CCA occlusions are often localized. Flow may be maintained in the ECA and ICA but must be reversed in one of the two vessels (58). Most commonly, retrograde flow in the ECA will supply the ICA (Fig. 2.29 A–E); occasionally, the opposite will be encountered. The astute sonographer, therefore, must always remain alert for the unusual possibility of reversed flow. Because scanning is performed from many directions and frequently displayed both above and below baseline, the "obvious" abnormality of flow reversal may be more easily overlooked than suspected.

In day-to-day practice we rely rather heavily on peak systolic velocity and the presence or absence of spectral broadening. Additional Doppler parameters, however, are also frequently essential in diagnosing rate-limiting lesions. The advantage of ratio measurements over peak systolic velocity lies in their ability to eliminate the effect of noncarotid variables. This is particularly useful, for example, in patients with high flow secondary to hypertension or low flow secondary to poor cardiac output.

Among the most widely used of these ratios is the comparison of ICA velocity to CCA velocity. Garth et al (24) actually rely more heavily on VICA-VCC than peak systolic velocity. Their excellent results indicate that a VICA-VCCA of greater than 1.5 strongly correlates with significant arterial compromise. Vaisman and Wojciechowski (59) evaluated a series of Doppler parameters including peak systolic velocity, VICA-VCCA, peak systolic velocity of the CCA, and the ratio of the right ICA to the left. Their study found the ratio of the velocity of one ICA to the other to be the most accurate variable in diagnosing hemodynamically significant ICA disease. They also demonstrated that the velocity in the common carotid artery is frequently altered when significant occlusion is present in the ICA. These latter two parameters seem to have attracted relatively little attention and do not seem frequently used. I would venture to say that at present, most laboratories rely primarily on peak systolic velocity and/or VICA-VCCA. Although other parameters may be less popular, the implications of the studies of Garth et al (24) and Vaisman and Wojciechowski (59) should be heeded. They found that the more parameters taken into account, the better the accuracy.

In general, one should use as much of the data from a duplex examination as possible and always integrate real-time findings with Doppler. The experienced operator will eventually become comfortable with certain parameters and rely less heavily on others. At times, however, the use of a host of duplex parameters, both real-time and Doppler, will be necessary to make the correct diagnosis.

Cerebrovascular Duplex Sonography: The Vertebral Artery

Before ending this chapter on cerebrovascular duplex, a brief discussion of the vertebral arter-

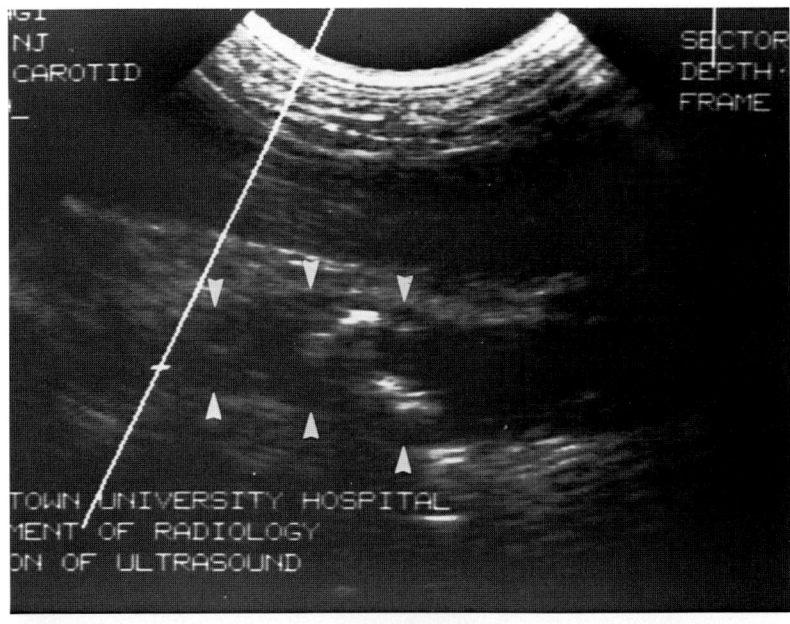

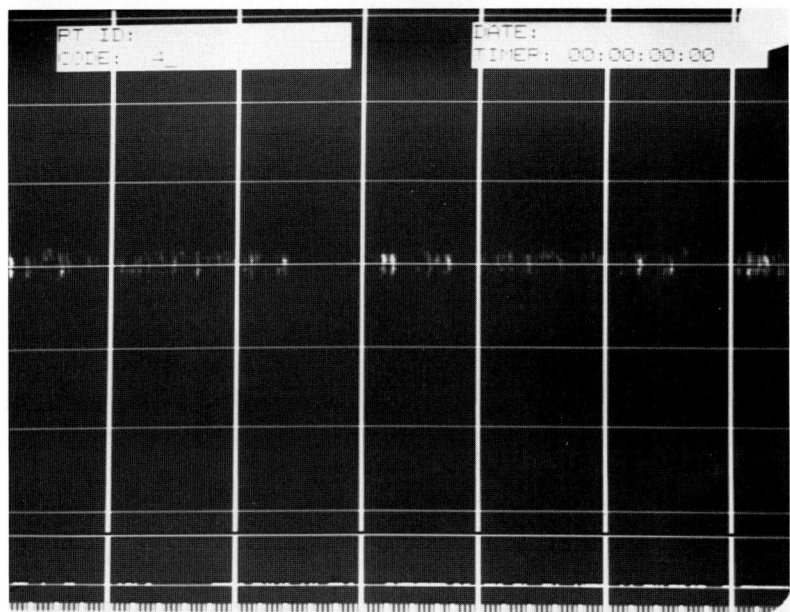

Fig. 2.28A–D. ECA-MCA bypass—Patient with known ICA occlusion who underwent bypass with anastomosis of superficial temporal artery to middle cerebral artery. Duplex scan performed because of recent episodes of confusion and dizziness. Origin of ICA occluded by large, soft, and calcific plaque (*arrowheads*); Doppler trace confirms absent flow (**A**, **B**). A patent ECA was identified and produced a diphasic trace (**C**). Anteriogram (**D**) shows unusual anatomy caused by surgical anastomosis.

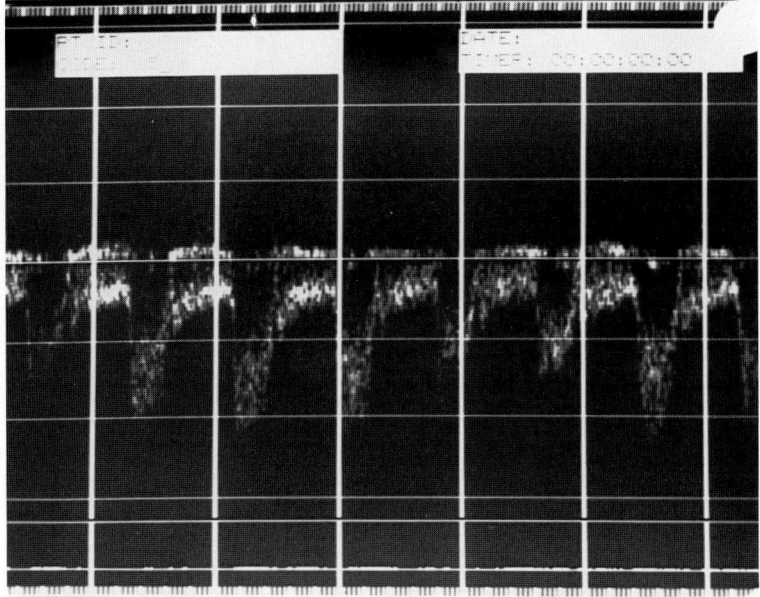

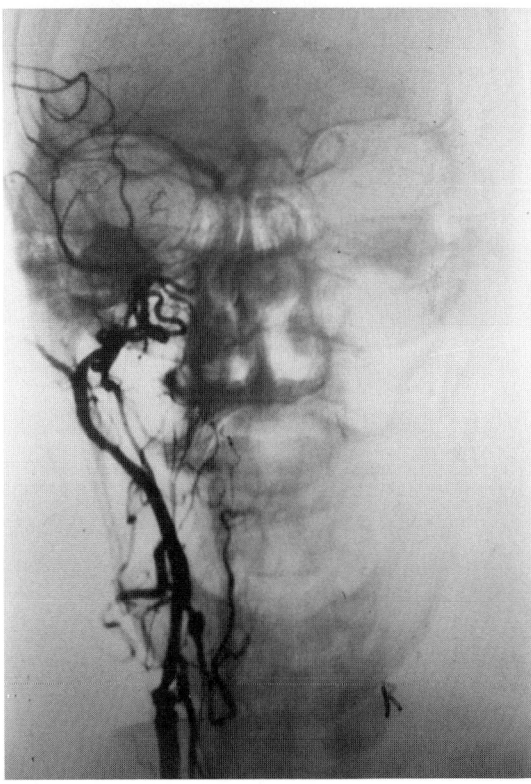

Fig. 2.28.

ies is warranted. The vertebral arteries form an integral part of the blood supply to the brain, particularly in the posterior fossa. They also serve as an essential collateral pathway in patients with carotid occlusive disease. The vertebral arteries may supply blood to the middle cerebral arteries via the posterior communicating/basilar portions of the circle of Willis. The vertebral arteries, however, have not been so closely scrutinized as the carotids. First, symptoms of vertebrobasilar insufficiency tend to be rather vague and poorly defined, compared with the obvious devastation produced by a middle cerebral artery infarction. In addition, there has been limited interest in surgical correction of vertebral lesions (60). The complex anatomy and often well-hidden location of the vertebral artery has not made it an attractive vessel for intervention. Finally, the many anatomic variations encountered in the normal vertebral arteries (33,61), coupled with the fact that they eventually join to form the basilar artery, render the diagnosis of vertebral disease quite difficult by any modality (Fig. 2.30 A–C). Even if a discrete stenosis or total absence is identified, it is frequently quite difficult to confidently make an association between a lesion and symptoms. We shall, therefore, limit our discussion to

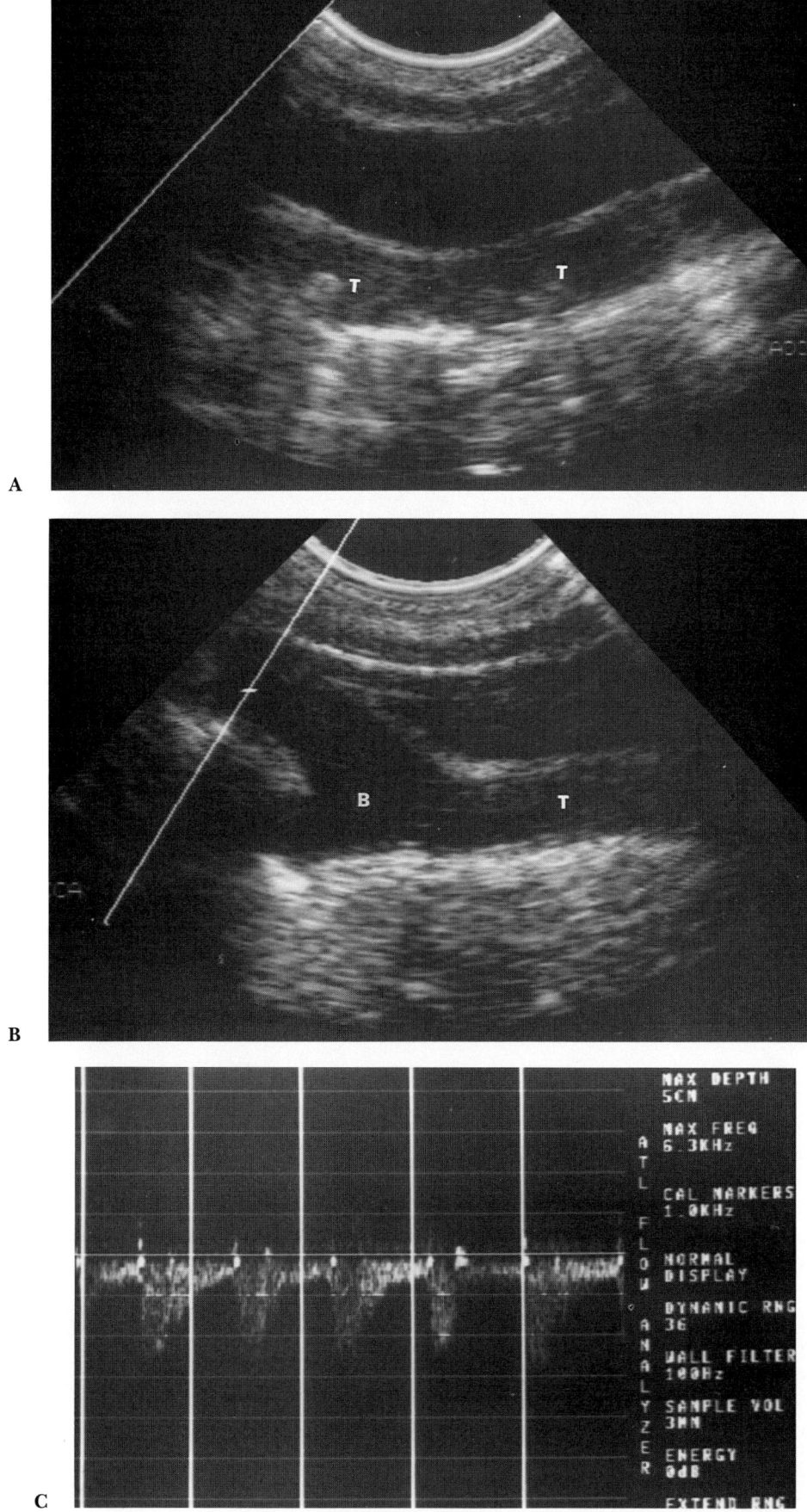

Fig. 2.29.

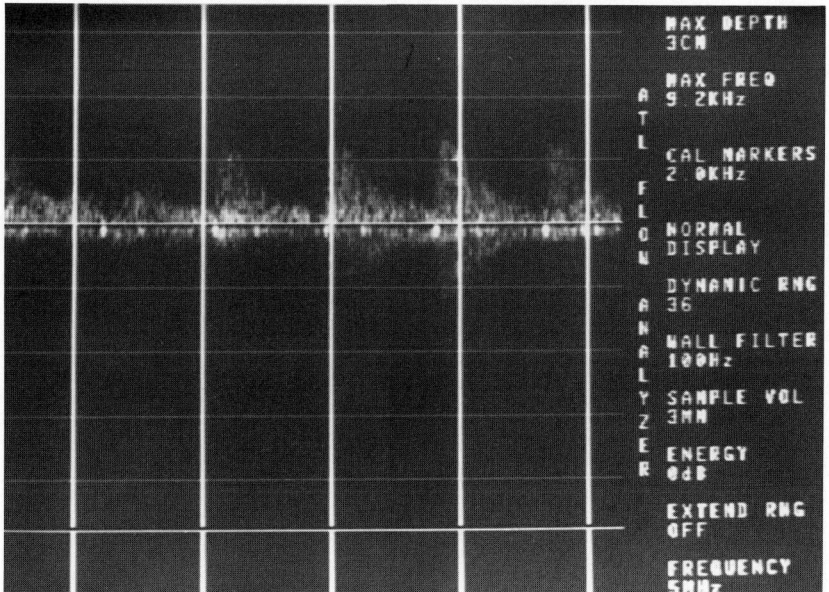

only two aspects of vertebral artery disease: segmental stenosis and subclavian steal syndrome.

The duplex characteristics of the normal vertebral artery have already been outlined in the section on scan techniques. Because stenoses beyond the immediate origins of these vessels are extremely uncommon, we will further limit our discussion to the area of the vertebral-subclavian junction. The normal vertebral artery serves a low-resistance vascular bed and should produce a diphasic signal that is usually of lower velocity than that found in the carotid of the same patient. A number of factors combine to make duplex evaluation of even proximal vertebral artery stenoses somewhat difficult. On the left, the vertebral artery originates from the subclavian in a rather low position. This low position often renders the proximal left vertebral artery difficult to visualize. On the right, although the subclavian-

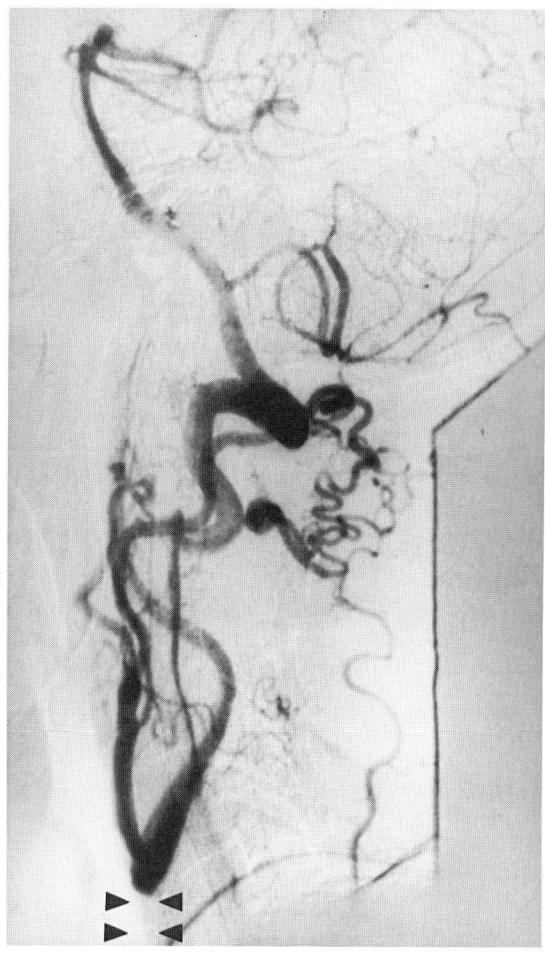

Fig. 2.29A–E. Total occlusion of CCA—Real-time images (**A, B**) show dense thrombus (T) filling CCA; bifurcation (B) remains anechoic. Doppler signals are obtained from both ICA and ICA. The signal in **C** is from ICA. Forward flow is present; trace is below baseline. **D.** From ECA, shows negative Doppler signal, indicating that flow in the ECA is reversed. Angiogram (**E**) confirms total occlusion of CCA (*arrowheads*) but patent ICA and ECA.

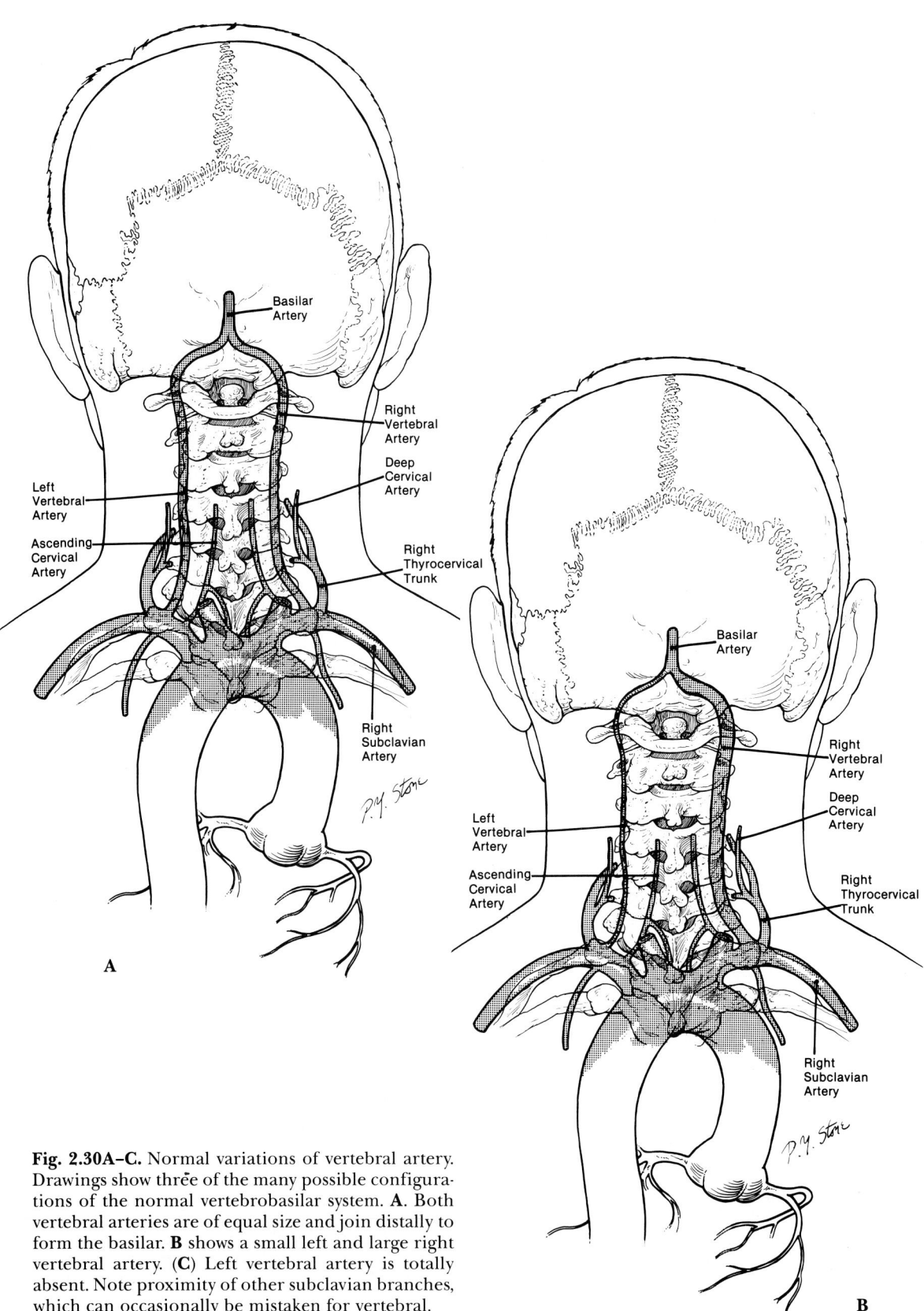

Fig. 2.30A–C. Normal variations of vertebral artery. Drawings show three of the many possible configurations of the normal vertebrobasilar system. **A.** Both vertebral arteries are of equal size and join distally to form the basilar. **B** shows a small left and large right vertebral artery. (**C**) Left vertebral artery is totally absent. Note proximity of other subclavian branches, which can occasionally be mistaken for vertebral.

2. Duplex Sonography of the Cerebrovascular System

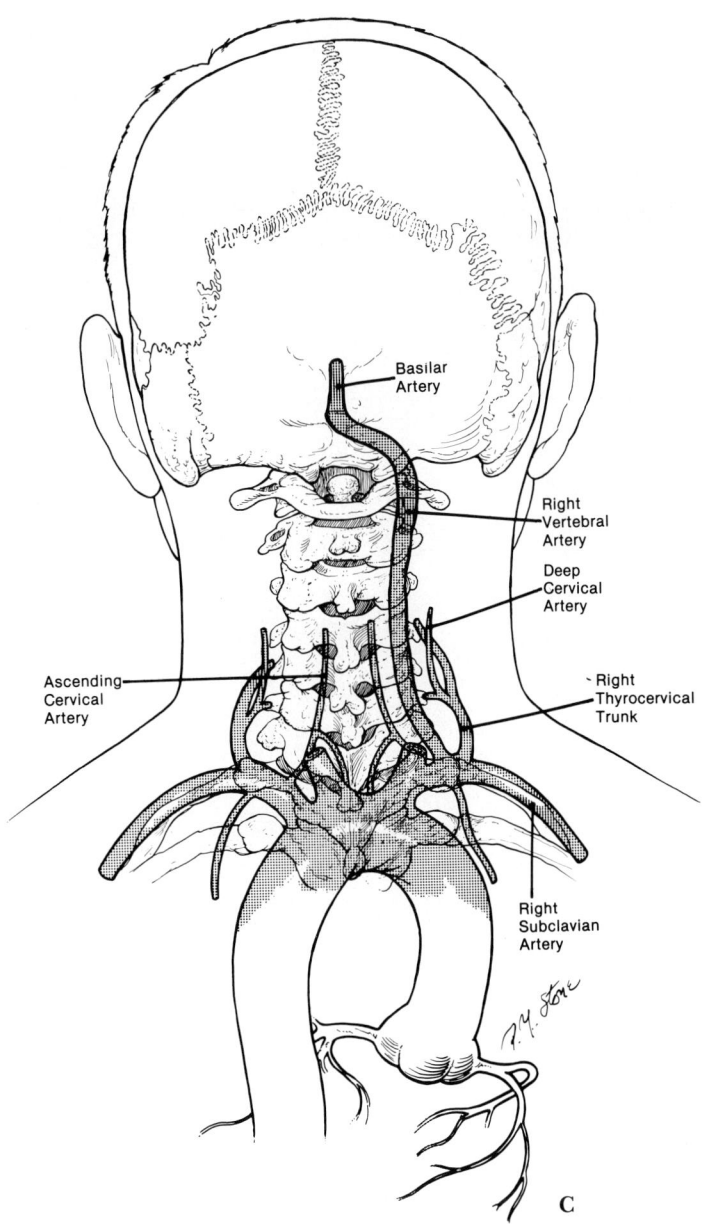

Fig. 2.30.

vertebral artery origin is usually visible, adequate adjustments of the Doppler angle are often impossible on the basis of anatomy alone. Any tortuosity at the vertebral origin on either side complicates matters considerably. In addition, flow in the vertebral artery is normally turbulent enough to fill in the sonic window, precluding the use of spectral broadening as a sign of vascular compromise. Finally, the extreme variability of the caliber of "normal" vertebral artery makes absolute velocity or even velocity ratios unreliable as indicators of stenosis. In general, the diagnosis of vertebral artery stenosis should only be entertained when a focal area of abnormal flow (increased peak velocity) is encountered compared with flow elsewhere in the same vessel. Visona and co-workers (32) determined that when scanning between 45 and 75°, peak systolic flow greater than 2 KHz indicates a 50 to 99% occlusion.

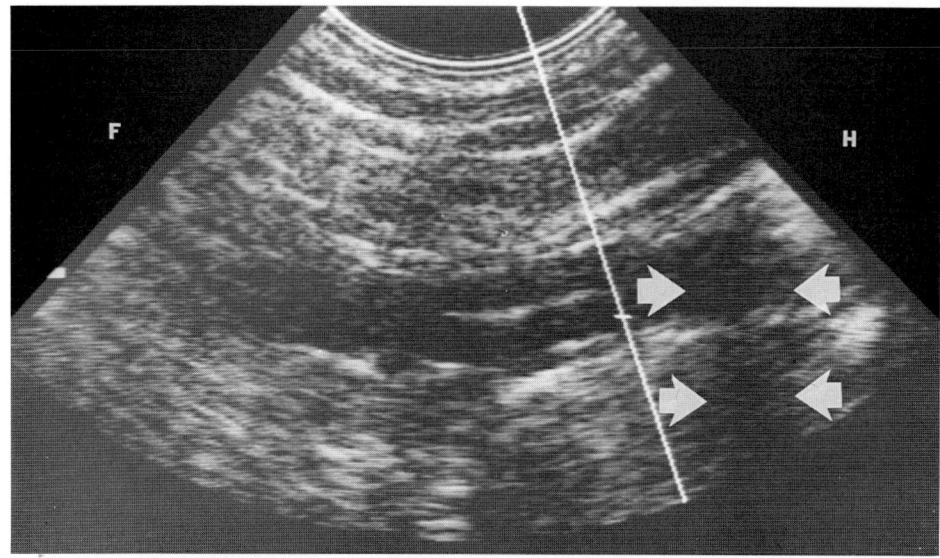

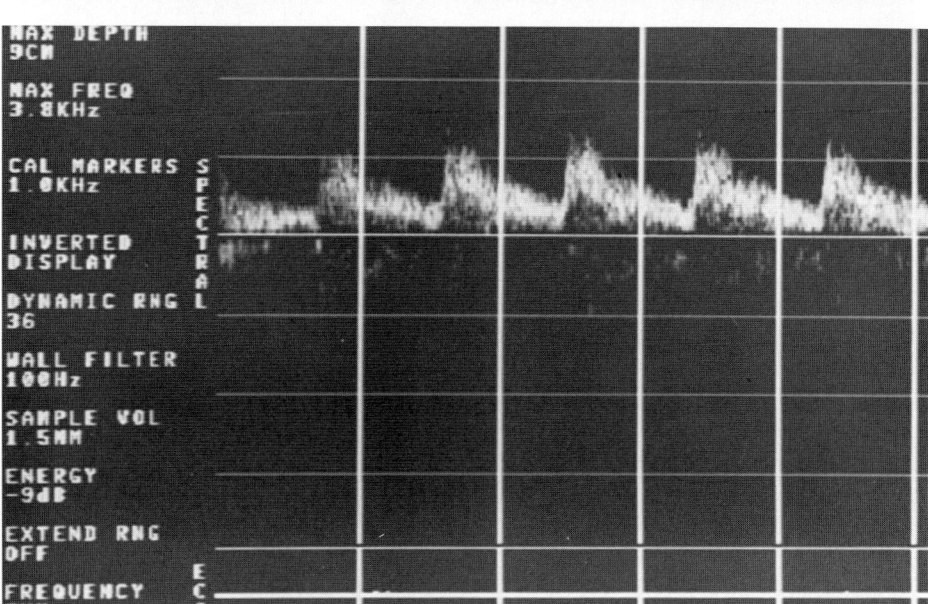

Fig. 2.31A–D. Subclavian steal syndrome—Two vessels course inferiorly from beneath area of shadowing (*arrows*) produced by cervical spine. Cursor is in more posterior of the two vessels; a waveform typical of the vertebral artery is identified (**B**). Signal is normal but positive deflection indicates that flow is toward the transducer. **A.** Left neck; patient's head toward right (H) and patient's feet to left (F). Superimposed digital subtraction arch arteriogram (**C**) shows normal flow in right (R) and left (L) carotids during early phase. Later, retrograde flow in left vertebral (*arrowhead*) fills subclavian artery (*arrow*). Proximal subclavian is occluded (*curved arrows*). **D.** Postoperative arteriogram; patient has innominate left subclavian bypass graft (G). Compliments of Dr. Dieter Schellinger, Department of Radiology, Georgetown University Hospital.

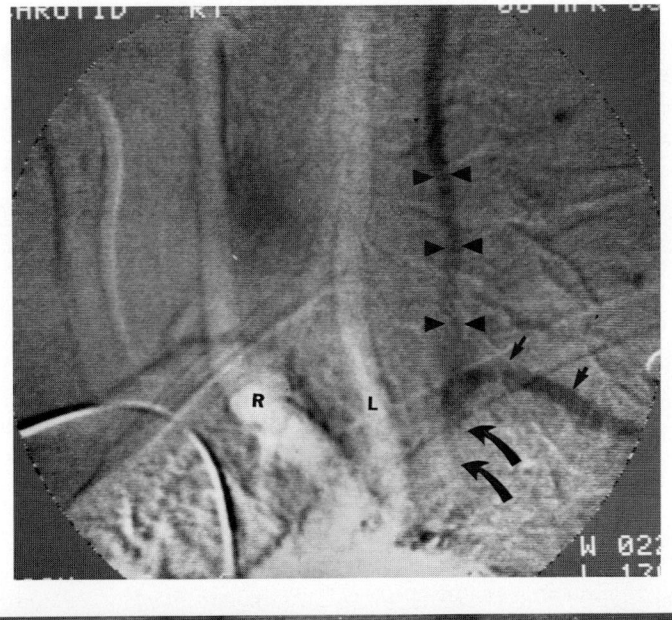

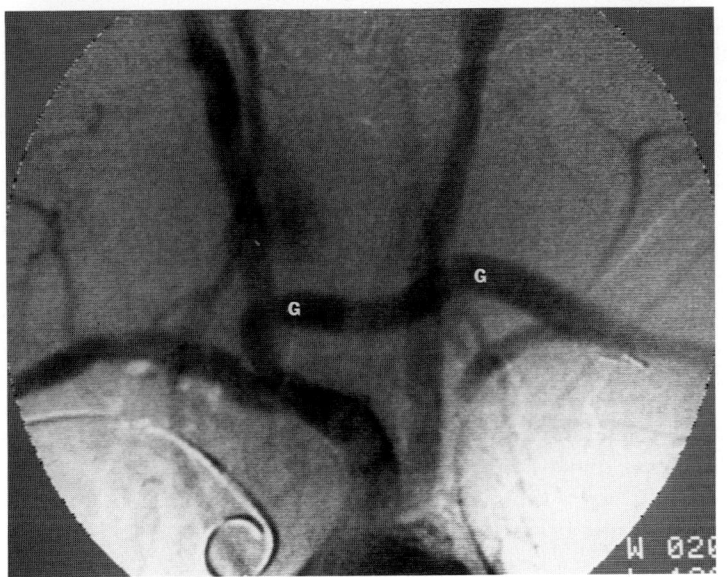

Fig. 2.31.

Although the duplex diagnosis of vertebral artery stenoses is difficult, duplex sonography is very helpful in the diagnosis of subclavian steal syndrome (62). In this situation, a narrowing or occlusion of the proximal subclavian artery blocks the normal blood supply to the arm and the vertebral artery serves as a collateral pathway around the stenosis. Flow in the vertebral artery is, therefore, reversed in direction. This complex physiology is usually clinically silent when the patient is at rest. The syndrome manifests itself when exercise of the affected arm causes decreased circulation to the brain by "stealing" blood via the vertebral collateral. Subclavian steal syndrome is usually relatively easily diagnosed with duplex sonography (Fig. 2.31). The sonographer, however, must take care to scan at an angle steep enough to produce a true representation of the direction of flow. Because of anatomy, one must often scan close to perpendicular to the axis of the vertebral artery. This may yield inconsistent results with regard to flow direction. A Doppler tracing with optimum angle (45 to 60°) must be used even if it means sampling from between vertebral bones. Demonstration of true flow reversal from any portion of the vertebral artery will allow the correct diagnosis.

Summary

Duplex scanning of the carotid arteries has become a well-established noninvasive technique over a relatively brief period. Although originally overshadowed by intravenous digital subtraction angiography, duplex has emerged as the modality of choice in many institutions, and its use is still growing. Although duplex is a rather technically demanding examination, its accuracy and total noninvasive nature make it an extremely attractive modality, particularly in a population at increased risk from contrast injection. The astute sonographer/sonologist will use all aspects of the duplex examination to their fullest. One must observe for numerous real-time abnormalities, paying particular attention to sometimes subtle changes of plaque echotexture and surface characteristics. In addition, the varied diagnostic characteristics of the abnormal Doppler signal must be identified both using auditory cues and the visible spectral display. Careful evaluation of this seemingly overwhelming array of parameters, however, will result in a degree of diagnostic accuracy that was thought impossible without a major interventional procedure just 10 years ago.

References

1. Cranley J: Presidential address: Stroke: A perspective. Surgery 91:537, 1982.
2. Callow A: An overview of the stroke problem in the carotid territory. Am J Surg 140::181, 1980.
3. Jacobs N, Grant E, Schellinger D, et al: The role of duplex carotid sonography, digital subtraction angiography, and arteriography in the evaluation of transient ischemic attack and the asymptomatic carotid bruit. Med Clin North Am 68:1423, 1984.
4. Strother C, Crummy A: Cervical artheriosclerosis—diagnosis in need of a clinical answer. Stroke 13:551, 1982.
5. Gorelick P, Caplan L, Hier D, et al: Racial differences in the distribution of anterior circulation occlusion disease. Neurology 34:54, 1984.
6. Eisenberg R, Nemzek W, Moore W, et al: Relationship of transient ischemic attack and angiographically demonstrable lesions of the carotid artery. Stroke 8:483, 1977.
7. Chiari H: Uber das Verhalten des Teilungswinkels der carotis communis bei der Endarteritis chronica deformans. Verh Dtsch Ges Pathol 9:326, 1905.
8. Hunt J: The role of the carotid arteries in the causation of vascular lesions of the brain, with remarks on certain special features of symptomatology. Am J Med Sci 147:704, 1914.
9. Fisher M: Occlusion of the internal carotid artery. Arch Neurol Psychol 65:345, 1951.
10. Fisher M: Transient monocular blindness associated with hemiplegia. Arch Ophthalmol 47:167, 1952.
11. Fisher M: Concerning recurrent transcerebral ischemic attacks. Can Med Assoc J 86:1091, 1962.
12. Fisher M: Occlusion-of the carotid arteries. Further experience. Arch Neurol Psychol 72:187, 1954.
13. DeBakey M: Successful carotid endarterectomy for cerebrovascular insufficiency. Nine-year follow-up. JAMA 123:1083, 1975.
14. Eastcott H, Pickering G, Rob C: Reconstruction of internal carotid artery in a patient with intermittent attacks of hemiplegia. Lancet 13:994, 1954.
15. Carrea R, Moins M, Murphy G: Surgical treatment of spontaneous thrombosis of the internal carotid artery in the neck: Carotid-caroideal anastomosis, report of a case. Acta Neurol Lat Am 1:71, 1955.
16. Hass W, Fields W, North R, et al: Joint study of extracranial arterial occlusion. JAMA 203:159, 1968.
17. Mani R, Eisenbert R, McDonald E Jr, et al: Complications of catheter cerebral arteriography: Analysis of 5000 procedures. I. Criteria and incidence. Am J Rad 131:861, 1978.
18. Earnest F IV, Forbes G, Saudok B, et al: Complications of cerebral angiography: Prospective assessment of risk. Am J Rad 142:247, 1984.
19. McDonald P, Rich N, Ciollins G, et al: Ocular pneumoplethysmography: Detection of carotid occlusive disease. Ann Surg 189:44, 1979.
20. Ginsberg M, Greenwood S, Goldberg H: Noninvasive diagnosis of extracranial cerebrovascular disease: Oculoplethysmography-phonoangiography and directional Doppler ultrasonography. Neurol 29:623, 1979.
21. Block S, Baltaxe H, Shonmaker R: Reliability of Doppler scanning of the carotid bifurcation angiographic correlation. Radiology 132:687, 1979.

22. Barber F, Baker D, Nation A, et al: Ultrasonic duplex echo-Doppler scanner. IEEE Trans Biomed Eng 21:109, 1974.
23. Blasberg D: Duplex sonography for carotid artery disease. AJNR 3:609, 1982.
24. Garth K, Carroll B, Sommer G, et al: Duplex ultrasound scanning of the carotid arteries with velocity spectrum analysis. Radiology 147:823, 1983.
25. Jacobs N, Grant E, Schellinger D, et al: Duplex carotid sonography: Criteria for stenosis, accuracy, and pitfalls. Radiology 154:385, 1985.
26. Wetzner S, Kiser L, Bezrah J: Duplex ultrasound imaging: Vascular applications. Radiology 150:507, 1984.
27. Fell G, Phillips D, Chikos P, et al: Ultrasonic duplex scanning for disease of the carotid artery. Circulation 64:1191, 1981.
28. Blackshear W, Phillips D, Chikos P, et al: Carotid artery velocity patterns in normal and stenotic vessels. Stroke 11:67, 1980.
29. Driesbach J, Seibert C, Smazal S, et al: Duplex sonography in the evaluation of carotid artery disease. AJNR 4:678, 1983.
30. Comerata A, Cranley J, Cook S: Real-time B-mode carotid imaging in diagnosis of cerebrovascular disease. Surgery 89:718, 1981.
31. Prendes J, McKinney W, Buonanno F, et al: Anatomic variations of the carotid bifurcation affecting Doppler scan interpretation. J Clin Ultrasound 8:147, 1980.
32. Visona A, Lusiani L, Castellani V, et al: The echo-Doppler (duplex) system for the detection of vertebral artery occlusive disease: Comparison with angiography. J Ultrasound Med 5:247, 1986.
33. Moosy J: Morphology, sites and epidemiology of cerebral atherosclerosis. *In* Milliken C (ed): Cerebrovascular Disease. Baltimore, Williams and Wilkins, 1986, p 1.
34. Anderson R, Powell D, Litak J: B-mode sonography as a screening procedure for asymptomatic carotid bruits. Am J Rad 124:292, 1975.
35. Cooperberg P, Robertson W, Fry P, et al: High resolution real-time ultrasound of the carotid bifurcation. J Clin Ultrasound 7:13, 1979.
36. Humber P, Leopold G, Wickborn I, et al: Ultrasonic imaging of the carotid arterial system. Am J Surgery 140:199, 1980.
37. James E, Earnest F IV, Forbes S, et al: High-resolution dynamic ultrasound imaging of the carotid bifurcation: A prospective evaluation. Radiology 144:853, 1982.
38. Wolverson M, Heiberg E, Sundaram M, et al: Carotid atherosclerosis high resolution real-time sonography correlated with angiography. AJR 140:355, 1983.
39. O'Donnell T, Erdoes L, Mackey W, et al: Correlation of B-mode ultrasound imaging and angiography with pathology findings at carotid endarterectomy. Arch Surg 120:443, 1985.
40. Bluth E, Kay D, Merritt C, et al: Sonographic characterization of carotid plaque: detection of hemorrhage. AJNR 7:311, 1986.
41. Reilly L, Lusby R, Hughes L, et al: Carotid plaque histology using real-time ultrasonography. Am J Surg 146:188, 1983.
42. Edwards J, Kricheff I, Riles T, et al: Angiographically undetected ulceration of the carotid bifurcation as a cause of embolic stroke. Radiology 132:369, 1979.
43. Eikelboom B, Riles T, Mintzer R, et al: Inaccuracy of angiography in the diagnosis of carotid ulceration. Stroke 14:882, 1983.
44. Perrson A, Robichaux W, Silverman M: The natural history of carotid plaque development. Arch Surg 118:1048, 1983.
45. Lusby R, Ferrell L, Ehrenfeld W, et al: Carotid plaque hemorrhage: Its role in production of cerebral ischemia. Arch Surg 117:1479, 1982.
46. Imparato A, Riles T, Gorstein F: The carotid bifurcation plaque: Pathologic findings associated with cerebral ischaemia. Stroke 10:238, 1979.
47. Imparato A, Riles T, Mintzer R, et al: The importance of hemorrhage in the relationship between gross morphologic characteristics and cerebral symptoms in 376 carotid artery plaques. Ann Surg 197:195, 1983.
48. Thiele B, Chikos P, Strandness D: Arteriography, the Gold Standard. Stroke (in press).
49. Roederer G, Langlios Y, Chan E, et al: Ultrasonic dulex scanning of extracranial carotid arteries: Improved accuracy using new features from the common carotid artery. J Cardiovasc Ultrasonography 1:373, 1982.
50. Atkinson P, Woodcock J: Doppler imaging of the extracranial cerebral arteries. *In* Doppler Ultrasound and Its Use in Clinical Measurement. New York, Academic Press, 1982, pp 146–162.
51. Withers C, Gosink B, Keightley A, et al: Duplex carotid sonography: Peak velocity measurement in quantifying internal carotid artery stenosis. Presented at Radiologic Society of North America, Chicago, Illinois, December 3, 1986.
52. Blackshear W Jr, Phillips D, Chikos P, et al: Carotid artery velocity patterns in normal and stenotic vessels. Stroke 11:67, 1980.
53. Phillips D: Flow velocity pattern in the carotid bifurcation of young presumed normal subjects. Ultrasound Med Biol 9:39, 1983.
54. Spencer M, Reid J: Quantification of carotid stenosis with continuous-wave (C-W) Doppler ultrasound. Stroke 10:326, 1979.
55. Berguer R, Hwang N: Critical arterial stenosis: A theoretical and experimental solution. Ann Surg 180:39, 1974.

56. Roederer G, Langlois Y, Jaeger K, et al: The natural history of carotid artery disease in asymptomatic patients with cervical bruits. Stroke 15:605, 1984.
57. Zweibel W, Crummy A: Sources of error in Doppler diagnosis of carotid occlusive disease. AJNR 2:231, 1981.
58. Blackshear W, Phillips D, Bodily K, et al: Ultrasonic demonstration of external and internal carotid artery patency with common carotid occlusion: A preliminary report. Stroke 11:249, 1980.
59. Vaisman V, Wojciechowski M: Carotid artery disease: New criteria for evaluation by sonographic duplex scanning. Radiology 158:253, 1986.
60. Thevenet A, Ruotolo C: Surgical repair of vertebral artery stenosis. J Cardiovasc Surg 25:101, 1984.
61. Meyer J, Lobe C: Stroke due to vertebrovascular disease. Springfield, Charles Thomas, 1965.
62. Walker D, Acker J, Cole C: Subclavian steal syndrome detected with duplex pulsed Doppler sonography. AJNR 3:615, 1982.

3
Cardiac Doppler

FREDERICK J. DOHERTY and KEVIN P. MCINERNEY

Two-dimensional echocardiographic evaluation of the heart has established itself as an invaluable tool in the noninvasive assessment of this organ in patients with suspected heart disease. Recent and rapid developments in Doppler technology have supplemented the two-dimensional echocardiographic examination, by augmenting the amount of clinical information available from ultrasonographic evaluation of the heart.

Two-dimensional echocardiography is uniquely capable of providing very detailed information about the anatomic, structural, and functional status of the heart and great vessels. Valvular lesions, wall motion abnormalities, chamber size, thrombi or tumors within the chambers, wall thickness, septal defects, and pericardial abnormalities are demonstrated, with high resolution, by two-dimensional ultrasonic imaging in a noninvasive way. Otherwise, comparable information can only be obtained in an invasive fashion, such as by cardiac catheterization. However, two-dimensional echocardiography is limited, in that it is incapable of providing important information about intracardiac blood flow dynamics, which, again, until recently, could only be obtained by cardiac catheterization. Modern Doppler echocardiographic equipment is now capable of noninvasively evaluating intracardiac blood flow dynamics; and information about the hemodynamics in specific cardiovascular problems is available now from Doppler, where it previously was only available by cardiac catheterization.

Combining high-resolution two-dimensional echocardiographic imaging with quantitative Doppler techniques has increased the diagnostic capabilities of noninvasive sonographic evaluation of the heart, and has opened up a new realm of clinical ultrasound applications, which relate to the demonstration of blood flow patterns within the heart and great vessels. This has resulted in a more complete and accurate noninvasive evaluation of cardiovascular disorders. Currently, Doppler evaluation of the heart is performed in three separate, but related, ways: pulsed-Doppler (PW), continuous-wave Doppler (CW), and the newly developed color Doppler flow mapping. These three ways provide different and complementary information, where the limitations of one form of Doppler evaluation are removed by the strengths of another form. Although the physics of Doppler ultrasound are explained elsewhere, the unique properties of the different types of Doppler are reviewed here pertaining to the way that they specifically influence the cardiac examination (Diagram 3.1).

Technical Aspects of the Cardiac Doppler Examination

Pulsed-Doppler

Pulsed-Doppler techniques are combined with high-resolution two-dimensional imaging. While being imaged simultaneously, specific sites throughout the cardiac chambers can be interrogated with pulsed-Doppler looking for normal and abnormal flow patterns. Intracardiac shunts, along with stenotic and regurgitant lesions can be evaluated in this fashion.

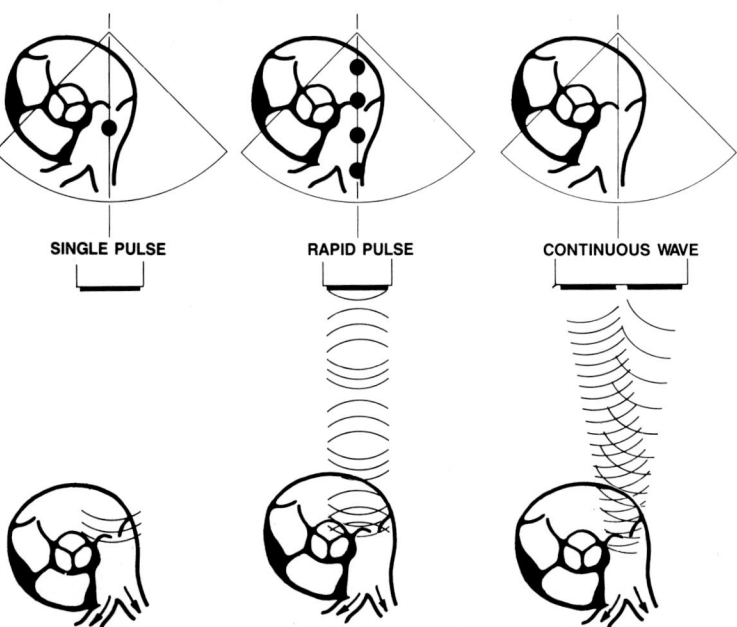

Diagram 3.1. Modes of Doppler interrogation. In single pulsed Doppler, a single range, or time gate, is established distal to the pulmonary valve, as shown here, and ultrasound information from that gate shown as the wavelets in the diagram below is processed for the Doppler shift. On the right hand panel for continuous Doppler, one transducer is sending and the other is receiving ultrasound from all along the line of site. Velocities from along the complete line of the right ventricular outflow tract are, therefore, summed into the resultant display. In the center panel, a rapid pulse, or high pulse repetition frequency Doppler, has been implemented. Individual sample volumes are shown with Doppler information being processed from gates with depths which are multiples of the depth of the first gate. This is illustrated by the position of 4 sample volumes in the upper panel and by the fact that ultrasound information is coming and going at the same time from within the tissue. The multiple sampling depths in the lower panel are also illustrated by the individual wavelet packets. Information may be coming back to the transducer from depths of either two, three, or four times the initial sample volume depth, returning from previous pulse bursts and having traveled and arrived back at the transducer at the same instant in time as the information from the first range gate from the pulse just sent. This allows implementation of rapid pulse repetition frequencies, since the device is not listening for the required period of time necessary to receive information from the fourth gate, but receives it back within the specified time gate period while functioning at four times the pulse repetition frequency. By permission of the American Society of Echocardiography. The Doppler Standards and Nomenclature Committee, August 1984.

The exact location, duration, and timing of low-velocity information can be evaluated.

Through the use of the "range gate," which is steerable throughout the two-dimensional image, only the Doppler signals in a particular area of interest are being analyzed (Fig. 3.1). Essentially, a movable small-windowed time frame is analyzed for Doppler shift signals along any ultrasonic interrogation path in the two-dimensional sector image. In the pulsed-Doppler mode, the advantage is that range resolution is obtained (1, pp 35–42). The velocity in a small-range cell at a variable depth along the ultrasound beam can be measured. The result is the ability to localize spatially an area of abnormal flow with great accuracy.

However, with pulsed Doppler, there is a limitation to the maximum velocity that can be measured. Because pulsed-Doppler uses a single crystal both to transmit and receive signals, the sampling rate, or pulse repetition frequency (PRF), is governed by the speed of sound in tissue and the depth of the sample volume. The deeper one interrogates, the lower that the PRF must be, as it takes longer for each individual pulse to be transmitted and received. For pulsed-Doppler accurately to measure returning frequencies, the PRF must be at least twice

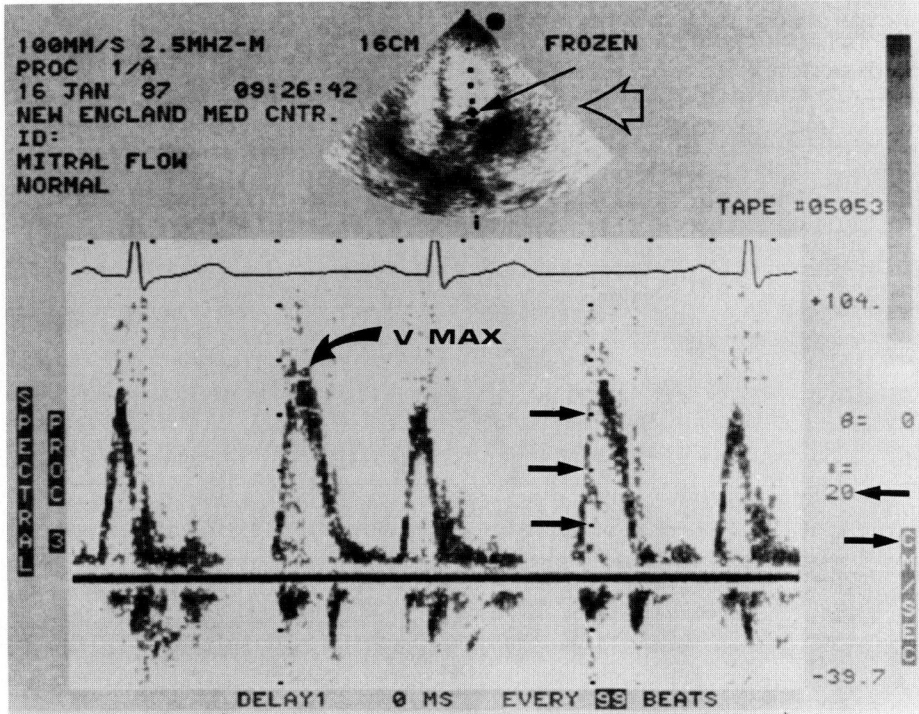

Fig. 3.1. Typical two-dimensional guided pulsed-Doppler tracing. This is an example of a normal flow velocity profile in the inflow portion of the left ventricle. In the center portion of the top of the illustration is a small two-dimensional sector image of a four-chamber view of the heart (*open arrow*). Within this image is a dotted line, extending deeply from the apex of the sector, which corresponds to the path of the pulsed-Doppler interrogation beam. This Doppler pathway, or cursor, can be steered anywhere from the left to the right of the image with a joystick or track-ball. The two small black triangles positioned approximately half way along the Doppler pathway outline the limits of the sample volume from which the pulsed-Doppler information is obtained. This is the range gate (*long black arrow*), which is also moveable over the Doppler pathway by the joystick, and can be expanded or narrowed from a wide to a very narrow depth range. In this example the sample volume is placed approximately 1 cm inside the left ventricle just beyond the mitral orifice to record diastolic mitral inflow. The lower half of the illustration shows a normal mitral flow profile obtained with pulsed-Doppler at the exact area represented in the two-dimensional image above. The calibration marks along the vertical axis are at increments of 20 cm/s (*short black arrows*). In this typical biphasic mitral flow, the maximum velocity (V max) is 0.9 m/s (*curved arrow*) in early diastole.

the frequency of the sound being measured (the Nyquist frequency limit). If the PRF is less than twice the returning frequency, "aliasing" or artifactual reversal of velocities occurs (Fig. 3.2) (2, pp 7–12). This is a drawback that is overcome by the ability of continuous-wave Doppler to measure maximum flow velocities without limit.

An attempt has been made in pulsed-Doppler to get around the limitation of aliasing in high-velocity flows at increasing depth from the transducer, by raising the Nyquist limit or by using a high PRF mode (Fig. 3.3). By increasing the pulse repetition frequency up to four times normal PRF, higher velocities can be measured without aliasing. By increasing the PRF, several ultrasound pulses will be traveling through the heart at one time, and, effectively, additional range gates are added at shallower depths from the original sample volume. The number of added range gates along the interrogating path is proportional to the depth of the sample volume being interrogated. This introduces a problem with "range ambiguity" (1, pp 39). By using high PRF the ability to localize in the pulsed-Doppler mode is lost, but the ability to measure higher velocities along the interrogat-

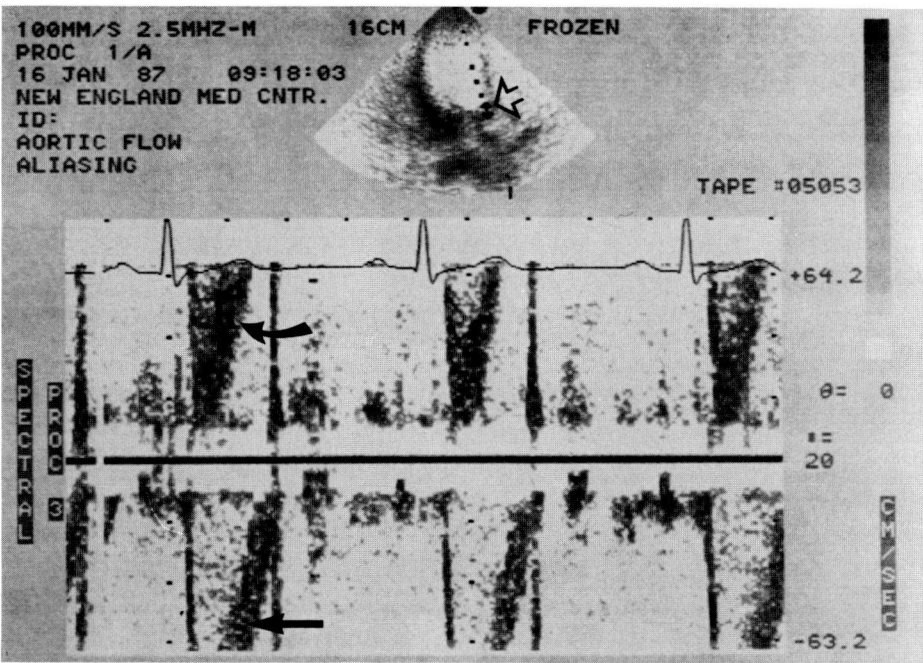

Fig. 3.2. Aliasing with pulsed-Doppler. This illustration shows the pulsed-Doppler sample volume placed just at the aortic valve orifice (*open arrow*) in an apical long axis view. On the pulsed-Doppler tracing below, "aliasing" or "wrap-around flow" is shown where the normal aortic flow away from the transducer in systole is too fast to be recorded completely below the zero line at this depth (*straight arrow*), and is aliased into the positive portion of the tracing (*curved arrow*) which is supposed to represent flow toward the transducer. Consequently, the velocity cannot be recorded here.

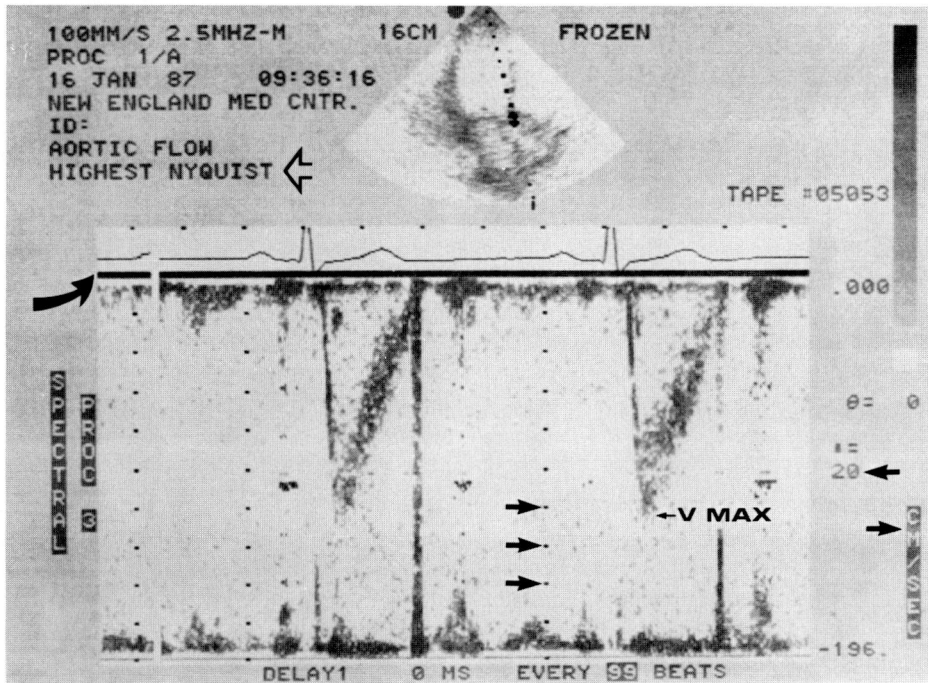

Fig. 3.3.

ing pathway is gained. However, because of a resultant loss of signal strength in the high PRF mode, conditions for optimal data acquisition are often only marginal with this technique.

Thus, pulsed-Doppler, combined with high-resolution two-dimensional imaging, is capable of discretely interrogating all areas of the cardiac chambers and identifying specific sites of abnormal flow patterns; but it is limited in its ability to measure high velocity flow patterns. Because of the finite size of the range gates, more time is required to position the beam to sample various portions of cardiac chambers for optimal flow interrogation (Fig. 3.4). Consequently, a pulsed-Doppler examination takes more time to perform than a continuous-wave Doppler examination. However, the pulsed-Doppler technique is superb for its ability to control the depth of high-velocity interrogation and to examine at multiple discrete sites. It is also helpful in situations where more than one high-velocity jet exists within one axial plane of the beam, such as in combined aortic valvular stenosis and hypertrophic cardiomyopathy (IHSS). In these situations pulsed-Doppler can easily resolve the spatial difference between the two separate lesions.

Continuous-Wave Doppler

Continuous-wave Doppler (CW) detects velocity information along the entire length of the sound beam, and easily records the highest velocities within the beam. With this technique, there is no simultaneous two-dimensional imaging, as there is with pulsed-Doppler. In a single housing, two transducer crystals are mounted side by side with a lens in front (1, p 36). One transducer is continously generating soundwaves, while the other is continuously receiving the reflected soundwaves. Signals returning from all depths, through which the ultrasound beam has passed, are being analyzed. With CW Doppler all velocities along the beam are observed; and, as opposed to pulsed-Doppler, there is no range resolution (Fig. 3.5). This is the major drawback to CW Doppler. It is incapable of spatially identifying where any given flow velocity is occurring along the ultrasound beam. In other words, it cannot localize flow velocity information. However, because of CW Doppler's essentially infinite pulse repetition frequently (PRF), it is capable of measuring very high velocities (Fig. 3.6). Continuous-wave Doppler allows for the evaluation of maximal velocity information. Intracardiac pressure information can be quantitated, such as the pressure gradient across stenotic valves or the drop across regurgitant valves.

The limitations and strengths of both pulsed-Doppler and CW Doppler make the use of both techniques complementary to each other in the cardiac examination. Continuous-wave Doppler can scan the entire heart quickly, searching for abnormal flow signals. With its ability to detect high-velocity flow patterns, CW Doppler lacks the range resolution of pulsed-Doppler. Pulsed-Doppler can easily localize the precise site of abnormal flow patterns; but it is limited in its ability to evaluate high-velocity lesions.

Color Flow Mapping

Recent technological advances have introduced a new two-dimensional color flow mapping system, which, noninvasively, maps intracardiac blood flow in a way that previously could only be done with angiography. The system basically uses pulsed-Doppler and performs flow analysis at multiple points along each scan line of echo data. Flow information is then color coded and displayed on a superimposed corresponding two-dimensional image. The result is an exciting and easily interpretable colored display of blood flow patterns within the cardiac chambers of a real-time two-dimensional echocardiogram (3). There is now a dynamic method for studying the spatial distribution of blood flow

Fig. 3.3. Raising the Nyquist frequency to resolve aliasing with pulsed-Doppler. In this example (same as Fig. 3.2), by raising the Nyquist limit (high PRF) (*open arrow*) and shifting the zero line (*curved arrow*), the highest detectable velocity at this depth is doubled. In this normal patient, a velocity of 1.3 m/s (V max) is recorded with pulsed-Doppler (calibration marks, 20 cm/s) (*short arrows*).

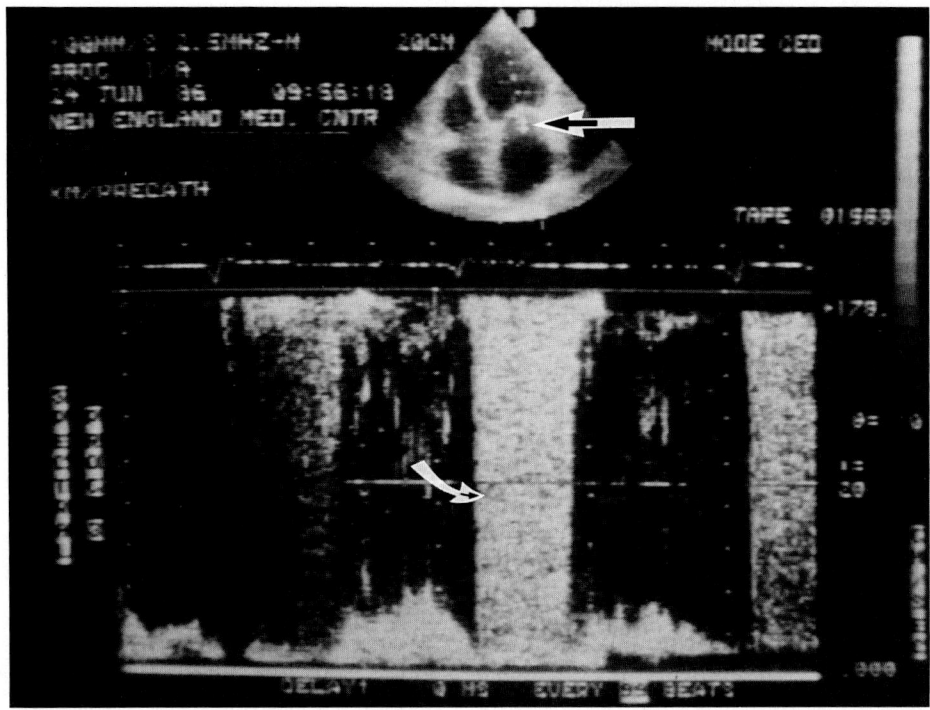

Fig. 3.4A–C. Two-dimensional guided pulsed-Doppler flow mapping—multiple sampling sites. In this example of a patient with severe mitral insufficiency, three different areas of an enlarged left atrium are sampled with pulsed-Doppler. In each example, the two-dimensional image at top is a four-chamber view from the apex showing an enlarged left atrium and left ventricle, and normally sized right-sided chambers. In each example, the negative systolic velocity of the regurgitant flow is too high to be measured at this depth with pulsed-Doppler and, hence, aliasing is seen in systole. **A.** Sample volume just on the atrial side of the mitral valve (*straight arrow*). Aliased flow in systole (*curved arrow*). **B.** Sample volume at the mid-atrial level (*long thin arrow*). **C.** Sample volume deep in the left atrium (*long thin arrow*).

velocities within the heart as has never before been seen, either invasively or noninvasively. Color flow mapping appears to have overcome the difficulty of defining the location and distribution of areas of normal and abnormal flow associated with valves, stenotic lesions, regurgitant lesions, and intracardiac shunts (4).

Positive Doppler shifts (flow towards the transducer) are displayed in shades of red through orange to yellow, whereas negative shifts (flow away from the transducer) are displayed in blue to blue-green. On the positive side, red indicates slower flow, orange represents average flow, and yellow corresponds to fast flow. With negative flow, slow velocities are displayed in dark blue, average velocities in bright blue, and fast velocities in blue-green. Increasing flow velocities are displayed with increasing brightness and intensity of the colors pushing toward bright white at maximum intensity. However, because this is essentially a pulsed-Doppler system, it suffers from aliasing, which produces multicolor mosaic patterns with shades of yellow-white to green on the flow map. In high-velocity situations the normal flow patterns can be tinged or even replaced with this yellow to green hue (Fig. 3.7).

Because of the large number of analyses that must be done at the numerous sites along each scan line, more time is needed for the generation of each line of echo data, and a price is paid in line density and, hence, resolution of the imaging system. Larger sector angles are accompanied by decreased line density, and the best line density in real-time flow mapping is obtained with narrower sector angles. Also, because of the increased time involved, full spectral analysis by fast Fourier transform tech-

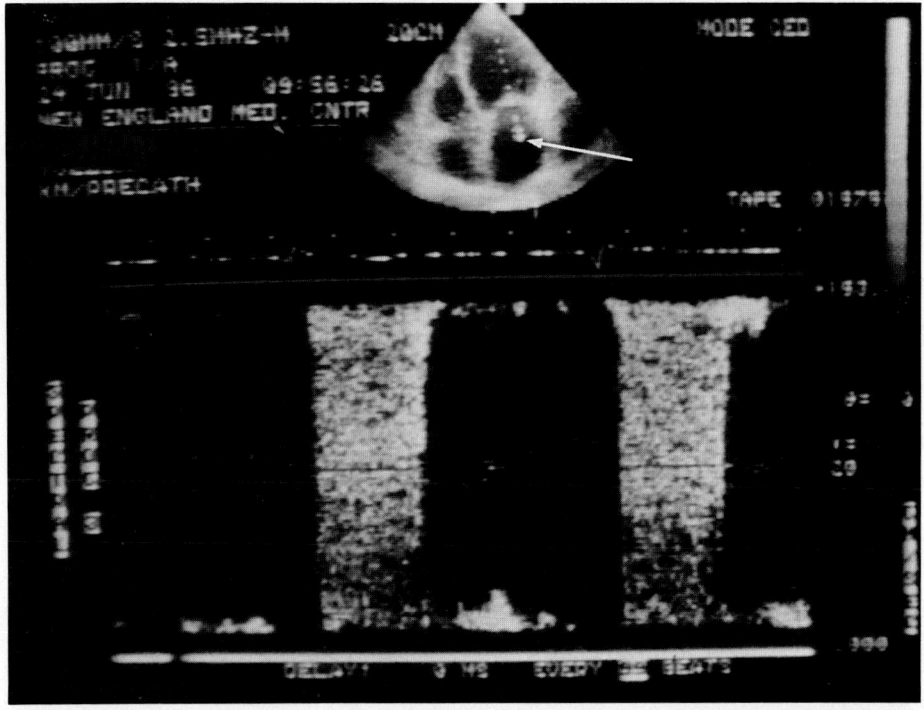

Fig. 3.4.

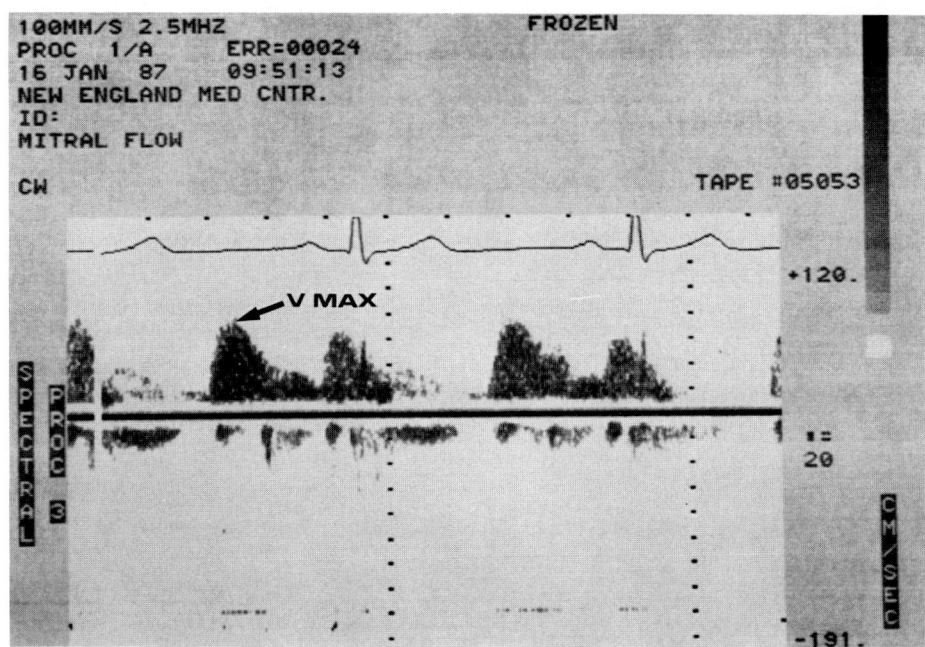

Fig. 3.5. Typical continuous-wave Doppler tracing. In this normal example of a mitral flow velocity recording obtained with continuous-wave Doppler, the characteristic biphasic profile is seen with a V max of 0.75 m/s (calibration marks, 20 cm/s).

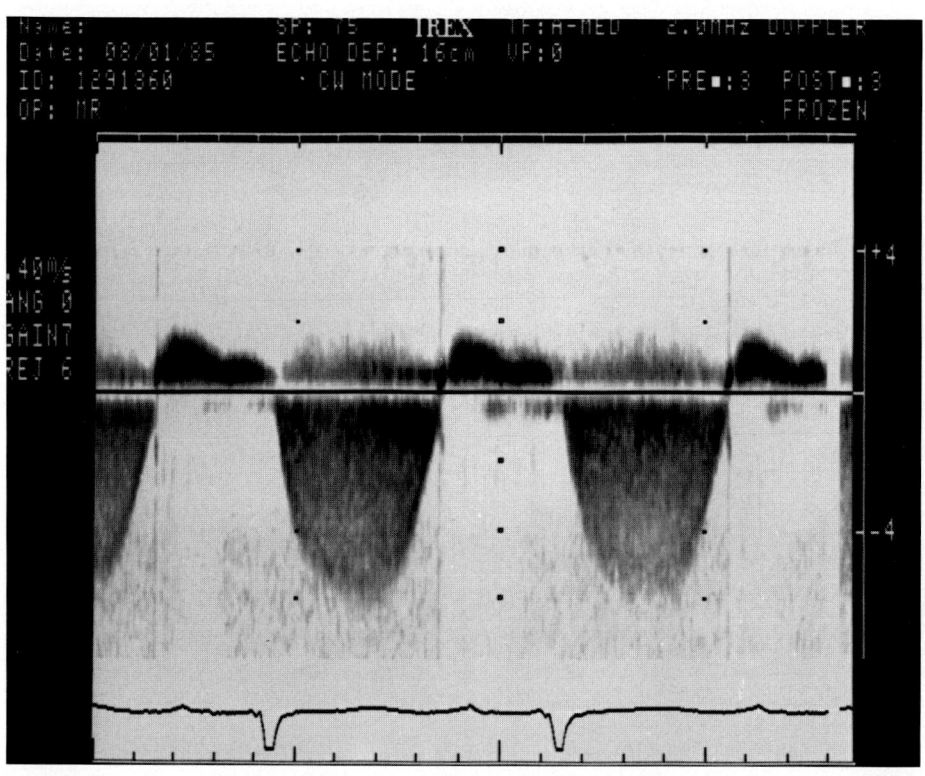

Fig. 3.6. Very high velocity flow recorded by continuous-wave Doppler. In this example of a patient with severe mitral insufficiency, a negative systolic flow with a V max of 6 m/s is measured (calibration marks, 2 m/s).

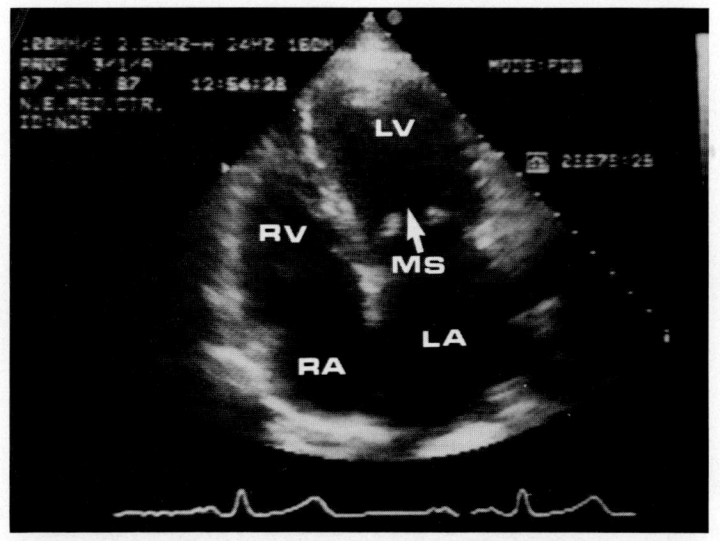

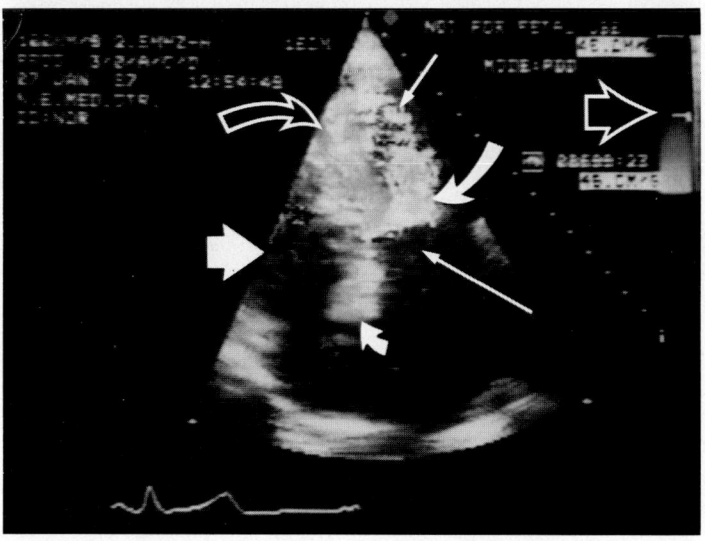

Fig. 3.7A,B. Typical color Doppler illustration. **A.** Black and white apical four-chamber view in a patient with mitral stenosis. Both the left atrium and left ventricle are enlarged; thickened, restricted mitral leaflets are seen (LA, left atrium; LV, left ventricle; RA, right atrium; RV, right ventricle; MS, stenotic mitral orifice). **B.** Color Doppler image in diastole in the same apical four-chamber view as in Fig. 3.7A. Positive flow toward the transducer is displayed in shades from dark red through orange to bright yellow-orange. This is shown on the color scale in the upper right-hand corner of the illustration. The darker red colors correspond to slow flow and the brighter yellow colors to fast flow (*broad open arrow*). Negative flow away from the transducer is displayed in shades of deep blue, for slow flow, through blue-green to bright light green, for fast flow (*broad open arrow*). The fastest flow detectable becomes so intense as to be displayed as white, and aliased flow is seen as a mosaic of colors. Because both positive and negative Doppler signals are displayed in aliased flow with pulsed Doppler, color Doppler likewise displays both positive and negative information, and the mosaic of intense multiple colors is obtained. In this example, forward flow in the left atrium is seen in red, being darker in the middle of the atrium, and going through orange to yellow as the blood speeds up as it goes through the narrowed mitral orifice (*long thin arrow*). The jet of blood curves somewhat laterally as it goes into the left ventricle. A large high velocity jet is seen, accelerating through the mitral orifice toward the apex (*short thin arrow*), which is an intense mosaic of colors primarily in white, bright yellow, or bright blue-green. The jet through the mitral valve into the apex is displayed as a mosaic of color because it represents aliasing of high-velocity flow. The intense blue-green flow just inside the valve is not reversed flow, but aliased flow (*long closed curved arrow*). A normal vortex of negative downward flow toward the aortic valve is seen in blue shades, hugging the ventricular septum (*long open curved arrow*). Higher flow velocities in this area are seen as light blue-green to white. Normal forward flow into the right ventricle from the tricuspid valve area is displayed as a red-orange jet (*broad closed arrow*). The small patch of blue on the right side of the atrial septum (*short closed curved arrow*) is partial detection of downward aortic flow, because of its close proximity in this view. For a color reproduction of this figure see frontmatter.

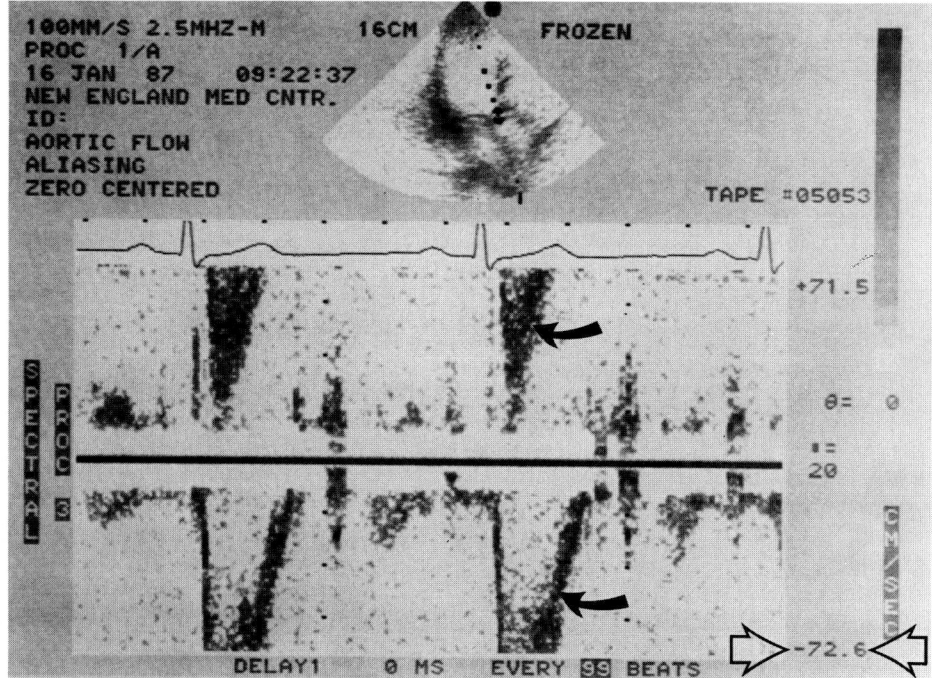

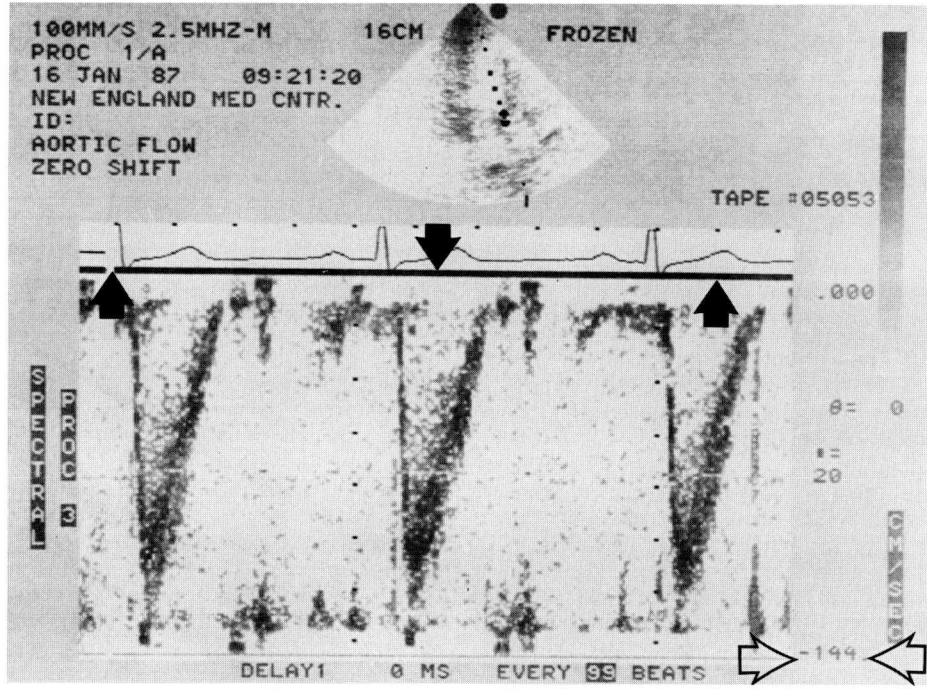

Fig. 3.8A,B. Shifting the "zero line" to resolve aliasing in a pulsed-Doppler recording. The sector image at top is an apical long axis view with the sample volume placed at the aortic valve orifice (calibration marks, 20 cm/s). **A.** Aliasing of pulsed-Doppler tracing (*curved arrows*) of normal systolic aortic flow velocity, which is too high to be recorded at this depth from the transducer with the zero line in the center of the tracing (*vertical arrow*). The maximum velocity that could be recorded in this situation is 0.72 m/s (*open arrows*). **B.** Raising the zero line to the top (*vertical arrows*) effectively doubles the scale here, and a negative systolic V max of 1.3 m/s is measured. Note on the scale that the maximum velocity that can now be recorded is 1.44 m/s (*open arrows*).

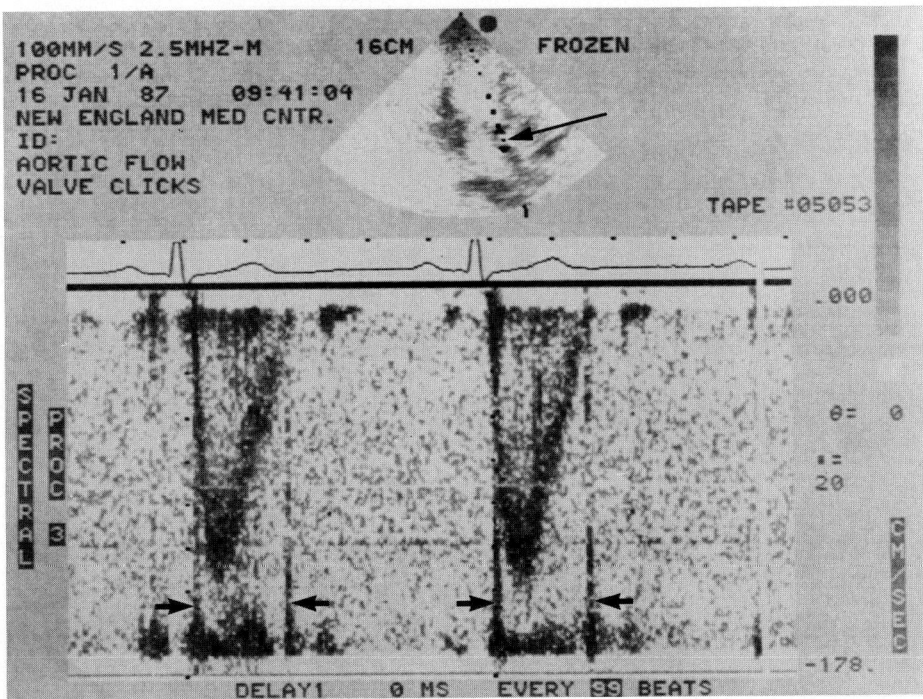

Fig. 3.9. Valve clicks on a Doppler tracing. In this illustration of normal aortic flow obtained at the aortic valve level (*long arrow*) with pulsed-Doppler, the movement of the valve leaflets is shown on the Doppler tracing as sharp high-amplitude spikes (*short arrows*) seen as aortic flow commences rapidly in early systole and just after it ceases at the end of systole.

niques cannot be done here. In essence a mean velocity of motion is depicted for all red cells encompassed in a sample volume, and the data that are obtained lack the precision of a full-power spectral analysis, as is seen with CW and pulsed-Doppler recordings (5).

Color flow mapping is changing the Doppler approach to the heart. Currently it can accurately display the flow abnormalities and allows for the exact placement of the Doppler cursor within a jet in order to measure the true velocity in the area in question. It greatly facilitates the accumulation of precise Doppler data.

Doppler Display

Both continuous-wave and pulsed-Doppler process and display the signals in the format of spectral analysis (ie, the breakdown of a complex waveform into its component frequencies by fast Fourier transform or Chirp Z methods). The display shows the Doppler frequency shifts on the vertical axis plotted against time on the horizontal axis of the graph. The range of velocities of positive and negative frequency shifts is typically displayed with the zero line of no flow positioned in the middle. However, it is possible to move the zero line to the top or bottom of the display to use the entire display to show one direction of flow. This effectively doubles the velocity limit of unidirectional flow (Fig. 3.8).

Flow toward the transducer is conventionally displayed in a positive direction above the zero line and flow away from the transducer is displayed in a negative fashion below the zero line. Normal laminar flow is displayed with a uniform range of frequencies, as all the blood cells are moving at a relatively similar velocity during the time they are examined. Laminar flow can be either flat in profile or parabolic in shape. Turbulent flow will be displayed with a wide range of frequencies, because the blood cells are moving with a wide range of different velocities at the site examined, and they are producing eddies and nonlaminar flow in multiple directions.

Valve motion is easily identified because valve movement gives strong reflections of high

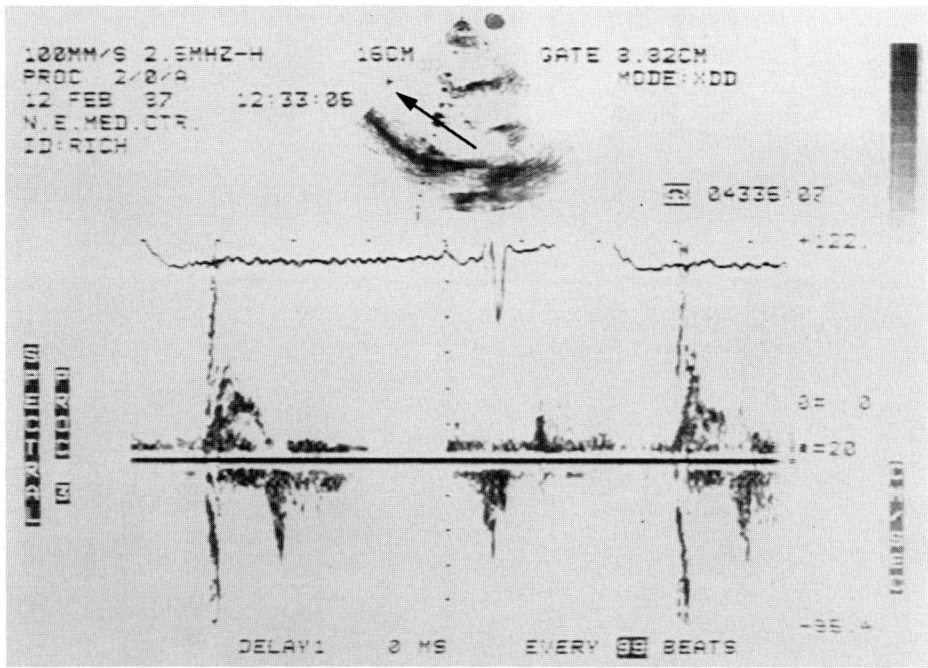

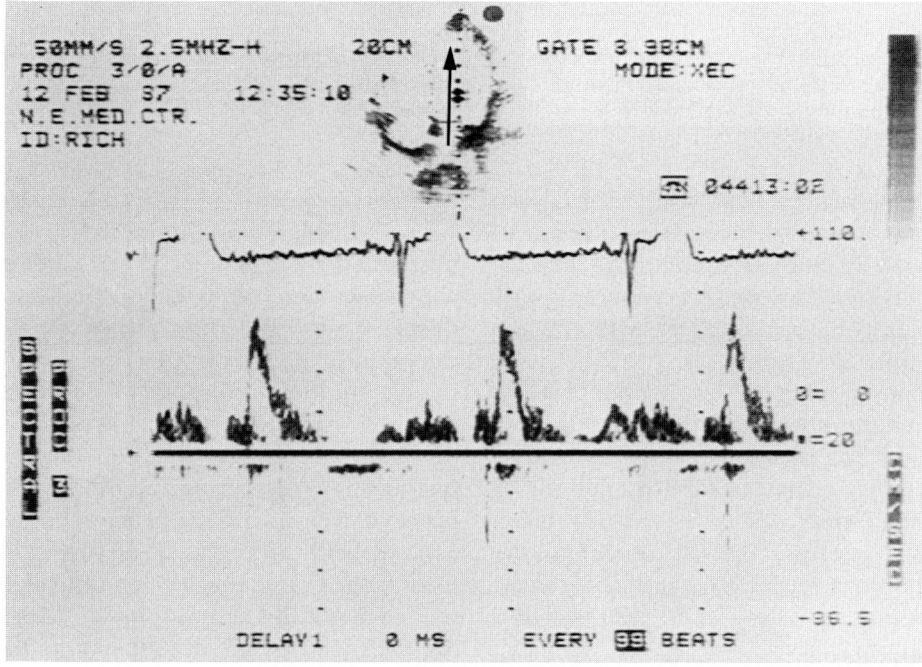

Fig. 3.10A,B. Effect of proper Doppler beam alignment in obtaining accurate velocity measurements. **A.** Pulsed Doppler tracing of normal mitral inflow in a parasternal long axis view. In this example, where the Doppler pathway is not directed along the direction of blood flow (*arrow*), a V max of 0.5 m/s is obtained, which is an underestimate (calibration marks, 20 cm/s). **B.** Pulsed Doppler tracing obtained from an apical four-chamber approach. This is the same individual as in part **A**, and, here, the pulsed-Doppler tracing correctly measures the V max of the mitral flow at 0.7 m/s, as the Doppler beam was directed parallel to the flow of blood (*arrow*) through the mitral valve (calibration marks, 20 cm/s).

amplitude and are heard as audible clicks, whereas the sound of blood flow is more continuous and less intense (Fig. 3.9) (1, p 59).

Doppler Examination

In the performance of a Doppler echocardiogram the normal ultrasound approach to the heart is somewhat altered. When examining the heart during a two-dimensional echocardiogram, structures are best imaged that are aligned at right angles to the ultrasound beam path, and are barely, if at all, seen when they are oriented parallel to the ultrasound beam path. This situation is reversed during a Doppler echocardiogram. The optimal Doppler signals are obtained with the ultrasound beam directed along the pathway of the blood flow velocity being sampled in a parallel fashion. This will accurately record the true maximum velocity of the blood flow in the area being sampled. The poorest Doppler signals are at a right angle to the interrogating ultrasound beam. The basic information obtained by Doppler relates to the direction and velocity of the flow. The best Doppler signal is often obtained with a less than optimal two-dimensional image. Theoretically there should be no Doppler shift detected at right angles to the ultrasound path in blood flow in normal individuals.

In performing a Doppler echocardiogram, blood flow velocity is evaluated from all possible acoustical windows. Maximal velocity information must be obtained where the ultrasound beam parallels the blood flow in the area being sampled. Because abnormal flow can occur along any possible vector, these situations require sampling from multiple sites to accurately localize discrete jets. Normal flow velocity generally can be measured along an assumed flow vector as directed by two-dimensional imaging guidance, in order to align the sampling pathway parallel with the direction of the flow velocity being analyzed in the selected range gate (Fig. 3.10).

Flow in the pulmonary artery is best examined from a parasternal short axis view at or just above the level of the aortic valve. As the pulmonary artery is usually well visualized from this approach, the Doppler beam can be optimally placed parallel to the flow vector in the pulmonary artery.

Both the mitral and the tricuspid valves are best evaluated from an apical approach, where the Doppler cursor is practically parallel to the flow of blood through each of these valves between the atria and ventricles.

The flow in the aorta also can be assessed from an apical approach, either from an apical long axis view, or from an apical "five chamber" view. Both views look up the barrel of the aorta in a similar fashion parallel to the flow of blood through this vessel. Flow in the various portions of the aortic arch can be evaluated from a suprasternal notch approach or form a right parasternal approach where the Doppler beam can be aligned parallel to the aortic flow vector.

Nevertheless, although the above positions offer windows for optimal transducer placement for maximal Doppler information in normal flow velocity situations, it must be restated that all acoustic windows are used to map the cardiac chambers to localize discrete sites of abnormal flow velocities.

Most normal adult patients can have a complete cardiac Doppler examination using the suprasternal notch, the left parasternal area, and the cardiac apex. These positions, and the corresponding two-dimensional images, with the different orientations of the heart within the sector, are shown in Diagram 3.2. Occasionally, nonstandard approaches to the heart must be used, and the right parasternal, subcostal, or left parasternal long axis views may be the best ways to obtain Doppler signals. In these situations, the angle of the ultrasound beam may not be parallel to the blood flow velocity being interrogated. Often good Doppler signals are found more easily when both the audible and visual components of the Doppler signal itself are used as a guide rather than the echocardiogram, and the operator's attention focuses on "finely tuning in" the best quality Doppler signal rather than closely following the two-dimensional image. The ability to develop an optimal Doppler signal, with both good quality sound and a technically fine spectral display, coupled with characteristic valve movements and flow profiles (as in "M mode" echocardiography), allows us to do a continuous-wave Doppler examination without two-dimensional imaging and find the characteristic flow veloc-

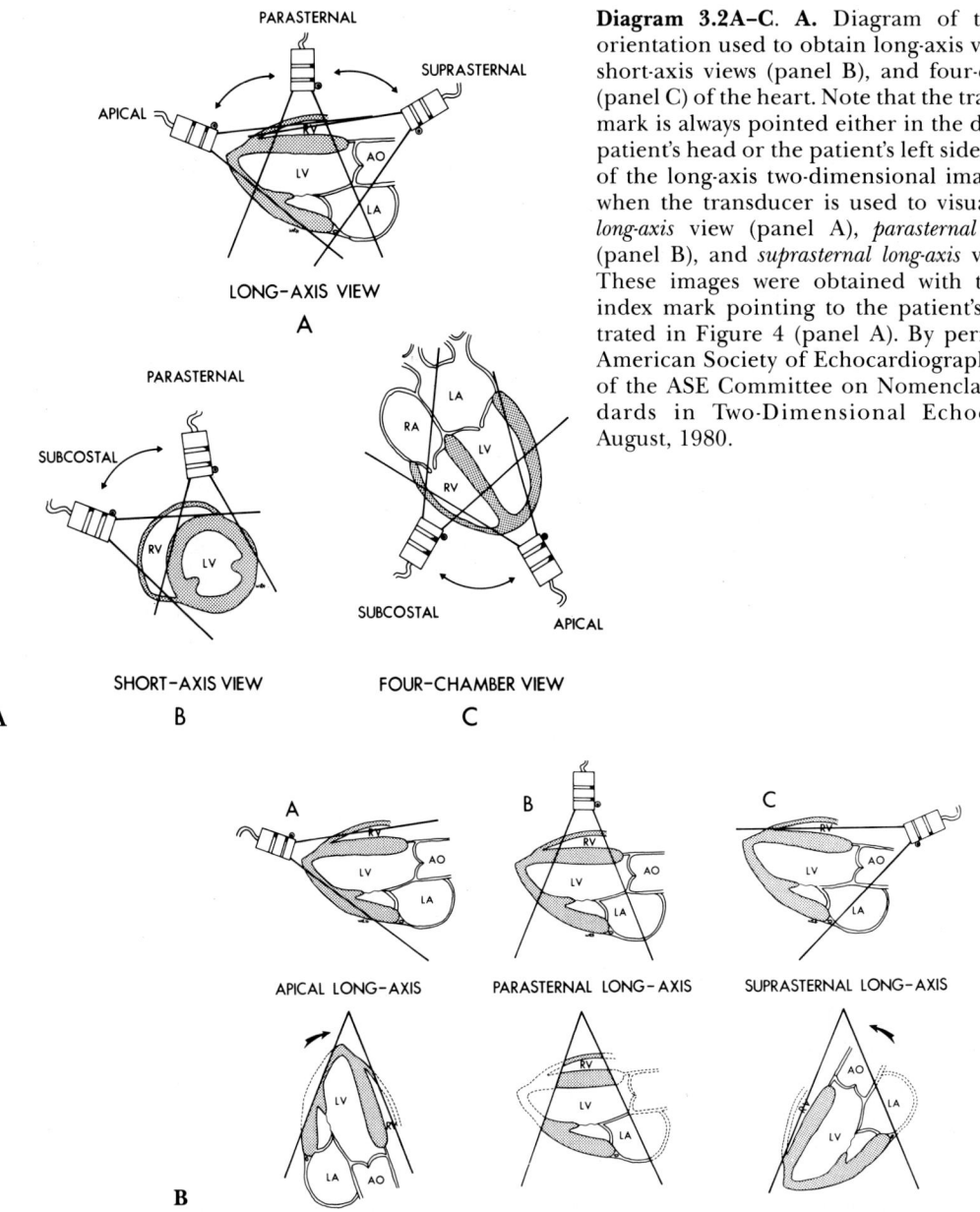

Diagram 3.2A–C. A. Diagram of the transducer orientation used to obtain long-axis views (panel A), short-axis views (panel B), and four-chamber views (panel C) of the heart. Note that the transducer index mark is always pointed either in the direction of the patient's head or the patient's left side. **B.** Illustration of the long-axis two-dimensional images that result when the transducer is used to visualize the *apical long-axis* view (panel A), *parasternal long-axis* view (panel B), and *suprasternal long-axis* view (panel C). These images were obtained with the transducer index mark pointing to the patient's head as illustrated in Figure 4 (panel A). By permission of the American Society of Echocardiography. The Report of the ASE Committee on Nomenclature and Standards in Two-Dimensional Echocardiography, August, 1980.

ity patterns throughout various portions of the cardiac chambers and great vessels. Then using pulsed-Doppler, the various flow velocity signals can be examined and localized spatially within the heart. In normal individuals, a pulsed-Doppler examination could be done without a CW Doppler study, because generally low blood flow velocities are being interrogated, and these low velocities can easily be measured within the limits of pulsed-Doppler. Finally, when applicable, color flow mapping is done to demonstrate in a pictorial fashion, specific flow patterns, such as leaks around prosthetic valves or complex lesions.

Equipment

Almost all current echocardiographic machines are made with complete echocardiographic capability. State-of-the-art phased array cardiac ultrasound scanners are equipped to perform M mode recordings, high-resolution two-dimen-

Diagram 3.2C. *(Top)* Diagram of the short-axis two-dimensional images that result when the transducer is used to visualize the *parasternal short-axis* view (panel A) and the *subcostal short-axis* view (panel B). These images were obtained with the transducer index mark pointing to the patient's left side as illustrated in Figure 4 (panel B). *(Bottom)* Illustration of the four-chamber two-dimensional images that result when the transducer is used to visualize the *apical four-chamber* view (panel A) and the *subcostal four-chamber* view (panel B). These images were obtained with the transducer index mark pointing to the patient's left side as illustrated in Figure 4 (panel C). Two options are included for each four-chamber view. In each case, option #1 is produced by activation of the image inversion switch which results in the near-signals of the image being inverted from the top to the bottom of the display. By permission of the American Society of Echocardiography. The Report of the ASE Committee on Nomenclature and Standards in Two-Dimensional Echocardiography, August, 1980.

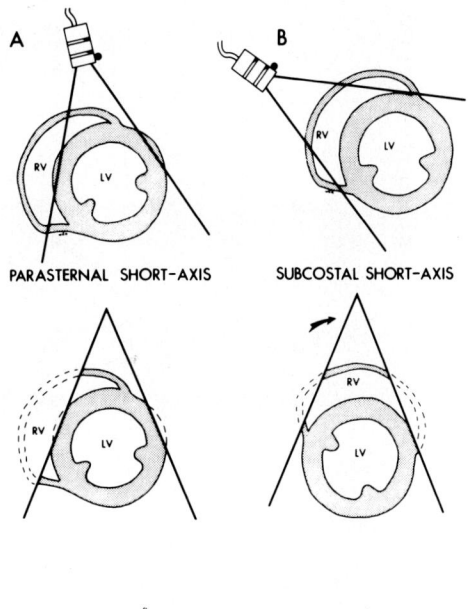

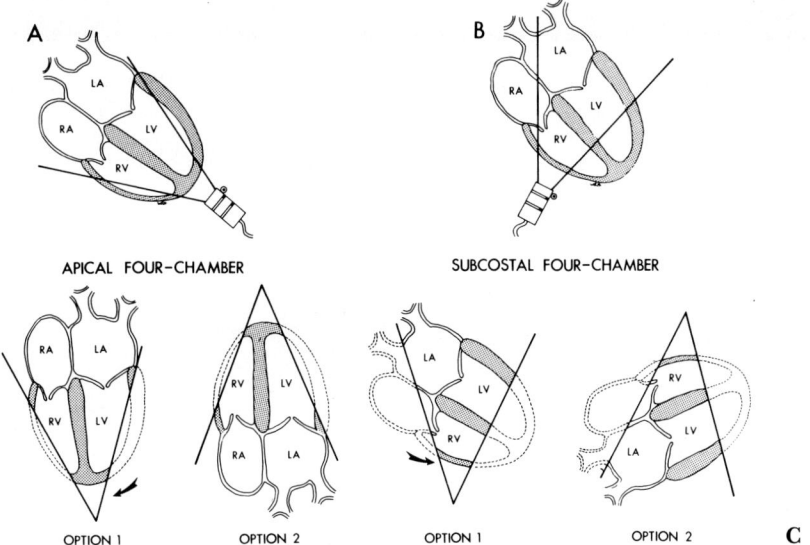

sional imaging, spatially guided pulsed-Doppler, and continuous-wave Doppler examinations of the heart, timed along with the electrocardiogram (EKG) in one portable unit. Many modern machines are now equipped with color flow mapping as well; almost all machines will offer this capability in the immediate future. A variety of interchangeable transducers allowing optimal echocardiographic information is used. Imaging (and pulsed-Doppler) transducers are generally in the standard 2 to 7.5 MHz range, where continuous-wave Doppler transducers are around 2 MHz in frequency. Images are recorded on videotape or Polaroid or they are printed on a strip chart recording on paper.

Normal Doppler Flow Patterns

In general the spectral analysis display of the Doppler frequency shifts obtained during Doppler examination of the heart is the same, whether the information is obtained from pulsed-Doppler or continuous-wave Doppler. Other than for the problem with aliasing, encountered in high-velocity flow situations, with pulsed-Doppler, the displayed waveforms

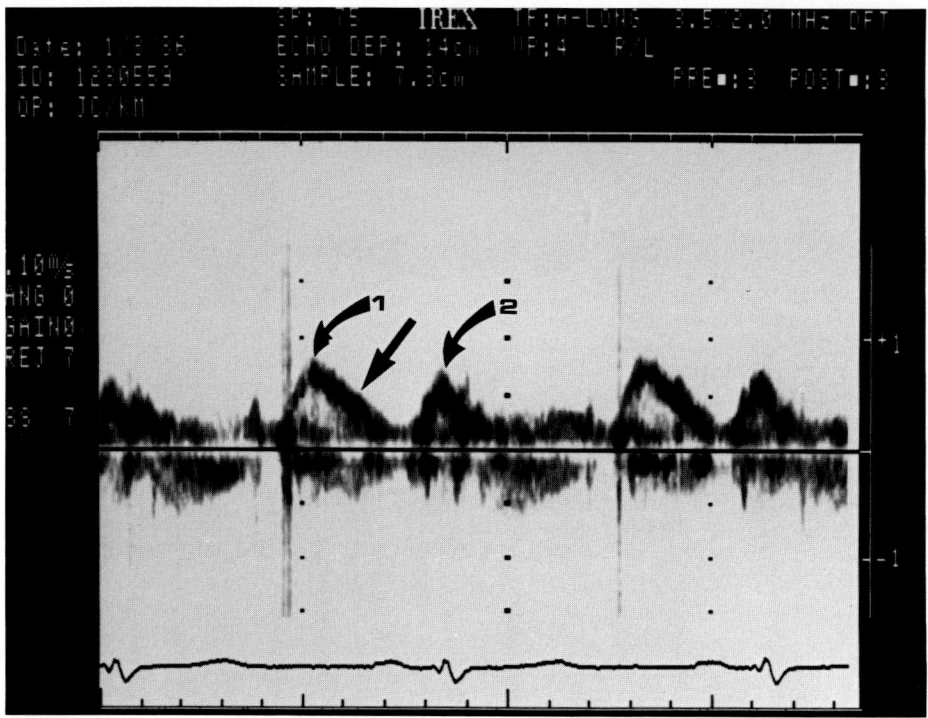

Fig. 3.11. Normal pulsed-Doppler tracing of left ventricular inflow. In this example, the typical mitral flow velocity profile is demonstrated. Its biphasic appearance is shown, with a higher peak in early diastole (*curved arrow 1*), that has a V max of 0.8 m/s, which is followed by a second lower peak later in diastole (*curved arrow 2*). Note the rapid deceleration of the mitral flow profile after the first peak (*straight arrow*). It effectively reaches the baseline in a period of no flow before the atrial contraction (calibration marks, 0.5 m/s).

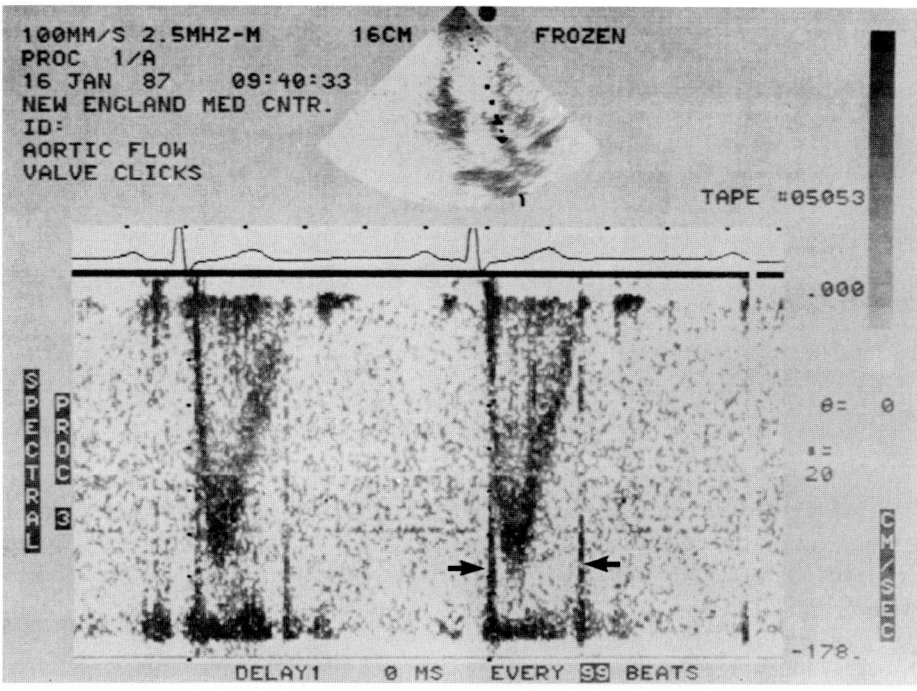

Fig. 3.12. Valve clicks on an aortic flow recording. The high-amplitude spikes (*arrows*) of the valve opening and closing are seen preceding and following the flow through the aortic valve in systole.

are essentially identical in both modalities. Whereas the pulsed-Doppler examination is done with two-dimensional image guidance, the Doppler flow patterns that are detected in various portions of the heart have characteristic and recognizable properties that are generally comparable with either pulsed- or continuous-wave Doppler techniques. In the following section, the characteristic Doppler flow profiles in normal adults will be reviewed, starting on the left side of the heart and then doing the same on the right side. The flow velocity curves in the left ventricle are examined in the inflow area, the middle of the ventricle, and the outflow area. The Doppler signals in the inflow area reflect flow across the mitral valve, and those in the outflow area measure aortic flow. On the right side, Doppler information obtained in the inflow area shows transmitral flow, and those from the outflow area are indicative of flow out through the pulmonic valve.

Table 3.1. Maximal Velocities Recorded by Doppler Ultrasound in Normal Individuals in Meters per Second

	Adults	Children
Mitral flow	0.9 (0.6–1.3)	1.0 (0.8–1.3)
Tricuspid flow	0.5 (0.3–0.7)	0.6 (0.5–0.8)
Pulmonary artery	0.75 (0.6–0.9)	0.9 (0.7–1.2)
Left ventricle	0.9 (0.7–1.1)	1.0 (0.7–1.2)
Aorta	1.35 (1.0–1.7)	1.5 (1.2–1.8)

From Hatle L, Angelsen B: Doppler Ultrasound in Cardiology (2nd ed). Philadelphia, Lea & Febiger, 1985, p 72; reprinted with permission.

Flow Velocity Curves in the Left Ventricle

From an apical approach, the left ventricular inflow area is evaluated for the blood flowing through the mitral valve from the left atrium. Forward diastolic flow in the left atrium is usually not recorded, although this can be seen at the entrance of the pulmonary veins into the back of the left atrium. The normal mitral flow velocity profile obtained from patients in normal sinus rhythm shows flow in a positive direction toward the transducer. This flow consists of two separate peaks (Fig. 3.11). The first peak represents the velocity of the flow in the phase of early diastolic filling. This peak is followed by a second, usually smaller, peak later in diastole, which corresponds to the increase in transmitral flow velocity after atrial contraction. As the sample volume is moved through the mitral valve area, the valve itself will be seen, heard, and recorded as high-amplitude clicks on the Doppler tracing. This situation is encountered whenever any of the cardiac valves are moving within the area being sampled (Fig. 3.12). In patients in atrial fibrillation, the mitral flow curve loses this second peak. In other atrial arrhythmias, such as atrial flutter, several mitral flow peaks may be seen corresponding to the multiple atrial contractions (1, p 60). The findings are similar to those seen in M mode echocardiography of the mitral valve. The maximal flow velocities recorded with Doppler ultrasound in normal adults range from 0.6 to 1.3 m/s (Table 3.1) (1, p 72).

While scanning from an apical approach, angling the transducer more medially and somewhat cephalad, the middle of the left ventricle, with both its diastolic inflow and systolic outflow patterns, will be examined. Positive doubly notched flow will be seen coming toward the transducer in diastole, corresponding to the mitral inflow into the left ventricle; uniphasic negative systolic flow, representing aortic flow out of the left ventricle, will be seen.

Continuing with still more medial and cephalad orientation of the transducer, the left ventricular outflow tract is interrogated. Only negative uniphasic flow away from the transducer in systole will be recorded (Fig. 3.13).

The same apical transducer position is used for color Doppler, although the left parasternal approach offers an excellent position for color flow mapping as well (Fig. 3.14).

Flow Velocity Curves in the Aortic Valve Area

Again, usually using an apical approach, the sample volume is placed in the left ventricular outflow tract. With two-dimensional image-guided pulsed-Doppler, the cursor is then progressively moved up through the aortic valves and into the proximal ascending aorta, beyond the aortic valve leaflets. A monophasic negative systolic flow velocity profile will be obtained representative of aortic flow velocity in the areas sampled. Maximal aortic flow veloc-

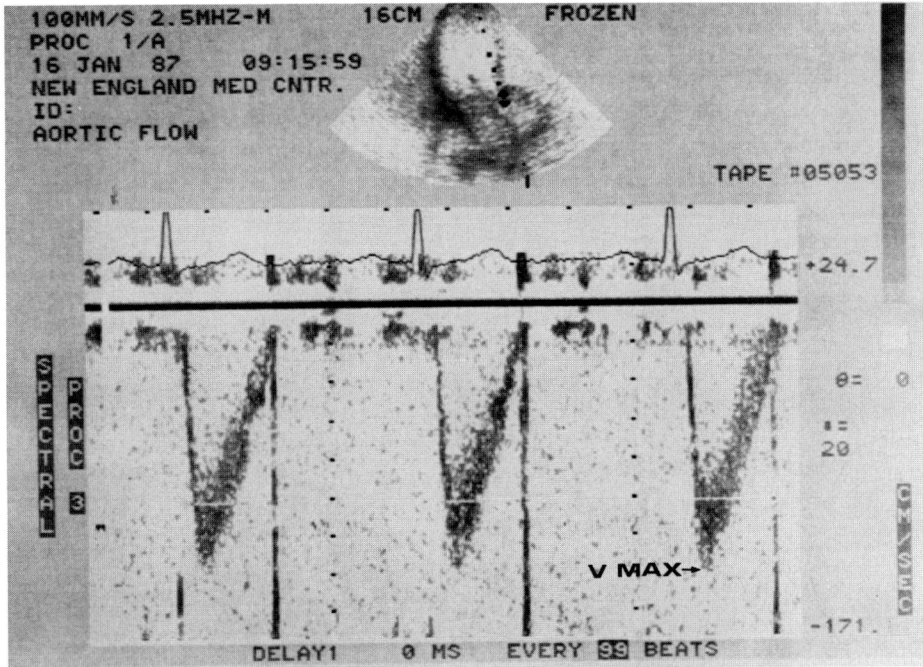

Fig. 3.13. Normal pulsed-Doppler tracing of left ventricular outflow. This is an example of a normal tracing obtained by pulsed-Doppler with the sample volume placed in the aortic valve area. Negative flow in systole away from the transducer is recorded, and a V max of 1.4 m/s is measured (calibration marks, 20 cm/s). Aliasing was present here until the zero line was shifted to the top of the scale.

ities recorded by Doppler in normal adults range from 1.0 to 1.7 m/s (Table 3.1). Because of the relationship between velocity and pressure in the Bernoulli equation, transvalvular pressure gradient can be calculated.

The commonly simplified formula for calculating the pressure gradient is:

$$\text{Pressure (P)} = 4 \times \text{maximal velocity}^2;$$
$$\text{or } P = 4 \, (V \max)^2$$

Using both pulsed- and continuous-wave Doppler in high-velocity aortic flow situations, the maximal aortic flow velocity can be accurately measured (Fig. 3.15).

Flow Velocity Curves in the Right Ventricle

As with the left side of the heart, the right ventricular inflow area is best seen using an apical approach. With the transducer, or sample volume, directed more medially from the mitral valve, the area around the tricuspid valve is interrogated. Like mitral flow, tricuspid valve flow has two peaks in diastole in a positive direction toward the transducer. However, normal tricuspid flow is of lower velocity than corresponding mitral flow. Normal tricuspid flow, as measured by Doppler, ranges from 0.3 to 0.7 m/s in adults (Table 3.1). The tricuspid valve also shows respiratory variability, with increase in flow through the tricuspid valve during inspiration (Fig. 3.16) (1, p 66).

In the middle of the right ventricle from an apical approach, with its mix of both inflow and outflow velocities, a positive doubly peaked inflow curve in diastole, and another positive monophasic flow curve in systole, corresponding to outflow, are seen.

Finally, if one angles the transducer more anteriorly, cephalad, and laterally into the right ventricular outflow tract, the flow switches to only a monophasic negative flow in systole.

In the right atrium, forward diastolic flow may be demonstrated in inspiration.

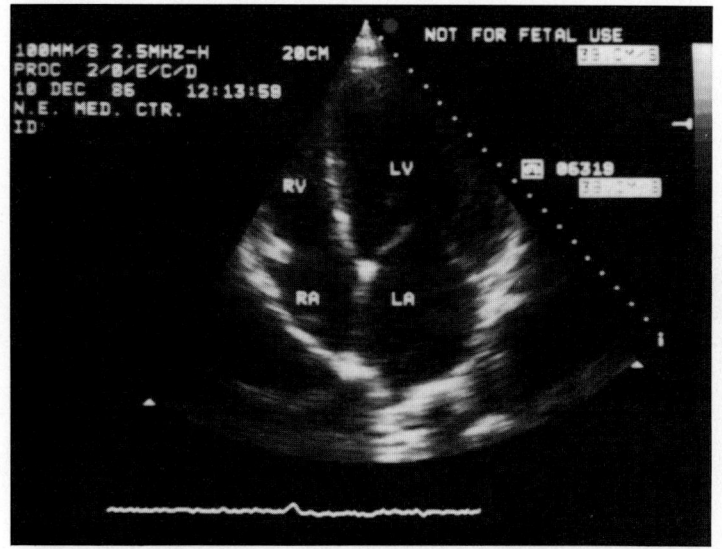

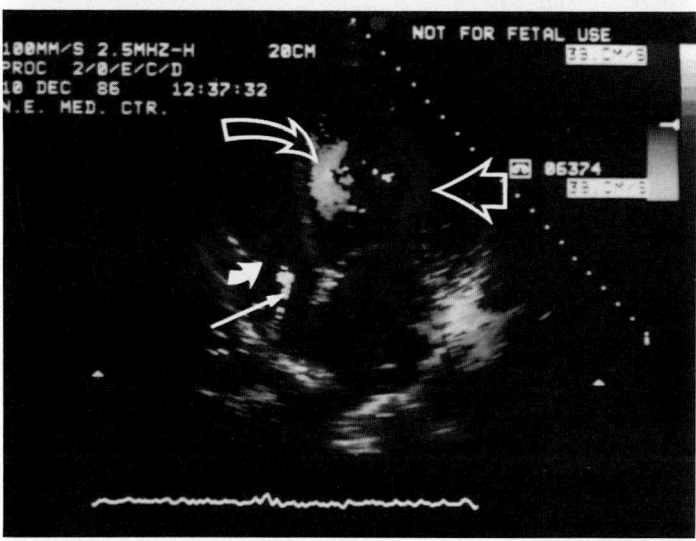

Fig. 3.14A–D. Normal left ventricular color Doppler images. **A.** Black and white apical four-chamber view of a normal heart. **B.** Early diastole. Normal forward positive flow is displayed in red and orange extending from the back of the left atrium toward the apex (*broad open arrow*). Areas of slightly higher velocity are seen in this jet in the left ventricle as areas of yellow to white. The normal downward vortex toward the aortic valve is seen along the septum in blue shades (*curved open arrow*). Right-sided forward flow is shown in red and orange (*short curved arrow*). The patch of blue (*thin arrow*) within this orange in the tricuspid area is partial imaging of normal downward flow out of the adjacent ascending aorta. **C.** Later in diasole. All the flow patterns shown in part **B** are again shown here. The velocities have all increased. The orange forward flow on both sides of the heart is now displayed with more yellow and white, indicating higher velocities. Note the higher velocities on the left side compared with the right. The patches of blue with the yellow-white areas of the left ventricular inflow represent aliasing (*arrow*). Note the acceleration in the downward vortex along the septum as blood approaches the aortic valve. This pattern is now displayed with brighter blue-green than in **B**. **D.** An apical long axis view of the left ventricle and left atrium in the same individual. The transducer has simply been rotated 90° at the apex. It offers a Doppler approach identical to the four-chamber view. A small patch of red is seen in the left atrium (*closed straight arrow*) probably representing pulmonary venous emptying, whereas the mitral valve leaflets are closed. Normal left ventricular outflow is demonstrated. Negative downward flow is shown in most of the anterior portion of the left ventricle in shades of blue (*open curved arrow*). This pattern extends through the aortic valve into the proximal ascending aorta. Note the increase in velocity in the subaortic region, hugging the upper septum and extending through the aortic leaflets. This is displayed as bright blue-green (*long thin arrow*), and shows the blood accelerating through the valve and actually outlining one of the sinuses of Valsalva (*short closed curved arrow*). For a color reproduction of this figure see frontmatter. (*See next page.*)

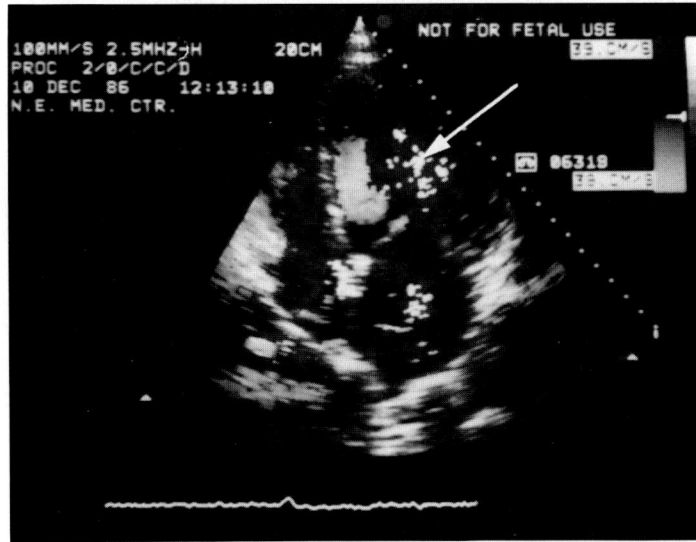

C

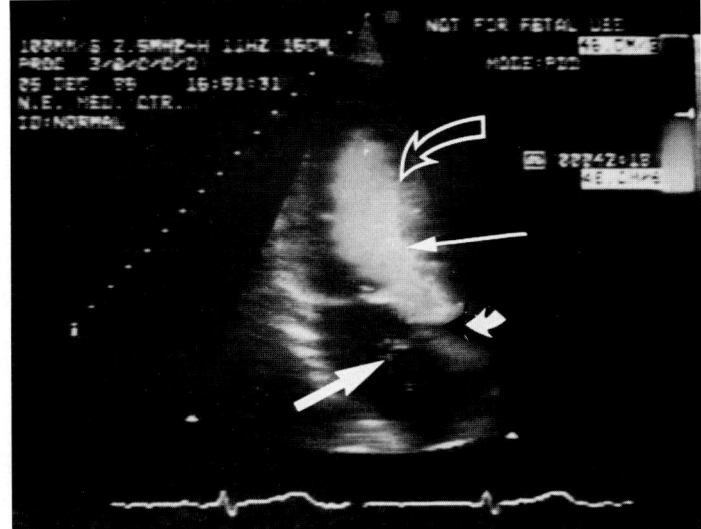

D

Fig. 3.14.

Flow Velocity Curves in the Pulmonary Valve Area

Flow velocity recordings in the pulmonary valve are best obtained from a left parasternal short axis approach. The pulmonary outflow tract is best seen from the fourth or fifth intercostal spaces, and the main pulmonary artery also can be evaluated from a window one or two interspaces higher. As in the left ventricle, the sample volume is moved through the right ventricular outflow tract, across the pulmonic valve, and into the main pulmonary artery. Negative low flow velocities away from the transducer will be recorded in systole. Normal pulmonic valve flow velocities recorded with Doppler ultrasound in adults are in the 0.6 to 0.9-m/s range (Table 3.1). In younger people, negative flow away from the transducer in late diastole probably represents diastolic flow into the pulmonary artery during atrial contraction, because of the low pressures that exist here (1, p 66). Pressure gradients can be calculated if desired (Fig. 3.17). The short axis view offers an excellent position for good color Doppler evaluation of the heart (Fig. 3.18).

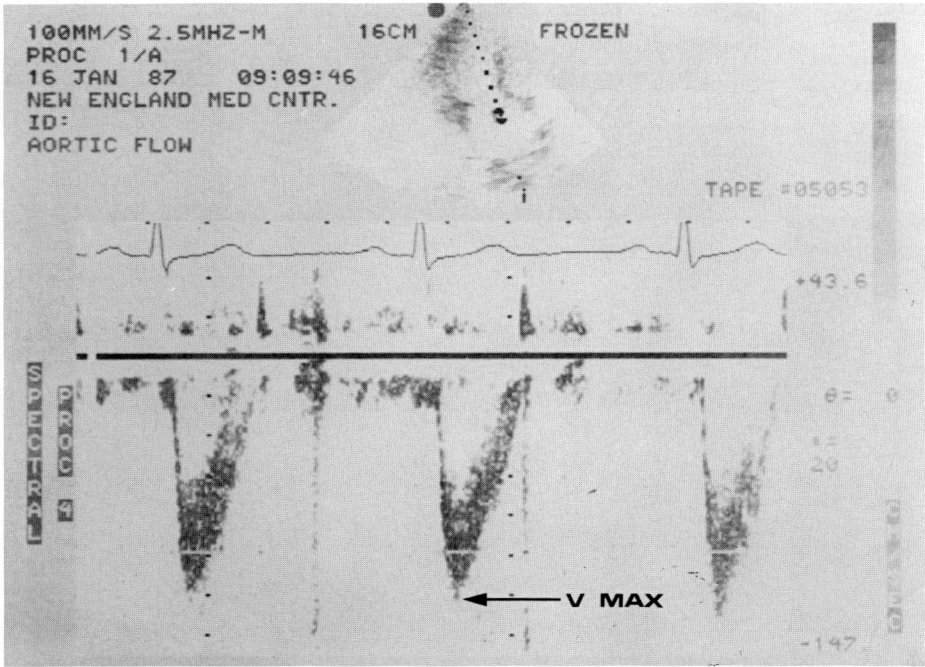

Fig. 3.15. Normal aortic flow. In this example, a V max of 1.2 m/s is obtained using pulsed-Doppler (calibration marks, 20 cm/s). Using the modified Bernoulli equation with V max = 1.2 m/s, the calculated pressure gradient across this normal aortic valve is 5.8 mm Hg.

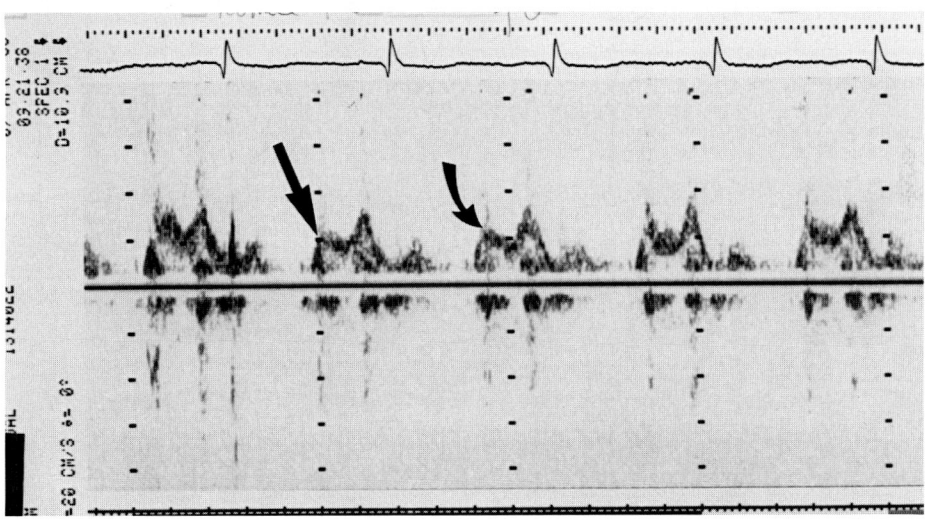

Fig. 3.16. Normal tricuspid flow. This is an example of normal flow obtained with pulsed-Doppler on the right ventricular side of the tricuspid valve. It has a characteristic biphasic appearance similar to the mitral valve. Note that the recorded velocities are lower than those obtained through the mitral valve (calibration marks, 20 cm/s). Note that the maximum flow across this tricuspid valve ranges over several heart beats from 0.2 m/s (*straight arrow*) up to 0.4 m/s (*curved arrow*). This represents normal respiratory variation of tricuspid blood flow.

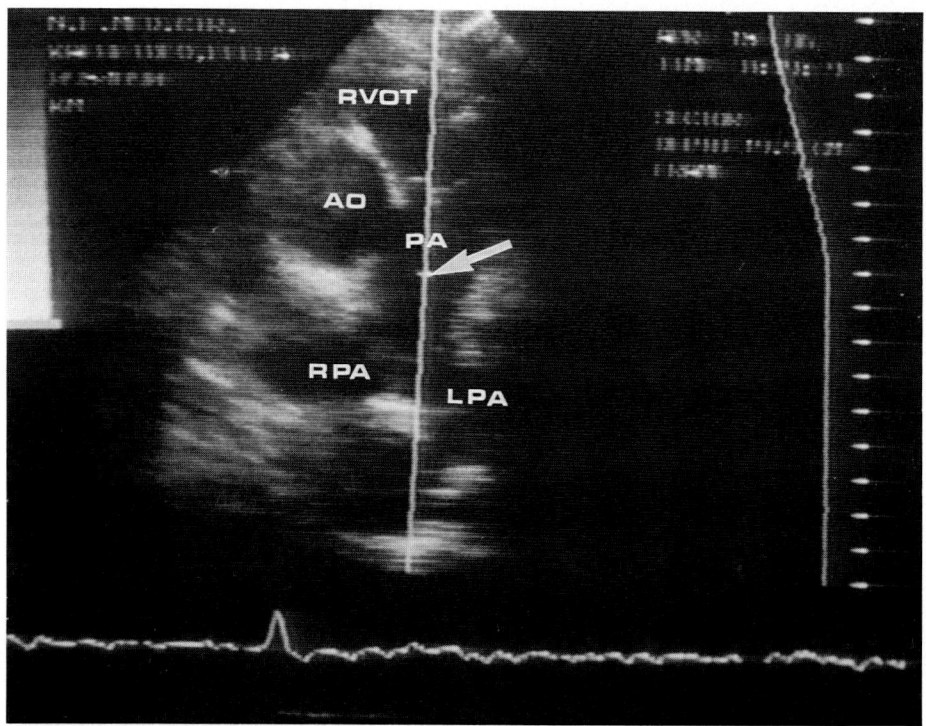

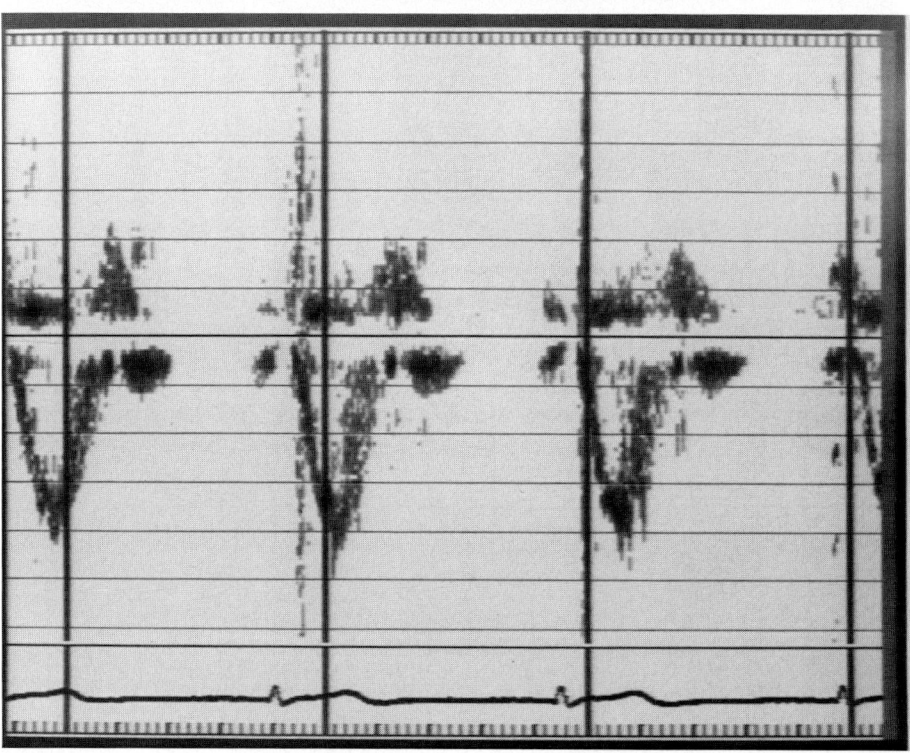

Fig. 3.17A,B. Normal pulmonic flow. **A.** Two-dimensional image of a short axis view of the pulmonary artery with the sample volume cursor placed in the main pulmonary artery (*white arrow*) (AO, aorta; RVOT, right ventricular outflow tract; PA, main pulmonary artery; RPA, right pulmonary artery; LPA, left pulmonary artery). **B.** Pulsed-Doppler tracing obtained from this site. A normal V max in the pulmonary artery of 0.9 m/s is shown (calibration marks, 20 cm/s).

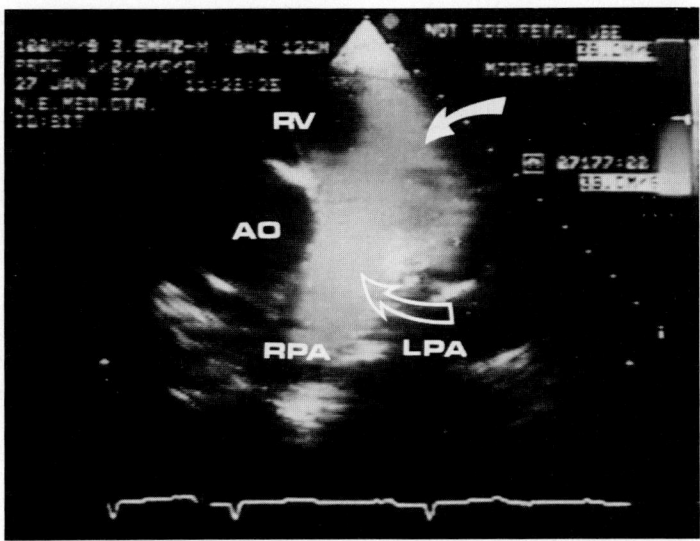

Fig. 3.18. Normal pulmonic flow. This is a short axis view of the right ventricular outflow tract obtained from the left parasternal approach. Normal downward negative flow is displayed in shades of deep blue, for slow flow in the right venticular outflow tract (*closed curved arrow*), to shades of bright blue-green, showing the blood flow as it acclerates through the pulmonic valve into the main pulmonary artery (*open curved arrow*), and down into the right pulmonary artery. No flow is shown in the left pulmonary artery in this illustration (AO, aorta; RV, right ventricle; LPA, left pulmonary artery; RPA, right pulmonary artery). For a color reproduction of this figure see frontmatter.

Doppler Assessment of Various Cardiac Abnormalties

In the following section the commonly seen cardiac lesions that best demonstrate the clinical importance of Doppler echocardiography will be reviewed. Because of the complementary roles and similarities of pulsed-Doppler and continuous-wave Doppler, along with the spatial presentation of color flow mapping, these various techniques will all be discussed together, placing various emphasis on particular techniques when the unique strengths of those techniques are called upon, such as the necessity to use CW techniques in high flow velocity situations. The organization of this section is lesion oriented rather than modality oriented.

Using pulsed-Doppler techniques, the spatial arrangement of flow signals can be accurately localized, and these flow velocity signals can be correlated temporally with intracardiac pressure and electrical events. Continuous-wave Doppler, on the other hand, allows for the accurate measurement of peak velocities in a specific flow pattern, which is extremely helpful in the diagnosis and quantification of specific valvular lesions. Finally, in many circumstances, the use of color flow mapping offers dramatic pictorial representation of the flow patterns in question. This is particularly helpful in characterizing flow phenomena caused by either normal or abnormal dynamics, surveying the heart to detect and localize multiple lesions, and quantitating regurgitant jets, along with determining the direction of a stenotic or regurgitant jet. Color flow mapping is also particularly helpful in the evaluation of valve prostheses and in localizing intracardiac shunts. It may soon be proven helpful in quantifying shunts (5).

As mentioned earlier, when performing a Doppler echocardiogram, blood flow velocity is evaluated from all acoustic windows whenever possible. It is also imperative to make every attempt to align the Doppler beam parallel to the flow velocity being interrogated in order to obtain the maximum velocity. Sometimes, because of technical reasons, this is not possible. Other approaches, different from the standard ones, must be used, and the frequency shift measured in an angled sampling beam, which is not truly parallel to the flow, must be angle

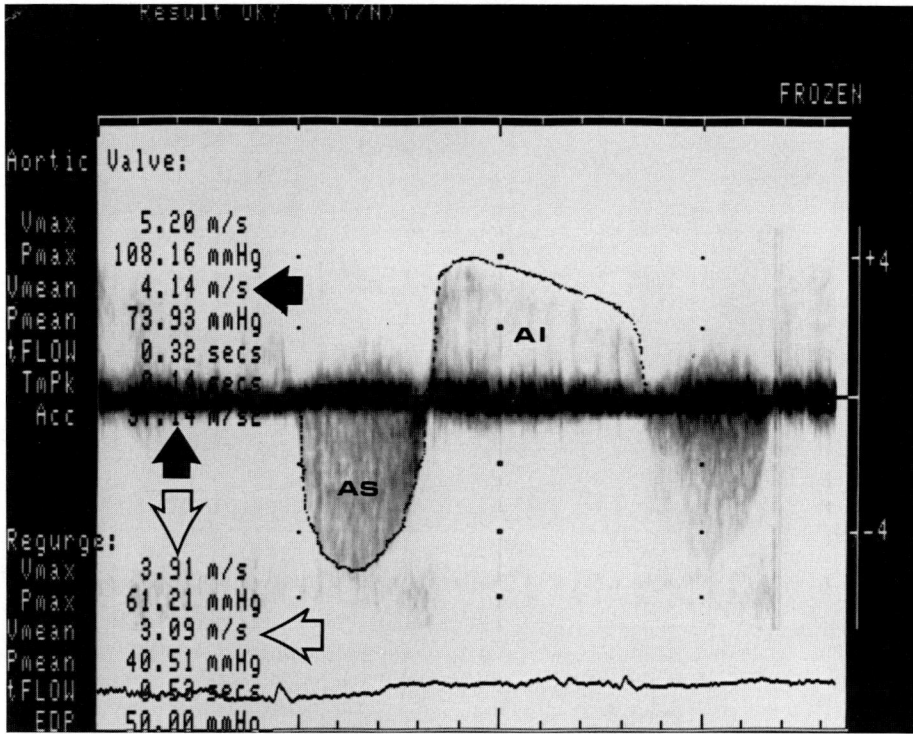

Fig. 3.19. Pressure gradient calculated from V max in continous-wave Doppler tracing. This is an example of a linear tracing of the Doppler flow velocity profile in a patient with both aortic stenosis (negative systolic flow, AS) and aortic insufficiency (positive diastolic flow, AI). Velocity and time measurements, as well as pressure calculations from the modified Bernoulli equation, are displayed on the left side of the image. The calculations for the aortic stenosis are displayed on the top portion of the left side (*solid arrow*), and those for the aortic insufficiency are displayed on the bottom portion of the left side (*open arrow*). The maximum velocity of the flow across the stenotic aortic valve is 5.2 m/s, which gives a pressure gradient of 108 mm Hg. The mean velocity of 4.1 m/s represents a pressure drop across the valve of 74 mm Hg. The display shown here unfortunately is confusing. Please note, that although the measurements and calculations are displayed in the top left of the image (above the zero line of the Doppler tracing), the Doppler tracing itself of the aortic stenosis is the negative one in systole below the zero line. As is shown, the velocity measurements across the regurgitant valve also can be used to obtain a pressure gradient here in diastole. Again, please note that although the data for the regurgitant valve are displayed at the bottom left, (below the zero line), the actual flow curve is the positive one in diastole above the zero line. The V max of the regurgitant lesion is 3.9 m/s.

corrected to the assumed path of the flow in the area being examined. When one encounters abnormal flow, there is no predetermined way to ascertain the true blood flow vector. In these situations, the abnormal flow must be examined at a multitude of sites from different approaches and axes to localize accurately discrete jets and the vectors of their flow and to map out the size of the abnormal flow patterns seen. This is especially true with regurgitant lesions, which can be seen in any one of a multitude of directions in relationship to the valve. Here again is a beautiful use for color flow mapping, which, by spatially orienting the blood flow, allows exact localization and quanitification of these flow abnormalities to be made quite simply.

Calculations

In abnormal flow velocity situations, two important calculations are used in the assessment of the Doppler signals: a modified Bernoulli equation for estimating pressure gradients across stenotic valves, and a pressure half-time equation for estimating the size of the opening of a stenotic mitral or tricuspid valve (2, p 25).

Bernoulli Equation

When obstruction to blood flow is present, the velocity of flow increases through the obstruction, and this increase in velocity is accompanied by a drop in pressure across the obstruction.

The Bernoulli equation is a hydraulic formula that relates velocity changes across an obstruction to the pressure gradient across the obstruction. With certain assumptions being made that neglect blood viscosity and inertial force factors (1, p 77), the Bernoulli equation can be simplified to estimate accurately the pressure gradient from the maximal flow velocity obtained in the Doppler tracing where:

Pressure gradient (PG, in mm Hg) = $4 (V max)^2$

For example, if the maximum velocity obtained through a stenotic aortic valve with continuous-wave Doppler (too high velocity situation for measurement with pulsed-Doppler because of aliasing) is 5.2 m/s (Fig. 3.19), then using the modified Bernoulli equation:

PG = $4 (V max)^2$, where V max = 5.2 m/s;

hen PG = $4 (5.2)^2$, and

PG = 4 (26) = 108

Thus, the pressure gradient across the stenotic aortic valve, shown in Figure 3.19, is 108 mmHg.

Mitral Pressure Half-Time

When blood flows passively through a stenotic valve (as with the atrioventricular valves), the opening size of the valvular orifice can be estimated from the amount of time it takes the initial peak velocity (and hence peak pressure gradient) to fall to a level corresponding to half the peak pressure gradient. This can be done from the tracing of the Doppler mitral flow velocity profile. Based on work done by Libanoffal and Rodbard (6,7), Hatle and others developed a method to assess the severity of mitral stenosis by measuring the duration of the velocity decline of the mitral flow profile during diastole. They found that in patients with mitral stenosis, the time from peak mitral flow velocity to the time when the mitral flow velocity reached one half its original level, was prolonged steadily, in the presence of increasing degrees of stenosis and obstruction to flow. Because of the relationship between velocity and pressure, this observation applies to pressure changes as well as velocity changes. The time in which the peak pressure reached a level equal to half its original value is the "pressure half-time." From the Bernoulli equation, it is known that the pressure gradient can be determined from squaring the velocity. The point on the downslope of the velocity of deceleration of the mitral flow, where a velocity is reached that corresponds to a pressure that is one half the original pressure when the maximum mitral flow velocity was reached (V max), can be located. This point where the pressure is halved is related to the square root of the velocity of blood flow. The point where half the original pressure is reached occurs when the original V max reaches a level equal to V max divided by the square root of 2. Because the square root of 2 is 1.4, the point where the velocity hits a level corresponding to one half the original pressure gradient is determined by dividing V max by 1.4. The pressure half-time is measured on the time scale on the horizontal axis, and it is the

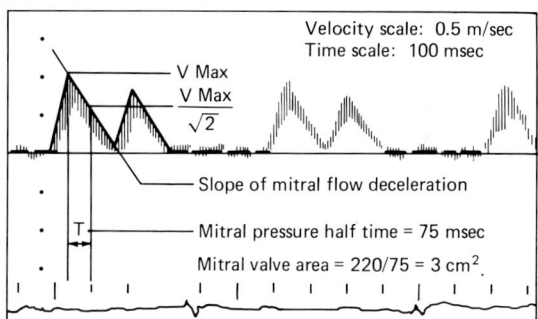

Diagram 3.3. In this diagram, a representative normal mitral flow is shown with a rapid downslope of deceleration. V max is 1 m/s, and the point where the original pressure is halved is where V max reaches a point where it equals V max/$\sqrt{2}$, or V max/1.4. This calculates to a velocity of 0.7 m/s. The time interval from a V max of 1.0 m/s to a velocity of V max/1.4 or 0.7 m/s is the mitral pressure half time, which measures 75 ms in this case. Since a pressure half time of 220 ms corresponds to a valve area of 1 cm^2, the mitral valve area is derived by dividing 220 by the measured mitral pressure half time. Here MVA = 220/75, which equals 3 cm^2. In this normal example where the mitral V max was 1.0 m/s, the measured pressure half time was 75 ms, and the calculated mitral valve area (MVA) is 3 cm^2.

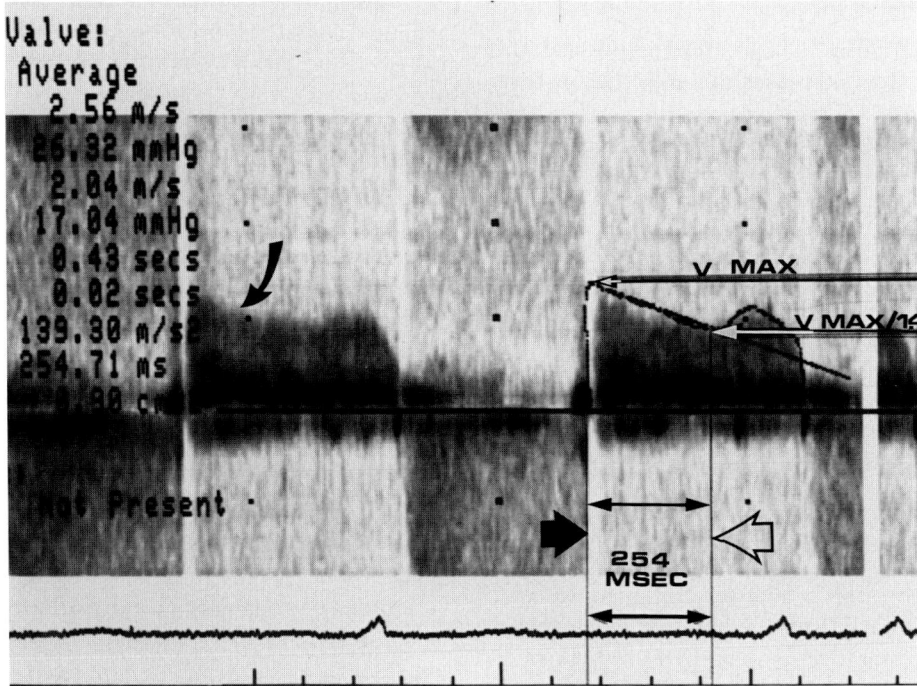

Fig. 3.20. Mitral stenosis with prolonged mitral pressure half-time. In this continuous-wave Doppler tracing from a patient with mitral stenosis, the V max of 2.56 m/s is elevated (top normal mitral flow is 1.3 m/s), and the downslope of the deceleration portion of the mitral flow curve is prolonged and shallower (*curved arrow*). The time interval (*horizontal double-headed arrow*) between V max (*solid arrow*) and the time point where V max/1.4 (*open arrow*) is reached is the mitral pressure half-time, which in this patient measures 254 ms. Please see Diagram 3 for an explanation of mitral pressure half-time. (Time calibration marks along the horizontal axis at the bottom of the graph are in 100-ms increments.) The calculated mitral valve area from the measured mitral pressure half-time is 0.90 cm² in this patient (MVA = 220/254).

time from when V max occurs until the time when V max/1.4 occurs, which is the velocity at which the original pressure gradient is halved. They found that a pressure half-time of 220 ms (milliseconds) corresponded to a valvular orifice area of 1 cm². By dividing 220 ms by the measured atrioventricular valve pressure half-time, an estimate of that atrioventricular (AV) valve's area can be calculated (8).

Summing up the above determination of pressure half-time centers around locating the velocity corresponding to half the original pressure gradient: V max occurs at time T-1 with pressure P; one-half P occurs at time T-2 when V 1/2 = V max/square root of 2, or V 1/2 = V max/1.4; and the time from T-1 to T-2 is the pressure half-time.

Therefore, the following equation is used to calculate the mitral valve area (MVA) once the mitral valve pressure half-time is determined from the Doppler tracing.

$$\text{MVA (in cm}^2\text{)} = \frac{220}{\text{pressure half-time (ms)}}$$

The gray-scale display of spectral analysis is converted to a simpler linear display of the spectral parameters plotting the velocity against time. The mitral pressure half-time is measured from the mitral Doppler tracing. Thus, any mitral pressure half-time that measures less than 220 ms will reflect a mitral orifice larger than 1 cm² (Diagram 3.3), and any one that measures greater than 220 ms will give a stenotic area less than 1 cm² (Fig. 3.20). In the example in Diagram 3.3, with a mitral pressure half-time of 75 ms, the mitral valve area is 220/75 or 3 cm². In the patient in Figure 3.20, the mitral pressure half-time measured 254 ms. Therefore,

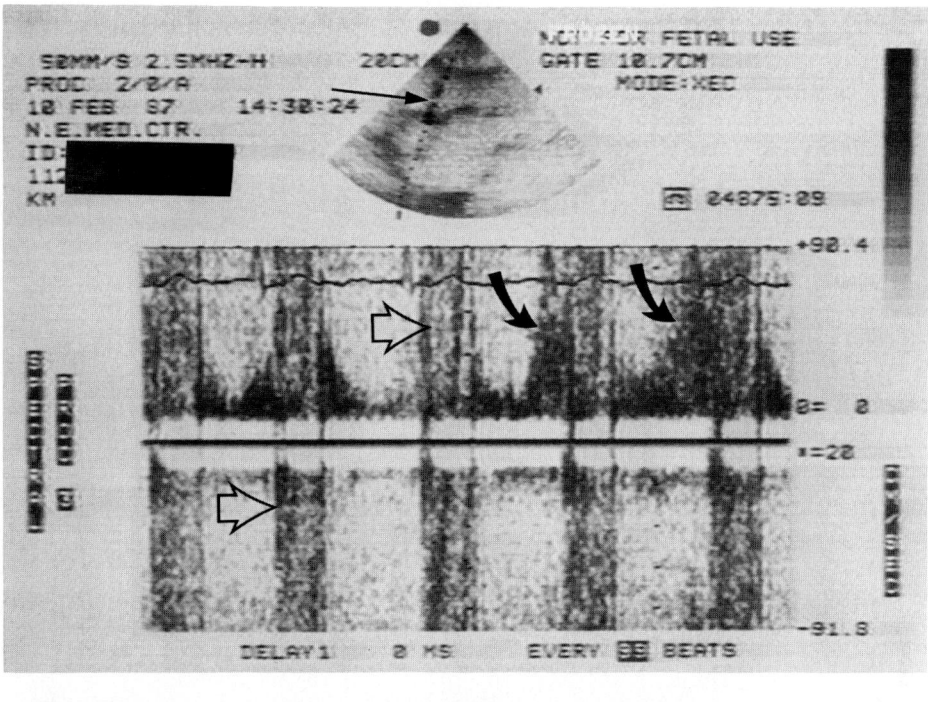
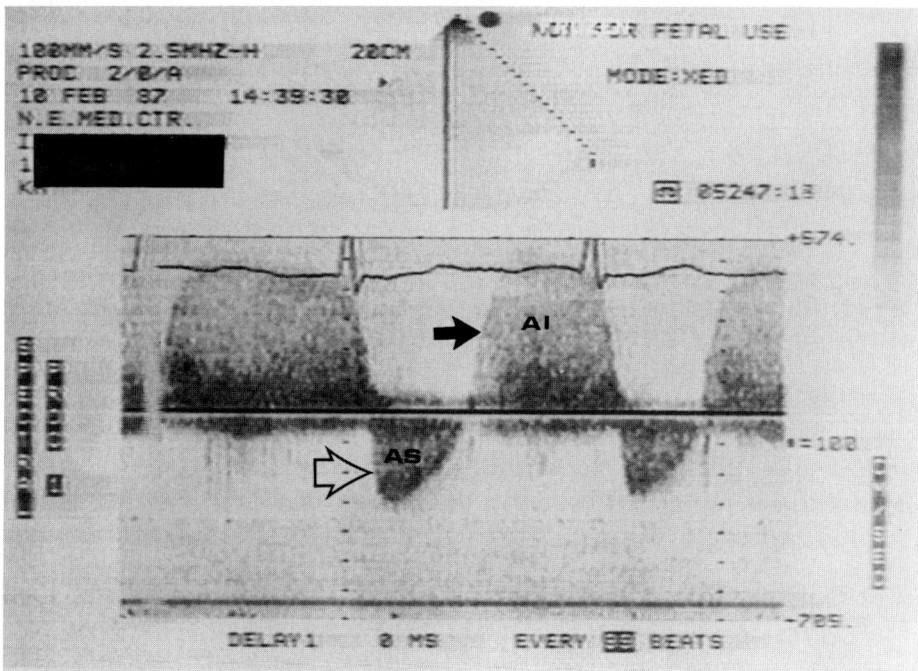

Fig. 3.21A,B. Pulsed and continuous-wave Doppler in aortic stenosis. **A.** Pulsed-Doppler tracing showing severe aliasing of systolic negative flow (*open arrows*), and some positive diastolic flow (*curved arrows*) at the aortic valve in a left parasternal view in a patient with aortic stenosis. The two-dimensional image on top shows the Doppler cursor in the orifice of the thickened valve (*long thin arrow*). The velocity of flow through the stenotic valve far exceeds the Nyquist frequency here, and the maximum velocity cannot be measured by pulsed-Doppler in this particular situation. **B.** Continuous-wave Doppler tracing obtained from an apical window shows a V max of 3 m/s, in a negative direction in systole (*horizontal broad open arrow*) of the flow through the aortic stenosis. The calculated pressure gradient here, using the modified Bernoulli equation, is 36 mm Hg. There is also a severe aortic regurgitant lesion here as well with a V max of 6 m/s seen as the large positive flow pattern throughout diastole (*horizontal broad closed arrow*).

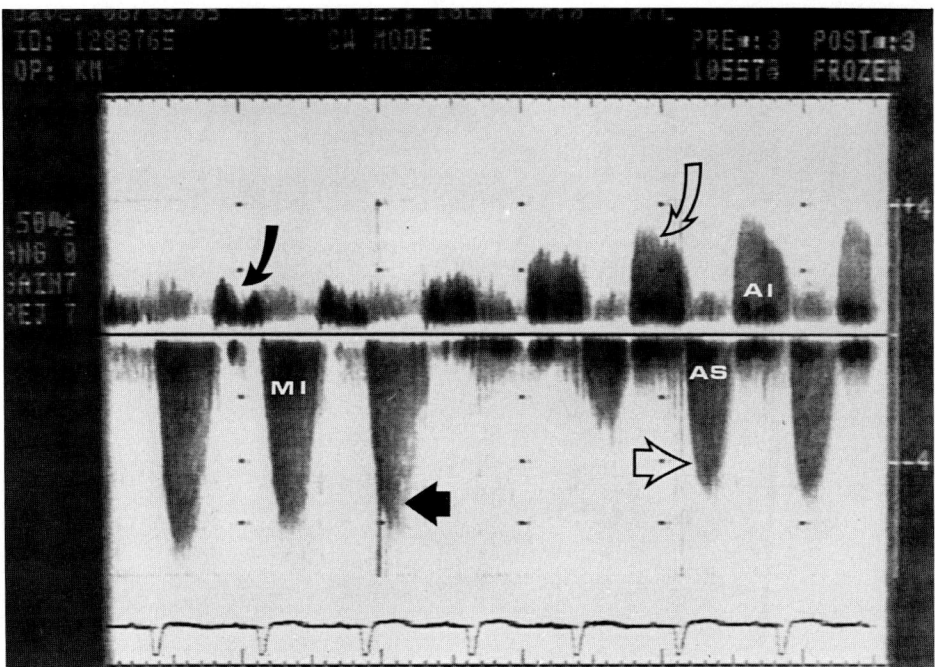

Fig. 3.22. Continous-wave Doppler in a patient with a combination of mitral insufficiency, aortic stenosis, and aortic insufficiency. In this tracing obtained from the apex, both the aortic stenosis and mitral insufficiency flow profiles are seen as similar patterns of systolic negative flow away from the transducer. Their velocities are, however, different. The tracing was started at the mitral valve and recorded as the transducer was angled in a slightly medial and cephalad direction to end in the direction of aortic outflow. On the left of the image the severe mitral insufficiency jet (*broad closed arrow*) is seen as the pronounced negative systolic flow with a V max of 7 m/s, and on the right of the image the high-velocity jet of aortic stenosis (*broad open arrow*) is also seen as a negative systolic tracing with a V max of 5 m/s (calibration marks, 2 m/s). Also on the left of the image can be seen mitral inflow, which is the doubly peaked diastolic positive tracing (*curved closed arrow*) with a V max of almost 2 m/s. This patient does not have mitral stenosis. The deceleration curve of the mitral flow after V max falls rapidly in a normal fashion. The higher flow velocity than normal is secondary to elevated flow volume because of the severe mitral regurgitant lesion. On the right of the image, the sharp systolic positive flow tracing (*curved open arrow*) with a V max of 3.8 m/s is the jet of aortic regurgitation.

the mitral valve area is estimated by dividing 220 by 254 to yield a value of 0.9 cm^2.

Abnormal Doppler Flow Patterns

Aortic Valve Pathology

Aortic Stenosis

The disappointment of the inability of two-dimensional imaging to assess the severity of aortic stenosis has been replaced by the acceptance of continuous-wave Doppler ultrasound's ability to quantitate the severity of this disease. Stenosis of the semilunar valves results in an increase in the velocity of blood flow across the valve (9). Using the modified Bernoulli equation, the accuracy of continuous-wave Doppler in the quantitation of transvalvular gradients has been demonstrated (10,11). Again, it must be noted that multiple sampling sites must be used to evaluate the stenotic jet through a deformed valve to record the highest velocity. Generally, in evaluating patients with aortic stenosis, the valve should be looked at from the apical, right parasternal, and suprasternal notch approaches. The highest velocity obtained from any of these areas would be used in the Bernoulli equation to determine the pressure gradient across the valve. Although the presence of aortic stenosis is shown with two-

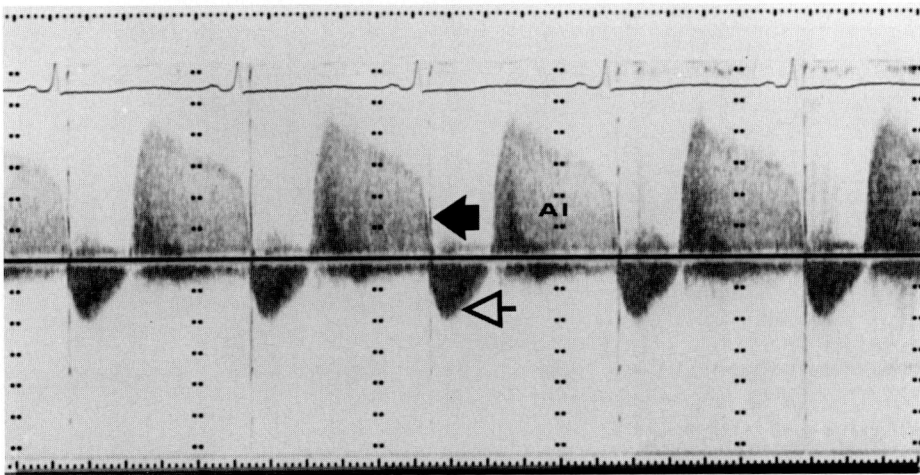

Fig. 3.23. Aortic insufficiency with continuous-wave Doppler. In this tracing obtained from an apical approach, diastolic positive flow (*closed arrow*) toward the transducer shows aortic insufficiency with a V max of 4.5 m/s. There is also elevated flow through the aortic valve of 2 m/s seen as a negative systolic deflection (*open arrow*). The elevated aortic flow here is secondary to the increased flow because of the severely regurgitant aortic valve (calibration marks, 1 m/s).

dimensional image-guided pulsed-Doppler, continuous-wave Doppler must be used to record the true maximum velocity. The direction of the Doppler frequency shift that is recorded in patients with aortic stenosis will be seen either in a positive (forward toward the transducer) or in a negative fashion (backward away from the transducer), depending on which window is used to interrogate the blood flow velocity across the valve. Thus, the high-velocity jet of aortic stenosis will be negative to the zero line on the Doppler recording obtained apically, and positive to the zero line from the right parasternal and suprasternal approaches (Fig. 3.21). Care must be used when performing CW Doppler not to confuse a jet of mitral regurgitation with one of aortic stenosis, especially from the apical position (Fig. 3.22). Careful beam positioning must be stressed and focused on to resolve the various abnormal flow patterns encountered in multivalvular disease when using a dedicated CW probe (12).

In the evaluation of aortic stenosis, the spatial localization and direction of the high-velocity jet is nicely demonstrated with color flow mapping.

Aortic Insufficiency

In the evaluation of patients with aortic insufficiency, Doppler examination appears to be a sensitive technique. Regurgitation results in detectable retrograde signals when the suspect valve is closed. In the Doppler tracings from aortic insufficiency, there are two important features. First, diastolic flow reversal is seen, either in the left ventricular outflow tract or in the ascending aorta, of a velocity greater than 2 m/s. Secondly, increased systolic forward aortic flow velocities, beginning in the left ventricular outflow tract in the range of 1.5 to 2.5 m/s are seen (2, pp 29–58). Again, these flows will be positive or negative depending on the window from which they were obtained. Nevertheless, the diastolic regurgitant flow is reversed from the normal systolic antegrade flow (Fig. 3.23).

In regurgitant lesions, flow mapping with either pulsed-Doppler or color Doppler are useful. One of the greatest advantages of color flow mapping is its ability to plot the direction of regurgitant lesions (Fig. 3.24).

The diagnosis of aortic insufficiency is best made using pulsed-Doppler recordings (13). A thorough sampling of multiple various sites in the recipient chamber is performed to determine the maximum velocity and direction of the regurgitant jet. In cases of aortic insufficiency, the left ventricle is mapped to determine the extent of the lesion. Beginning at the level of the aortic valve plane, if a regurgitant diastolic jet is seen up to 2 cm into the left ventricle

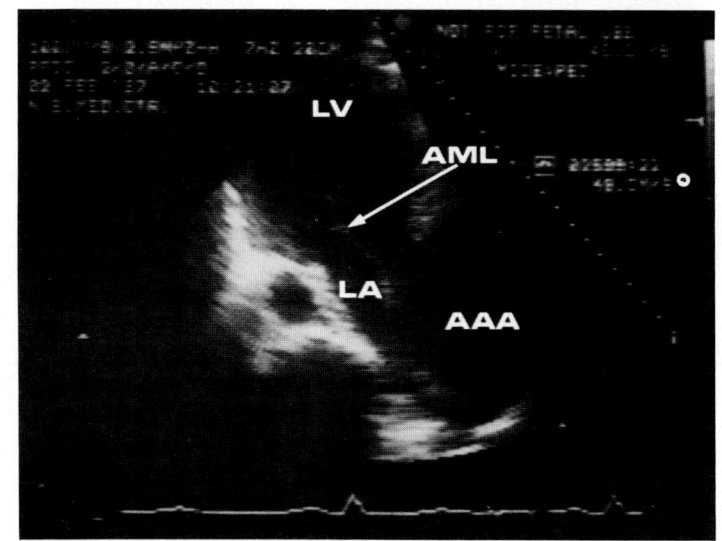

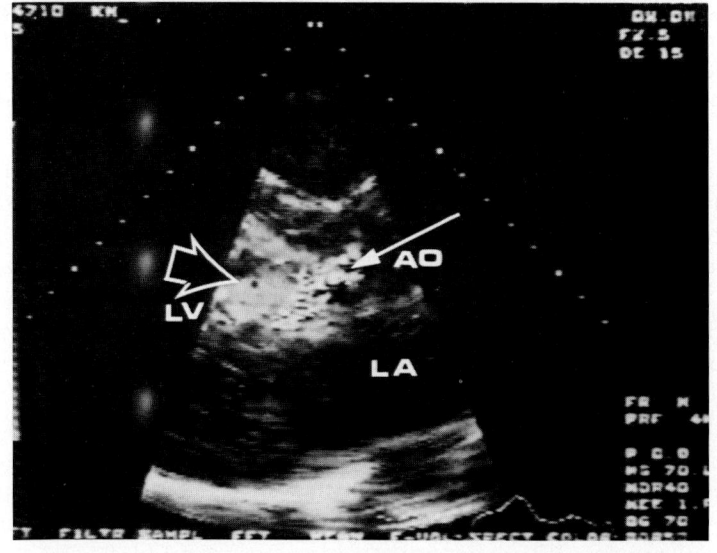

Fig. 3.24.

below the aortic valve, then the lesion is considered mild. A regurgitant jet that extends beyond 2 cm and continuing up to the level of the papillary muscle level is considered moderate. Severe aortic insufficiency exists when the diastolic reversed jet reaches a level beyond that of the papillary muscle (Fig. 3.25) (2, pp 29–58).

There have been attempts made to evaluate regurgitant lesions by assessing the forward flow distal to the valve in question. In the absence of stenosis, increased forward flow is further evidence of the hemodynamic significance of the incompetent valve. Studies have been done that quantify forward and regurgitant flow with Doppler ultrasound in an attempt to estimate the regurgitant fraction (14).

It is important to be aware of other conditions, in addition to aortic insufficiency, that can cause reversal of flow in the aorta. These are patent ductus arteriosus and aorticopulmonary or aorticosubclavian shunts (1, p 107).

Mitral Valve Pathology

Mitral Stenosis

In the presence of mitral stenosis, a pressure gradient between the left atrium and left ventrical develops, which is related both to the flow across the valve and to the size of the valve opening. In the evaluation of mitral stenosis, Doppler ultrasound obtains information about the severity of the disease by estimating the valvular orifice size, through the pressure half-time formula, and by calculating the transmitral pressure gradient, from the Bernoulli equation using the maximum velocities obtained. In a normal mitral valve, the Doppler tracing shows a maximum flow velocity of approximately 1 m/s; the deceleration of the flow velocity profile, after the period of early diastolic filling, is rapid. By contrast, patients with mitral stenosis exhibit opening maximum mitral flow velocities greater than 1 m/s along with a much slower rate of deceleration in the flow velocity profile after early diastolic filling (2, pp 59–76).

Doppler recordings in mitral stenosis are best made from an apical approach where the highest velocity of the mitral flow can be measured by continuous-wave Doppler (Fig. 3.26). Coincident mitral regurgitation is also searched for from this area (Fig. 3.27). Once satisfactory Doppler tracings are obtained, the pressure gradient across the valve and the valve orifice size are calculated from the Bernoulli and pressure half-time equations, respectively.

Finally, when applicable, color flow mapping spatially can show the stenotic jet through the mitral valve. This is helpful in the documentation of a single stenotic lesion with or without a coexisting regurgitant abnormality (Fig. 3.28).

Again, it should be reiterated that care must be taken to position the ultrasound beam parallel to the pathway of the blood flow through the stenotic valve, to measure the true maximum velocity of flow with continuous-wave Doppler. With the normal maximum mitral flow velocity at approximately 1 m/s, patients with mitral stenosis exhibit transmitral flow velocities greater than 2 m/s. The mitral flow velocity profile then decelerates slowly, and with the increase after atrial contraction, it usually has a velocity still greater than 1 m/s at the end of diastole. With an

---

Fig. 3.24A–C. Aortic insufficiency. **A.** Black and white apical long axis view of a dilated left ventricle and massively dilated ascending aorta. This patient, with an aneurysm of the ascending aorta, had severe aortic insufficiency (LV, left ventricle; AML, anterior mitral leaflet; LA, left atrium; AAA, ascending aortic aneurysm). **B.** Color Doppler image in diastole. Normal mitral inflow is seen in the left atrium extending into the posterior portion of the left ventricle, and is displayed in red to yellow-orange shades (*closed arrow*) corresponding to the positive forward motion of blood. The coincident jet of severe aortic regurgitation is displayed in the anterior portion of the left ventricle adjacent to the septum. It is displayed in a mosaic of blue-green, yellow, orange, and white (*open arrow*), representing turbulent high-velocity aliased flow, and not downward negative flow. **C.** Mild aortic insufficiency. This illustration is from a different patient with a small jet of aortic insufficiency. In this long axis parasternal view, the sector angle has been narrowed to increase the line density and image quality. The regurgitant aortic jet in diastole is shown as an area of blue and blue-green (*open arrow*) in the subaortic region of the left ventricle. A small discrete high-velocity jet is shown as a bright mosaic of color (*long thin arrow*), indicating aliased high flow originating from the center of the closed aortic valve leaflets (AO, ascending aorta; LA, left atrium; LV, left ventricle). For a color reproduction of this figure see frontmatter.

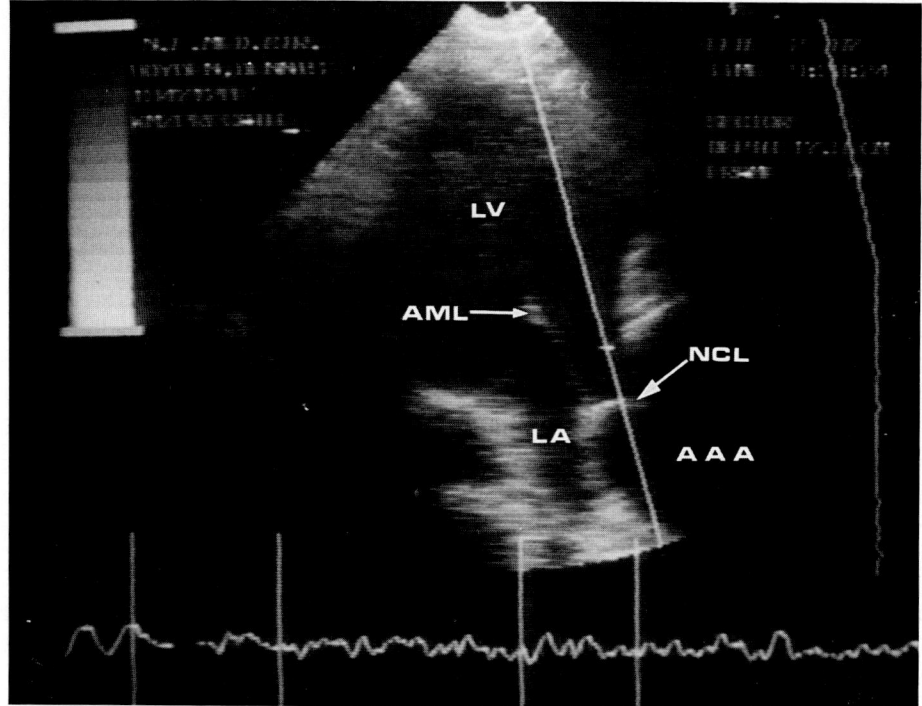

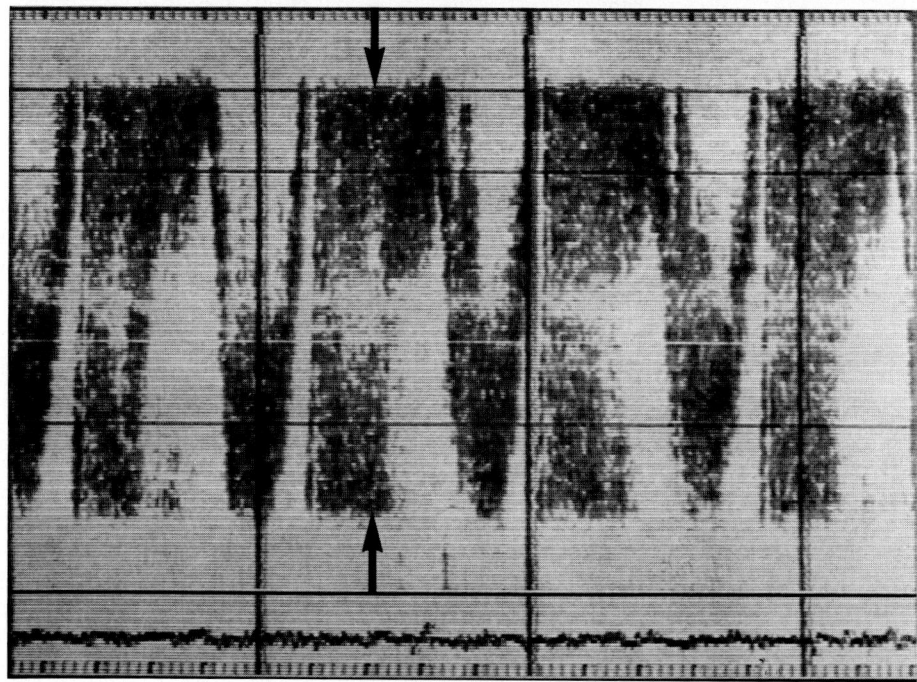

Fig. 3.25A–D. Mapping the degree of aortic insufficiency with pulsed-Doppler. **A.** Two-dimensional apical long axis view of the left ventricular outflow tract, with the Doppler cursor positioned just below the aortic valve, in a patient with a huge aneurysm of the ascending thoracic aorta (LA, left atrium; AAA, ascending aortic aneurysm; NCL, noncoronary leaflet of aortic valve; AML, anterior leaflet mitral valve; LV, left ventricle). **B.** Pulsed-Doppler tracing obtained at the site shown in part **A.** Severe aliasing of diastolic flow (*straight arrows*) represents the high-velocity jet of aortic insufficiency (calibration marks, 20 cm/s). **C.** Two-dimensional apical view with the Doppler sample volume just beyond the level of the papillary muscles (*long thin arrow*). **D.** Pulsed-Doppler tracing obtained at the site shown in part **C** shows continual, but less, aliased diastolic flow (*curved arrows*) indicative of severe aortic insufficiency extending beyond the level of the papillary muscles.

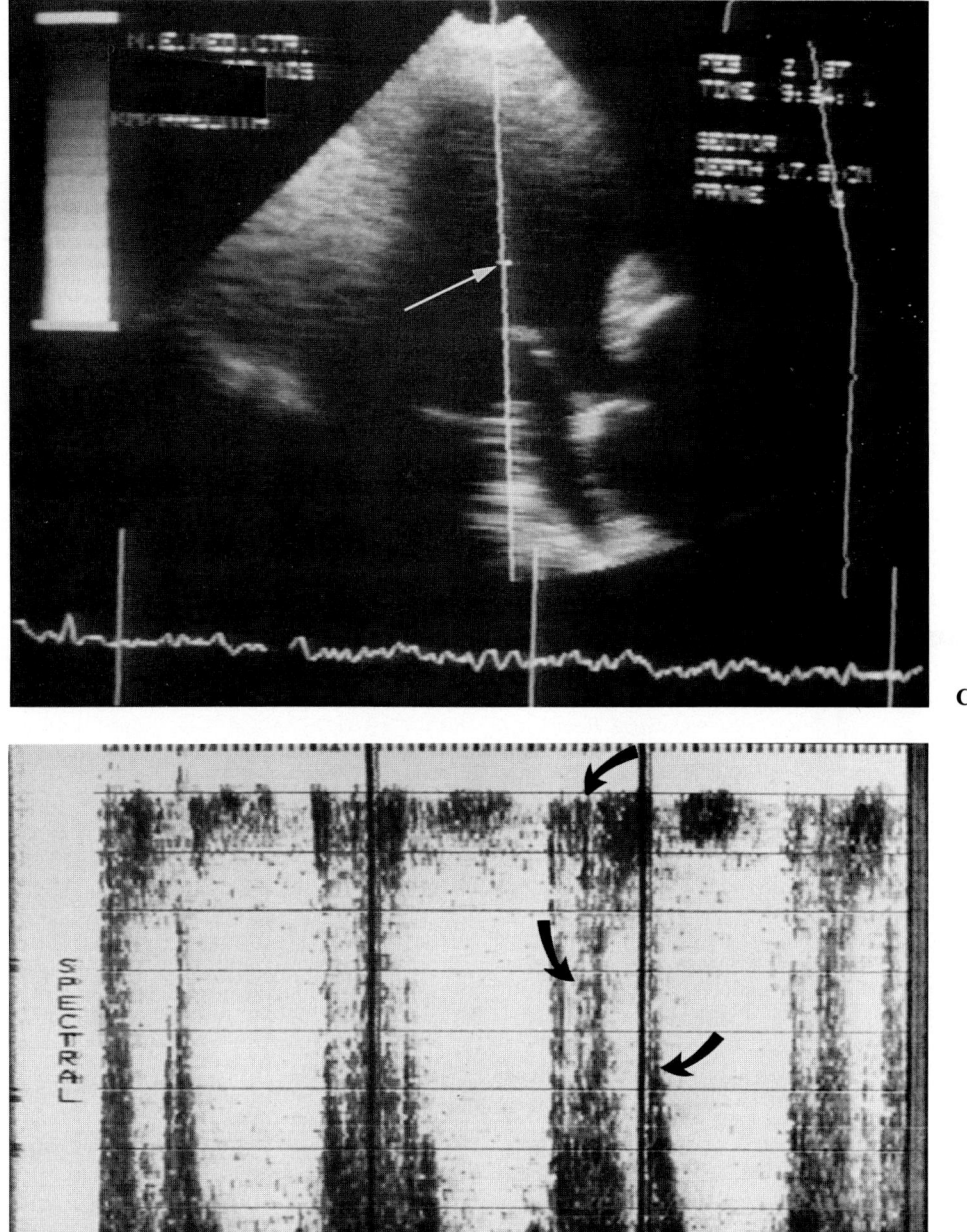

Fig. 3.25.

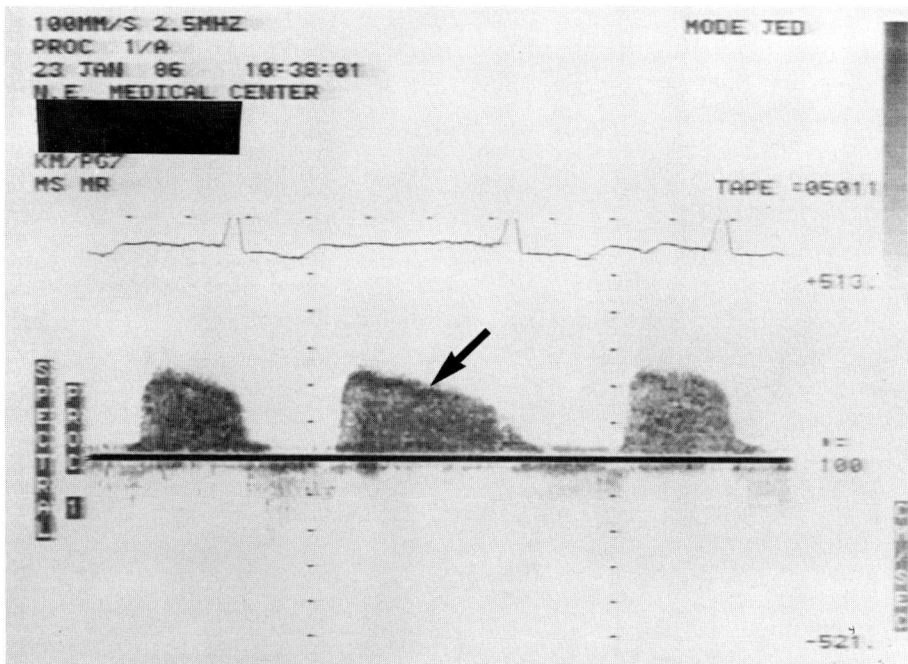

Fig. 3.26. Mitral stenosis with continuous-wave Doppler. This tracing shows increased mitral flow with a V max of 2.5 m/s (calibration marks, 1 m/s). The pressure half-time in this patient is obviously prolonged with the long, slow, almost horizontal deceleration curve of mitral flow (*arrow*), and no visualization of a second peak corresponding to the atrial contraction.

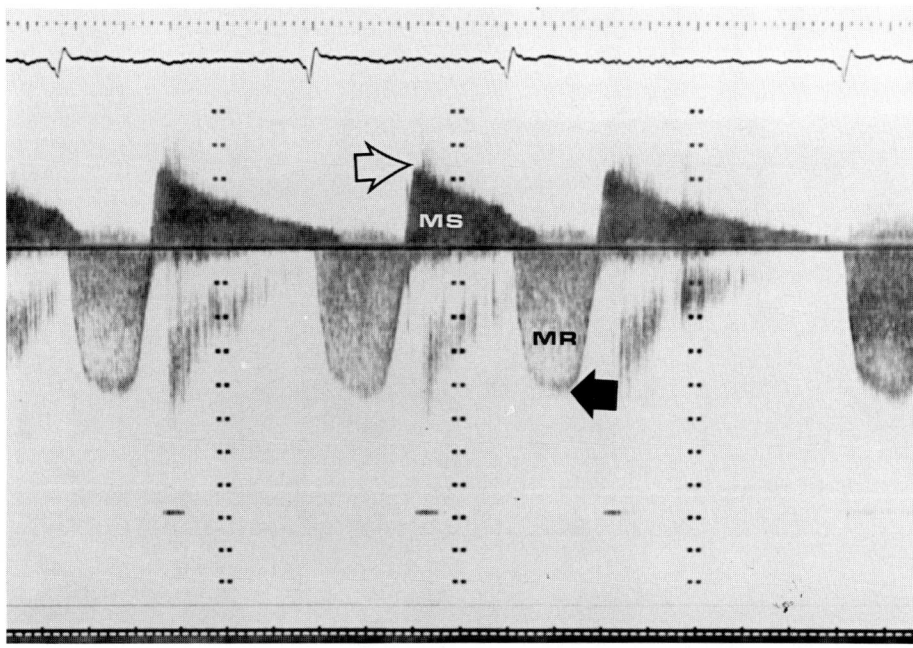

Fig. 3.27. Both mitral stenosis and mitral insufficiency with continuous-wave Doppler. Here, the negative systolic flow of mitral insufficiency with a V max of 4.5 m/s is seen (*closed arrow*) in a patient who also has mitral stenosis. The jet of mitral stenosis (*open arrow*) shows elevated flow velocity of 2.6 m/s and a prolonged half-time as evidenced by the slow deceleration curve.

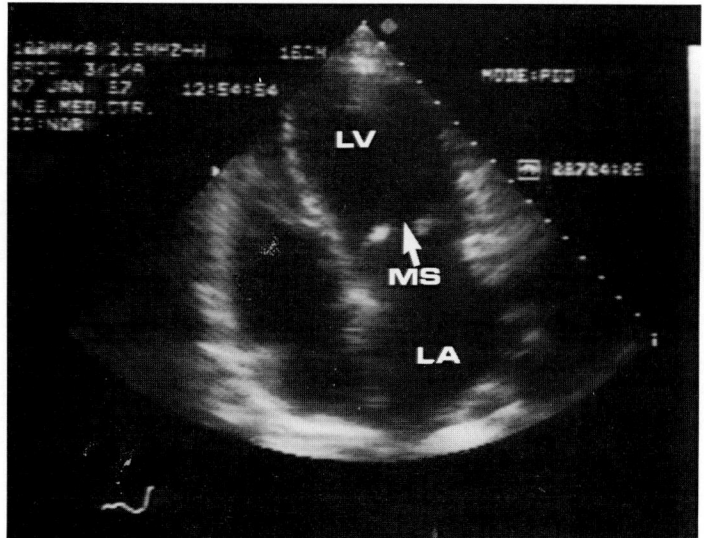

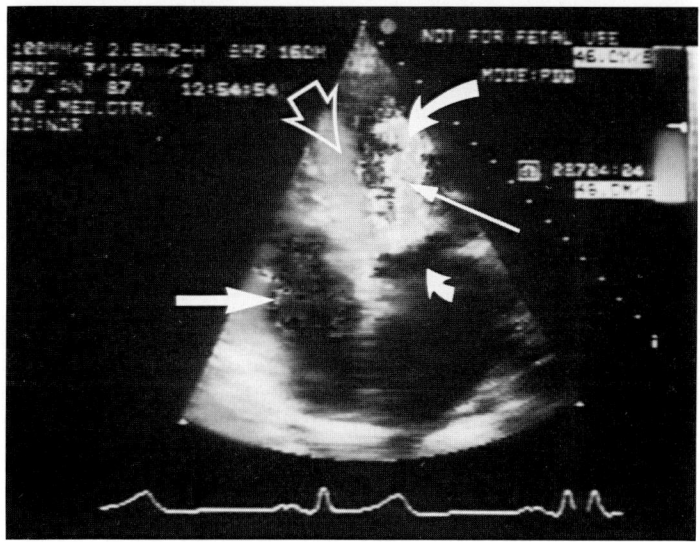

Fig. 3.28A,B. Mitral stenosis. **A.** Black and white apical four-chamber view in a patient with mitral stenosis. Both the left atrium and left ventricle are enlarged, and the mitral valve leaflets are thickened with restricted motion (LA, left atrium; LV, left ventricle; MS, stenotic mitral orifice). **B.** Color Doppler image of mitral stenosis in diastole. Normal forward right atrial flow is shown in red and orange (*straight closed arrow*). The normal downward diastolic vortex adjacent to the septum is seen in shades of deep blue to a slightly lighter blue (*straight open arrow*). The high-velocity jet of mitral stenosis is seen in the lateral aspect of the left ventricle, extending from the mitral orifice close to the apex (*long curved closed arrow*). It is displayed in a variety of colors but is clearly distinct from the normal negative vortex against the septum. Here, the bulk of the stenotic jet is displayed in bright orange to bright yellow. The central portion of the jet shows the fastest velocities, and is displayed in a bright mosaic of yellow-blue-green shades (*long, thin arrow*), representing very high velocity aliased flow, bordered by white, representing the highest flow properly recorded in this pulsed-Doppler system. Note the slowdown and backup of blood on the atrial side of the mitral valve as blood piles up here before it is squeezed through the narrowed opening (*short closed curved arrow*). Also note both the similarity and the difference of the appearance of the normal downward vortex adjacent to the septum and the aliased abnormal high-velocity jet of mitral stenosis going in the opposite direction. Both patterns are displayed with much blue. The normal blue flow is more homogeneously deep blue to blue-green. The abnormal aliased blue flow is brighter, yellower, and less homogeneous. For a color reproduction of this figure see frontmatter.

increased heart rate, the atrial contraction may occur so early in diastole that the second peak of the mitral flow profile may no longer be seen, and the decline in velocity in early diastole no longer exists (1, p 78).

Mitral Insufficiency

As was done in the left ventricle in the presence of aortic insufficiency, multiple sites in the left atrium are mapped with pulsed-Doppler to evaluate the regurgitant jet flowing in a retrograde fashion through the mitral valve in systole when the mitral leaflets are closed. The severity and direction of the mitral insufficiency is then assessed. Mitral insufficiency is defined by Doppler ultrasound as systolic velocities of 2 m/s or more across the mitral valve from the left ventricle into the left atrium (2, pp 59–76). Sampling different areas of the left atrium, which is the recipient chamber in mitral regurgitation, and noting the areas of disturbed flow allow an estimate of the size of the flow disturbance area. Once the high-velocity jet has been found, it should be tracked back into the left atrium. Beginning at the level of the plane of the valve, the sample volume is moved further backward in the left atrium until a systolic flow abnormality is no longer evident.

Mitral regurgitation is graded as mild, moderate, or severe. Mild mitral insufficiency exists only at or just below the valve plane. Moderate insufficiency exists when the regurgitant jet reaches the midatrial level, and severe regurgitation is present when the flow abnormality is seen in the distal portions of the left atrium (Fig. 3.29) (2, pp 59–76; 15).

Again, multiple sites are used to interrogate the regurgitant jet, as these jets can occur in any direction with respect to the valve. Parasternal long and short axis, as well as apical and subcostal views, should be used. Often, with patients with mitral regurgitation, there is accompanying cardiac enlargement both in the ventricles and atria. Sometimes, the heart may be too big to map the left atrium with pulsed-Doppler from an apical approach, and in these cases mapping of abnormal flow is usually best accomplished from a left parasternal approach (1, p 117). Continuous-wave Doppler can obtain the true maximum flow velocity from the apex.

Again, here is an excellent application for color flow mapping to picture the spatial disturbances of the blood flow from the regurgitant mitral valve (Fig. 3.30).

Also, after a regurgitant lesion is detected with pulsed-Doppler, it should be evaluated with continuous-wave Doppler to record the true direction and highest velocity of abnormal flow. This is usually best done from an apical approach (Fig. 3.31).

Pulmonic Valve Pathology

Pulmonic Stenosis

With the transducer in the second or third left intercostal space in a transverse plane, slight medial and cephalad angulation will usually interrogate the pulmonic valve jets in patients with pulmonic stenosis. Also a subcostal approach often is useful in this lesion. Usually, continuous-wave Doppler will record the highest velocity in the jet, and pulsed Doppler will be used to localize the site of the lesion (Fig. 3.32).

Increased flow velocities also are seen in the pulmonary artery in patients with increased right-sided flow as in significant left-to-right shunts and with significant pulmonary regurgitation. In these cases, flow velocity is increased on both sides of the pulmonic valve: both in the right ventricle and in the pulmonary artery. In pulmonic stenosis, on the other hand, the flow velocity increases only distal to the valve. The velocity of blood in the right ventricle is normal with simple pulmonic stenosis (1, p 98).

Pulmonic stenosis is rare outside the pediatric age group. It can be either valvular or infundibular, as in tetralogy of Fallot; the proper site of the obstruction can be accurately localized with pulsed-Doppler. As with the aortic and mitral valves, the pressure gradient across whatever lesion (valvular or infundibular pulmonic stenosis), which causes right ventricular outflow obstruction, can be measured by using the Bernoulli equation.

In the above example of the CW Doppler tracing in the patient with pulmonic stenosis shown in Figure 3.32C, the maximum velocity recorded was 4 m/s. Using the Bernoulli equation:

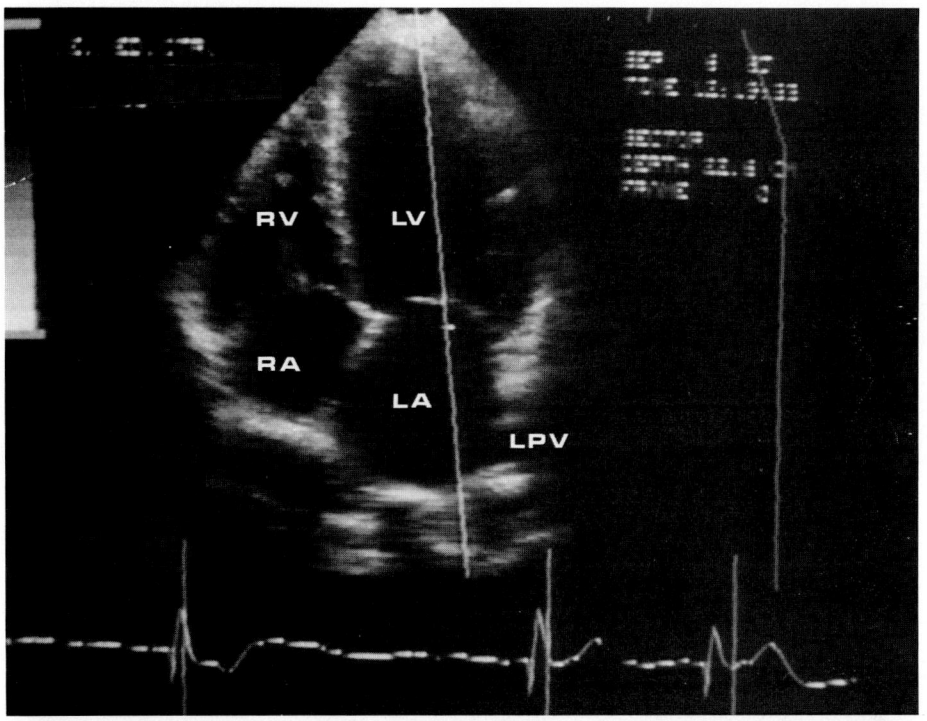

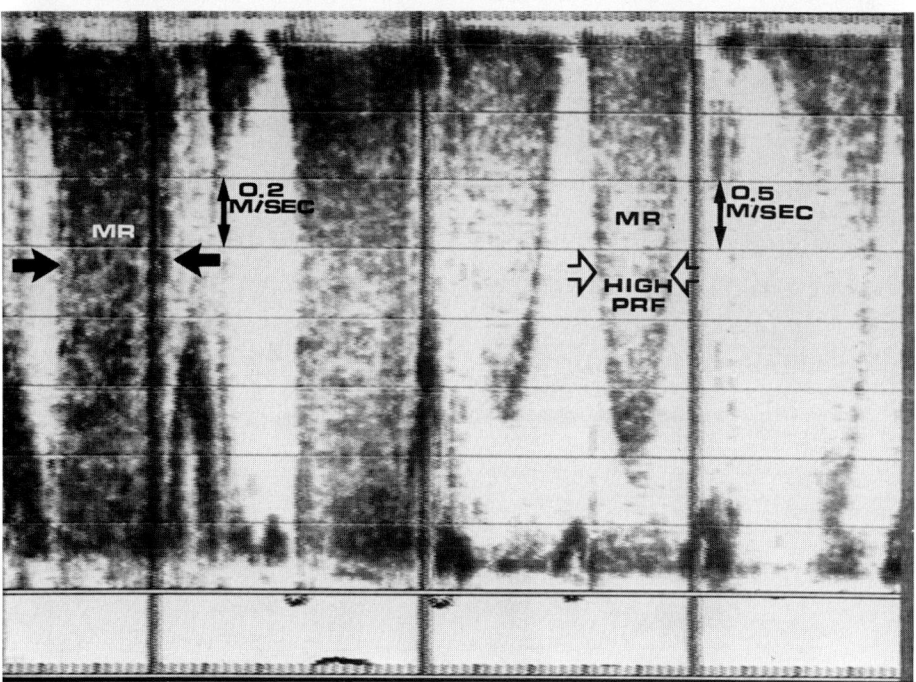

Fig. 3.29A–F. Mapping severe mitral insufficiency with pulsed-Doppler. The patient does not have mitral stenosis. **A.** Apical four-chamber view with sample volume placed just inside the atrial aspect of the mitral valve. The right-sided chambers are normally sized. The left-sided chambers are significantly enlarged (RV, right ventricle; RA, right atrium; LV, left ventricle; LA, left atrium; LPV, left pulmonary vein). **B.** Pulsed-Doppler tracing taken at the site shown in part **A** showing aliased flow in systole from the severe mitral insufficiency (*closed broad arrow*) on the left side of the image. On the left side of the image, the calibration marks in the normal pulsed-Doppler mode are in increment of 20 cm/s. While the tracing was being recorded, the pulsed-Doppler was changed to the high PRF mode, which is seen in the right of the image as the sharp negative systolic deflections without aliasing (*open broad arrow*). Now that the equipment is in the high PRF mode, the calibration scale has changed to increments of 50 cm/s. The aliased flow seen on the left is barely able to be measured by pulsed-Doppler at this depth when switched to high PRF. The V max of the regurgitant mitral jet is 4 m/s. *(Continued.)*

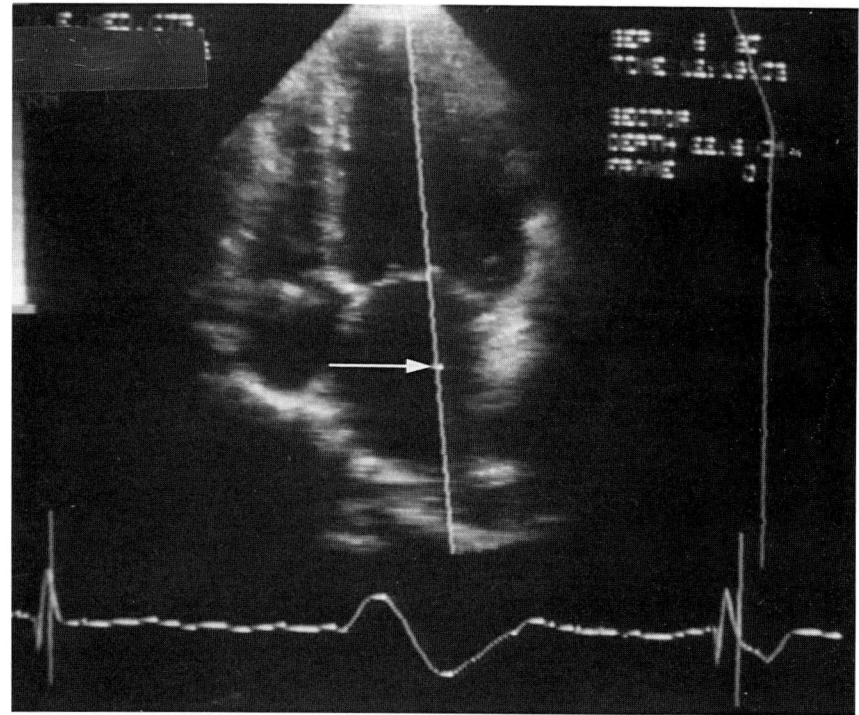

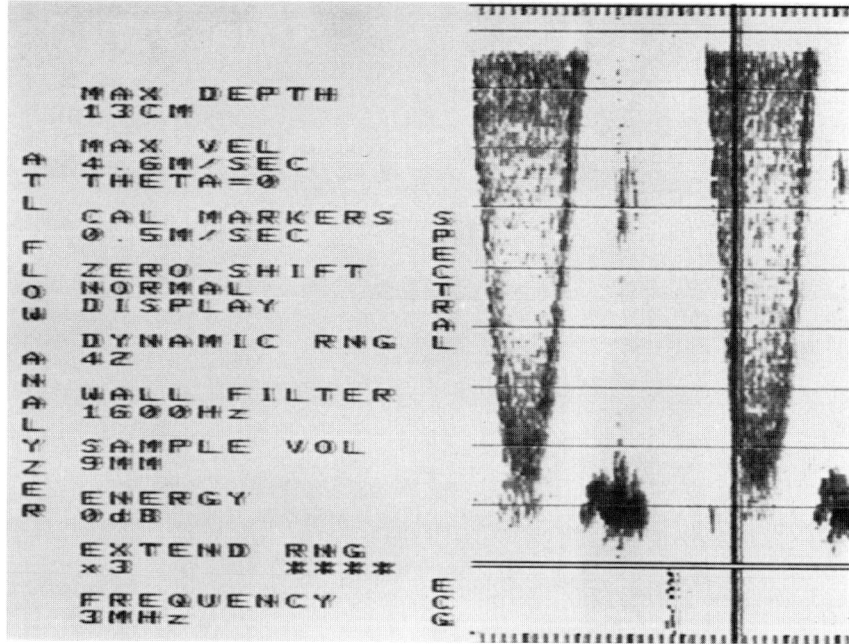

Fig. 3.29C. Apical four-chamber image with the sample volume placed in the middle of the left atrium (*long thin arrow*). **D.** Pulsed-Doppler tracing in high PRF mode (calibration marks, 50 cm/s) measuring a V max of 4 m/s at the mid-atrial level shown in part **C. E.** Apical four-chamber image with the Doppler cursor placed near the back of the very enlarged left atrium (*long thin arrow*). **F.** Pulsed-Doppler tracing in regular mode (calibration marks, 20 cm/s) showing a persistent regurgitant jet of 0.8 m/s at the back of the left atrium at the level shown in part **E**. This represents severe mitral insufficiency.

3. Cardiac Doppler

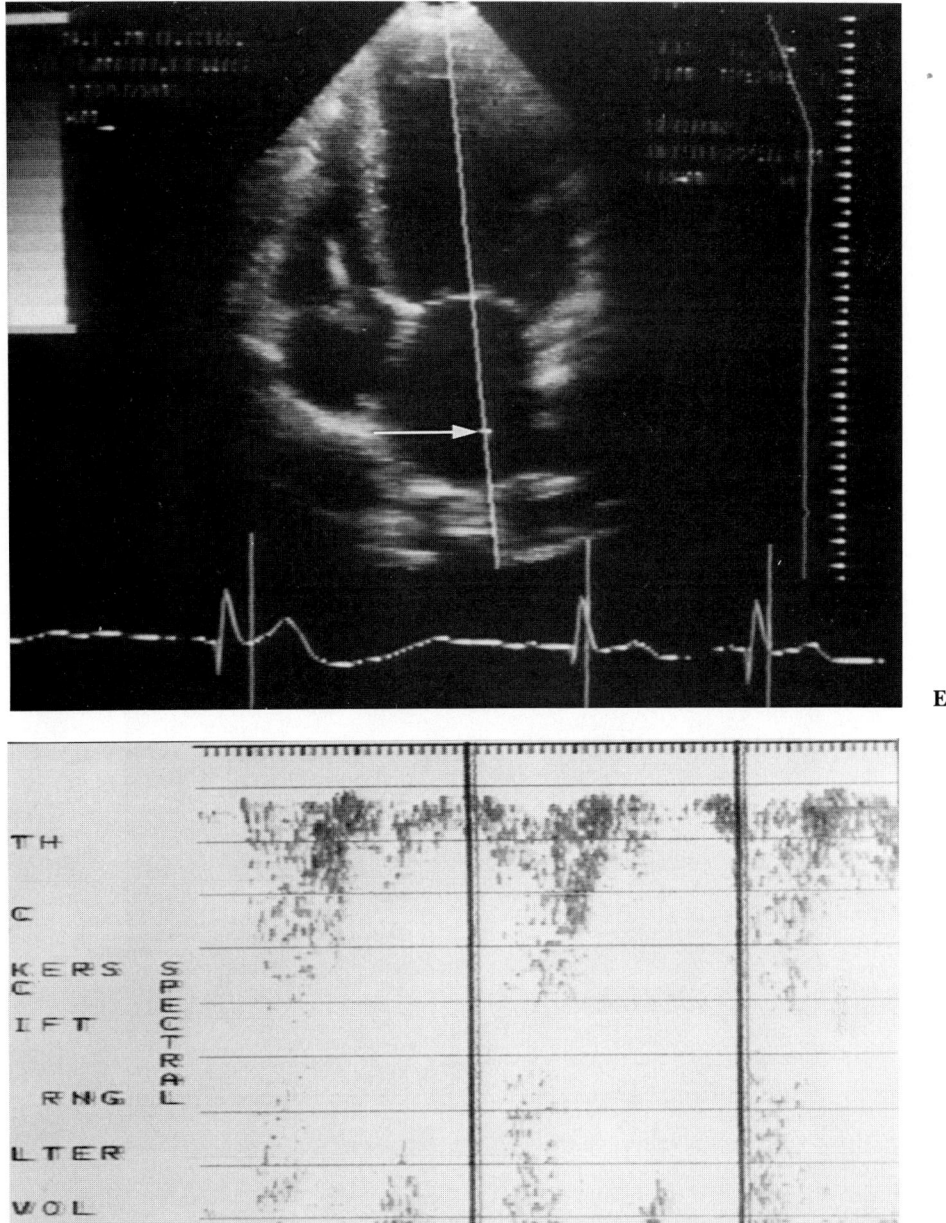

Fig. 3.29.

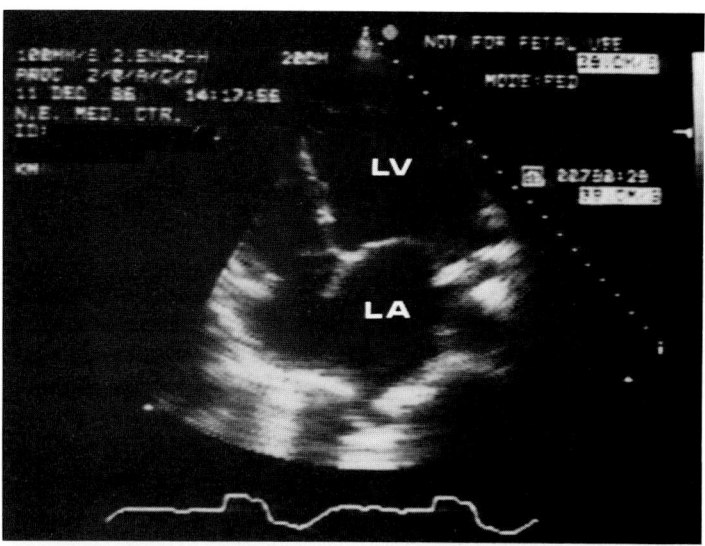

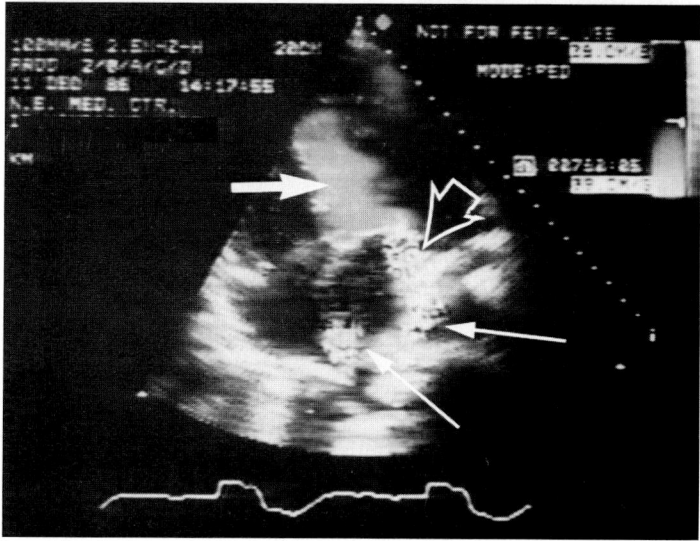

Fig. 3.30A–D. Mitral regurgitation. **A.** Black and white apical four-chamber view of a patient with mitral regurgitation. An enlarged left atrium and left ventricle are seen here (LA, left atrium; LV, left ventricle). The right-sided chambers are normally sized. The mitral valve leaflets appear normal. **B.** Color-Doppler image in systole. Normal downward negative left ventricular outflow is seen extending along the left side of the ventricular septum up to the immediate subaortic area (*closed straight arrow*). This is displayed as deep blue with some normal acceleration of flow shown by the lighter blue-green closer to the aortic valve and septum. The abnormal high-velocity regurgitant jet (*open straight arrow*) into the left atrium, through the closed mitral leaflets in systole, is shown as a bright mosaic of blue, green, yellow, and white traveling along the lateral aspect of the left atrium all the way to its posterior aspects. When the jet reaches the back wall of the left atrium, it appears first to turn medially and then it turns forward along the atrial septum (*long thin arrow*) going toward the mitral valve. It changes from aliased blue-green to yellow, and then to red as it finally slows down in the left atrium close to the mitral valve. **C.** Another color Doppler image in systole, showing how easily color flow mapping can be used to guide the placement of the Doppler cursor if one wants to do a tracing of the flow velocity profile. In this example, the Doppler cursor is directed exactly through the center of the jet of mitral insufficiency (*short broad closed arrow*), which extends to the back wall of the left atrium. **D.** Continuous-wave Doppler tracing obtained along the path shown in part **C**. Severe mitral insufficiency with a V max of 4.3 m/s is measured (calibration marks, 1 m/s). For a color reproduction of this figure see frontmatter.

3. Cardiac Doppler

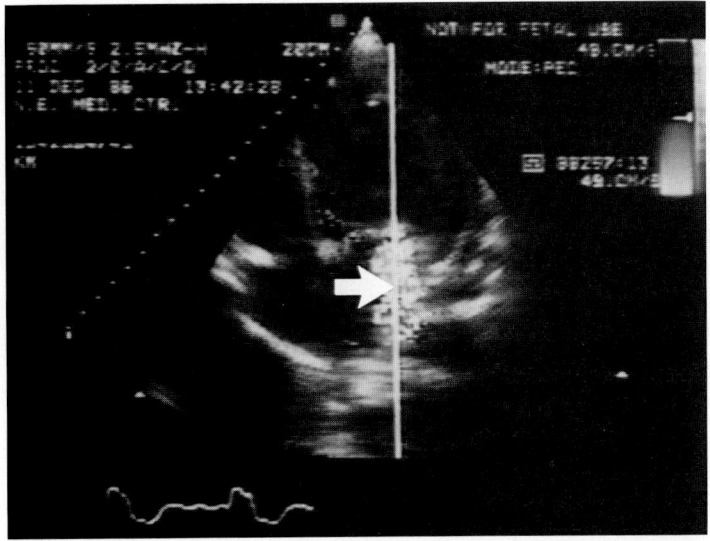

c

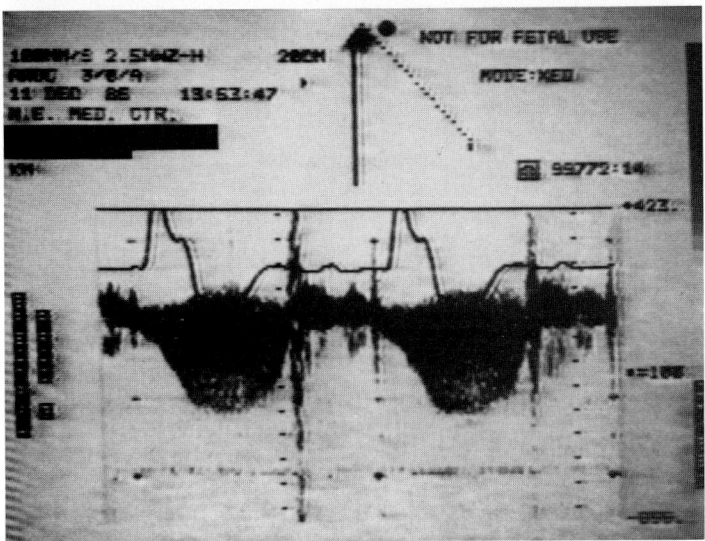

D

Fig. 3.30.

PG = 4 (V max)² and with (V max) = 4 m/s;

PG = 64 mmHg

Thus, the estimated pressure gradient across this stenotic pulmonic valve is calculated from the CW Doppler measurement as 64 mmHg.

Evaluating the disturbance to the blood flow in right ventricular outflow tract obstruction is another fine use for color flow mapping.

Pulmonic Insufficiency

In a fashion similar to what was described with aortic valvular insufficiency, the regurgitant jet received by the right ventricle in diastole is mapped at various sites below the pulmonic valve to assess the severity of the pulmonic insufficiency (Fig. 3.33).

The diastolic pressure drop across the regurgitant pulmonic valve, from the pulmonary artery to the right ventricle, can be calculated with the Bernoulli equation, using the maximal velocity of the regurgitant diastolic jet. Generally, the greater this velocity, the higher will be the pulmonary artery diastolic pressures.

With significant pulmonic insufficiency, there will be a moderate increase in systolic flow velocity both in the right ventricle and in the

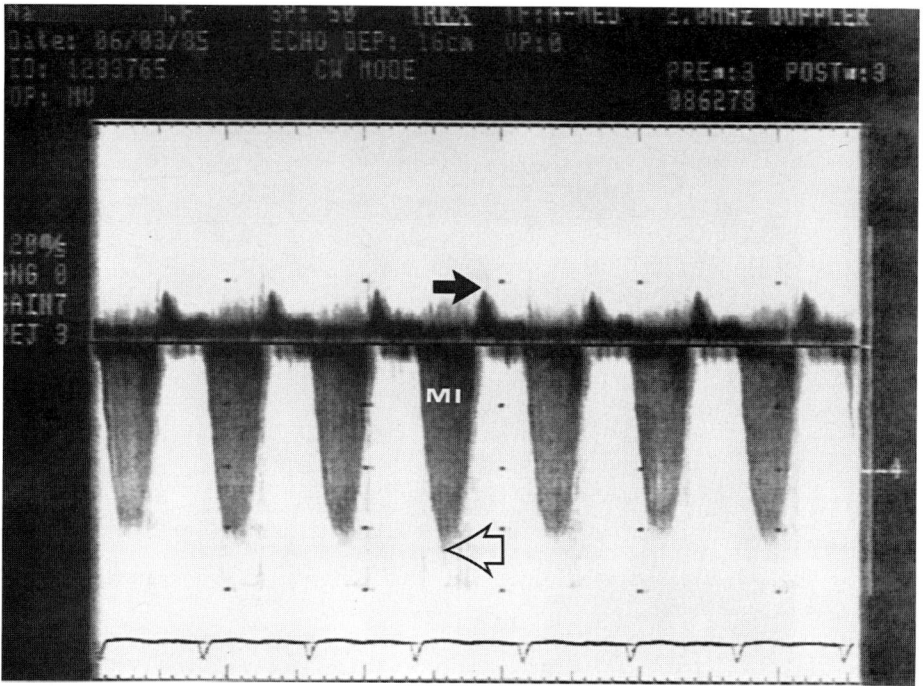

Fig. 3.31. Mitral insufficiency with continuous-wave Doppler. From an apical approach, this high-velocity jet of mitral insufficiency (*open arrow*) is easily recorded as a negative systolic deflection with a V max of 5.2 m/s (calibration marks, 2 m/s). This patient does not have mitral stenosis. Slightly elevated mitral inflow with a V max of 1.9 m/s, secondary to the increased flow from the severe mitral regurgitation, is seen as a positive diastolic flow curve (*closed arrow*). Note that the mitral inflow deceleration is rapid.

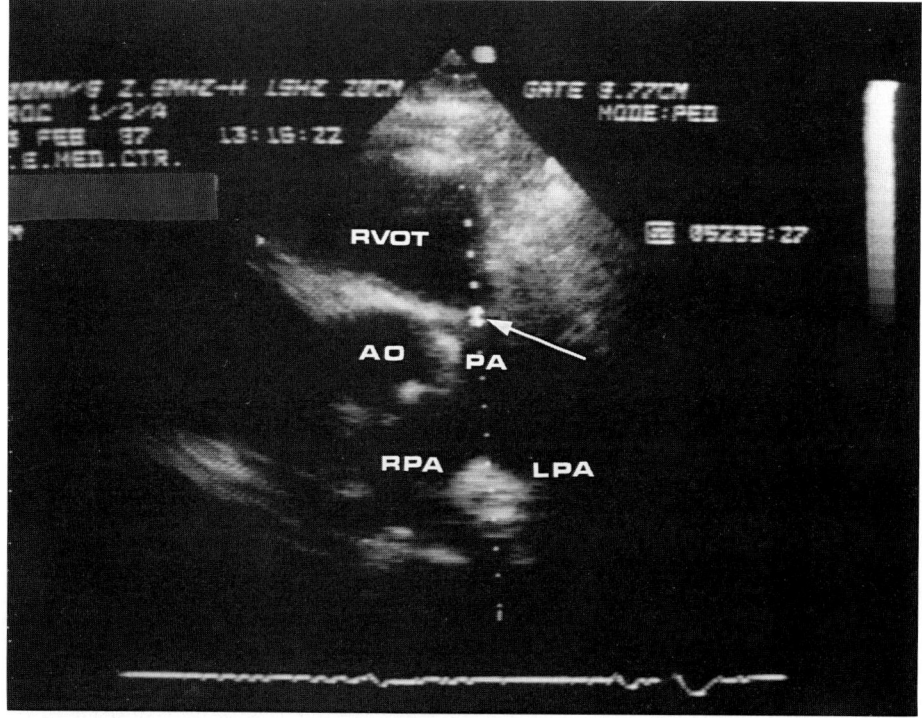

Fig. 3.32.

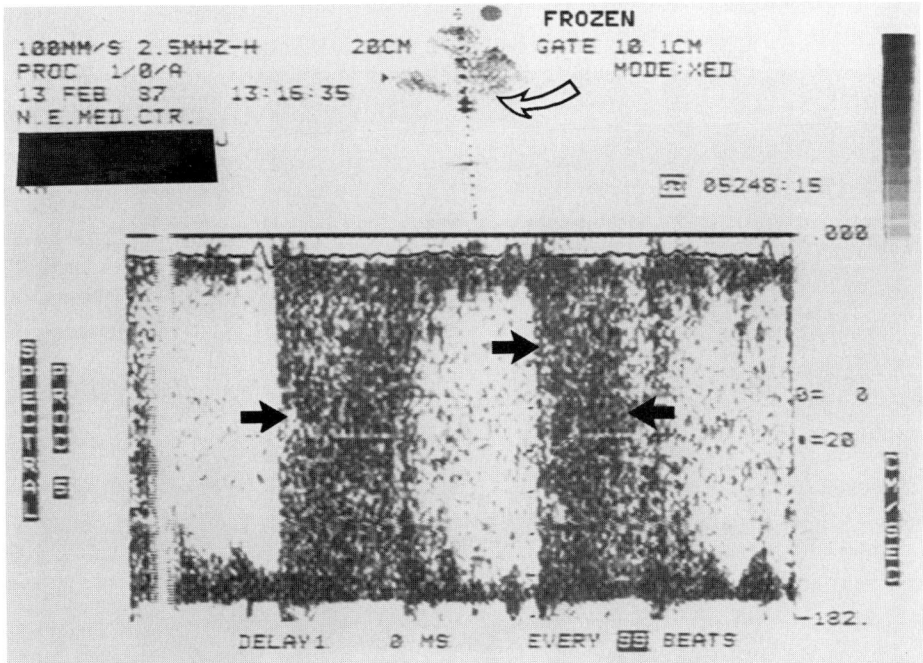

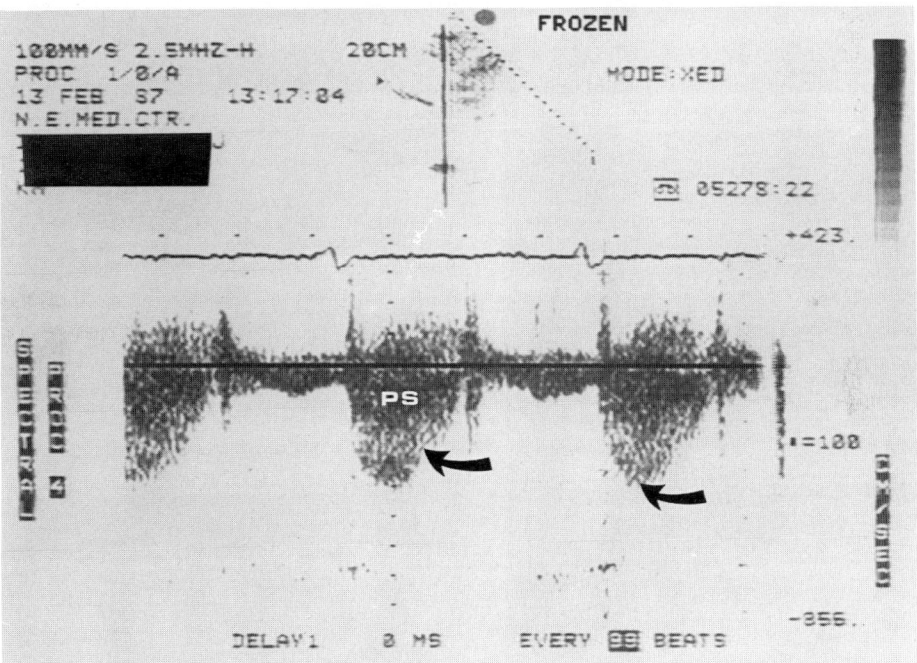

Fig. 3.32A–C. Pulmonic stenosis. **A.** Short axis two-dimensional image of the pulmonary artery region in a patient with pulmonic stenosis. The Doppler sample volume is placed in the main pulmonary artery, just beyond the thickened and domed pulmonic valve (RVOT, right ventricular outflow tract; PA, main pulmonary artery; RPA, right pulmonary artery; LPA, left pulmonary artery; AO, aortic outflow area). **B.** Pulsed-Doppler tracing obtained at the site shown in part **A**. High-velocity flow in systole is seen as severely aliased flow (*solid arrows*). The two-dimensional image is poorly seen at the top of the illustration (*open curved arrow*). This is often the case with simultaneous imaging while performing a pulsed-Doppler examination, where the settings on the equipment may be changed to optimize Doppler information and there may be a simultaneous and resultant loss of the quality of the displayed and minified two-dimensional image. However, two-dimensional imaging is being used for guidance of Doppler only at this point, and a good operator will focus on the sound and the quality of the waveform of the Doppler signal. Meticulous high-resolution two-dimensional imaging already has been done before the Doppler examination. **C.** Continuous-wave Doppler tracing of the pulmonic flow in the same patient showing a strong negative systolic flow pattern (*closed curved arrows*) with a V max of 4 m/s. Using the modified Bernoulli equation, the pressure gradient across this severely stenotic valve is 64 mm Hg.

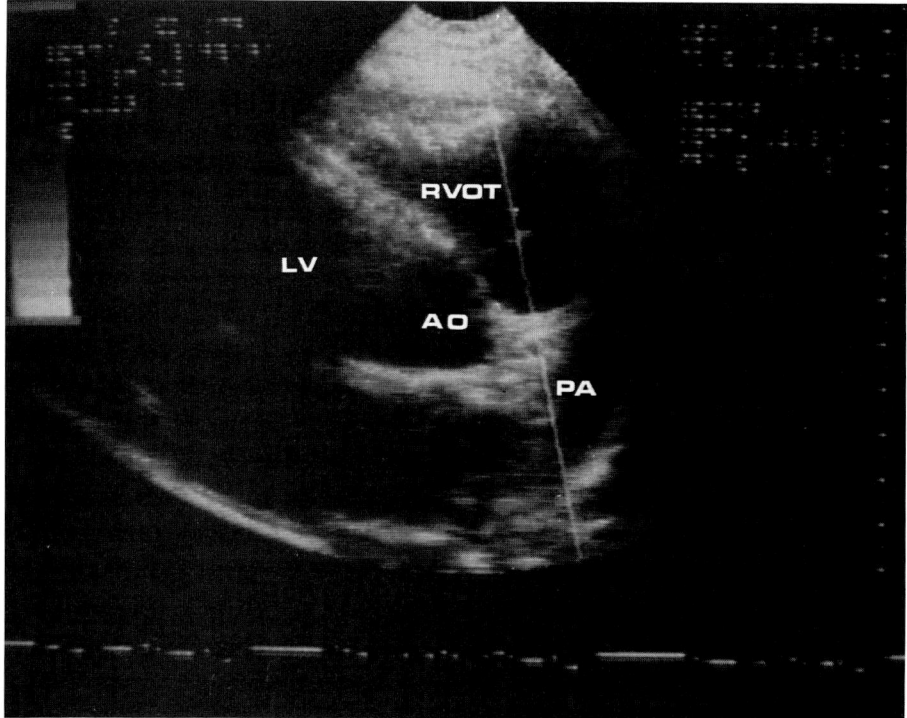

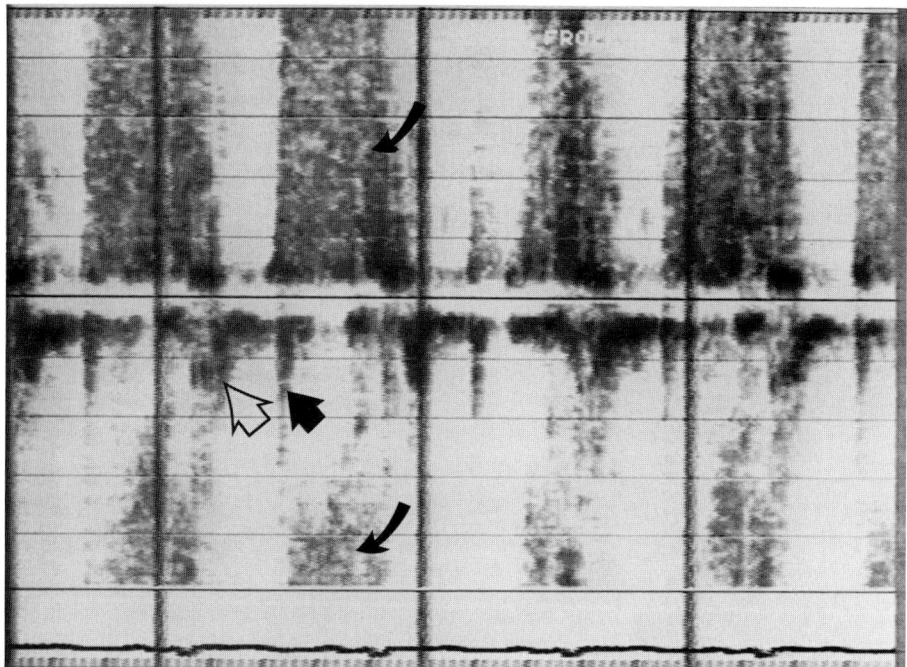

Fig. 3.33A,B. Pulmonic insufficiency with pulsed-Doppler. **A.** Short-axis two-dimensional image of a dilated right ventricular outflow tract and main pulmonary artery, with the Doppler cursor placed just under the pulmonary valve leaflets at the closed orifice (LV, left ventricle; AO, aorta; PA, main pulmonary artery; RVOT, right ventricular outflow tract). **B.** Pulsed-Doppler tracing obtained at the site shown in part **A** demonstrating high-velocity aliased flow in diastole (*curved arrows*). The opening (*open broad arrow*) and closing (*closed broad arrow*) clicks of the pulmonic valve also are seen.

pulmonary artery (1, p 109). Patients with pulmonary hypertension exhibit varying degrees of pulmonary regurgitation, which is mapped only in the right ventricle below the pulmonic valve; it is not seen either in the pulmonary artery or at the level of the pulmonic valve (1, pp 109–111). Patients with pulmonary hypertension also may show certain alterations in the profile characteristics of the waveforms obtained in the pulmonary artery in systole (16).

The evaluation of pulmonic insufficiency is often difficult, as the sensitivity of Doppler ultrasound is able to demonstrate small amounts of pulmonic and tricuspid regurgitation in normal individuals. Because of the frequency of this finding, clinical pulmonic insufficiency should only be considered when the flow disturbance as tracked by pulsed-Doppler is recorded deeper than 1 cm below the pulmonic valve in the right ventricular outflow tract (Fig. 3.34) (2, p 79).

Tricuspid Valve Pathology

Tricuspid Stenosis

Evaluation of the tricuspid valve is similar to that of the mitral valve because they both lie in the same plane. Medial angulation from the apex will put the Doppler beam in a line fairly parallel to the flow of blood from the right atrium into the right ventricle. The tricuspid valve, similar to the pulmonic valve, is also well seen from the short-axis left parasternal view, but usually one interspace lower than the pulmonic valve. The subcostal approach offers additional access to the tricuspid valve area.

In tricuspid stenosis, findings similar to those seen with mitral stenosis, are found, but they are less striking. The maximal velocity recorded through a stenotic tricuspid valve will not be as high as in mitral stenosis. However, it will be moderately increased and clearly above normal, accompanied by the characteristic slow deceleration curve as seen in mitral stenosis. Increases in transmitral flow velocity with inspiration are greater in individuals with tricuspid stenosis than in normals (1, p 103). As with other valves, a multitude of approaches and sampling sites, with interchangeable use of pulsed- and continuous-wave Doppler, as well as color flow mapping, are used in the evaluation of tricuspid valve stenosis. Using the Bernoulli equation, the pressure gradient across the stenotic valve can be calculated from the maximum velocity of tricuspid flow. Also, in patients with tricuspid stenosis, the valve opening area can be calculated, using the same pressure half-time formula as used in mitral stenosis.

Tricuspid Insufficiency

Again, the situation is essentially similar to that encountered with the mitral valve. Tricuspid insufficiency is the most common tricuspid valvular disease, and the systolic regurgitant flow velocity abnormalities received in the right atrium are plotted with pulsed-Doppler (Fig. 3.35) and with color flow mapping (Fig. 3.36). Very high velocity jets are measured with continuous-wave Doppler (Fig. 3.37). Pressure gradients may be calculated from the maximum velocity of abnormal flow recorded. The calculations of the pressure drop across the tricuspid valve measured by Doppler, have been shown to correlate well with those obtained at cardiac catheterization (17).

Tricuspid insufficiency is best evaluated from the apex, or from the left parasternal approach. The subcostal approach also may be used. Again, multiple sites from multiple approaches are used to map out the regurgitant jet's direction and to assess the severity of the insufficiency. Information regarding degrees of tricuspid regurgitation can be obtained by evaluating the superior vena cava from a suprasternal approach, or the inferior vena cava along with the hepatic veins from a subcostal approach (18). Like mitral insufficiency, tricuspid insufficiency is also accompanied by increased diastolic forward flow velocity through the tricuspid valve to handle the increased load here. The severity of tricuspid insufficiency, when mapped by pulsed-Doppler in the right atrium, is graded at mild within 1 cm of the tricuspid valve, moderate from 1 to 3 cm of the valve, and severe if the regurgitant jet extends beyond 3 cm into the right atrium from the tricuspid valve. Patients with Ebstein's anomaly, with their apically displaced tricuspid valve, usually offer dramatic findings of severe

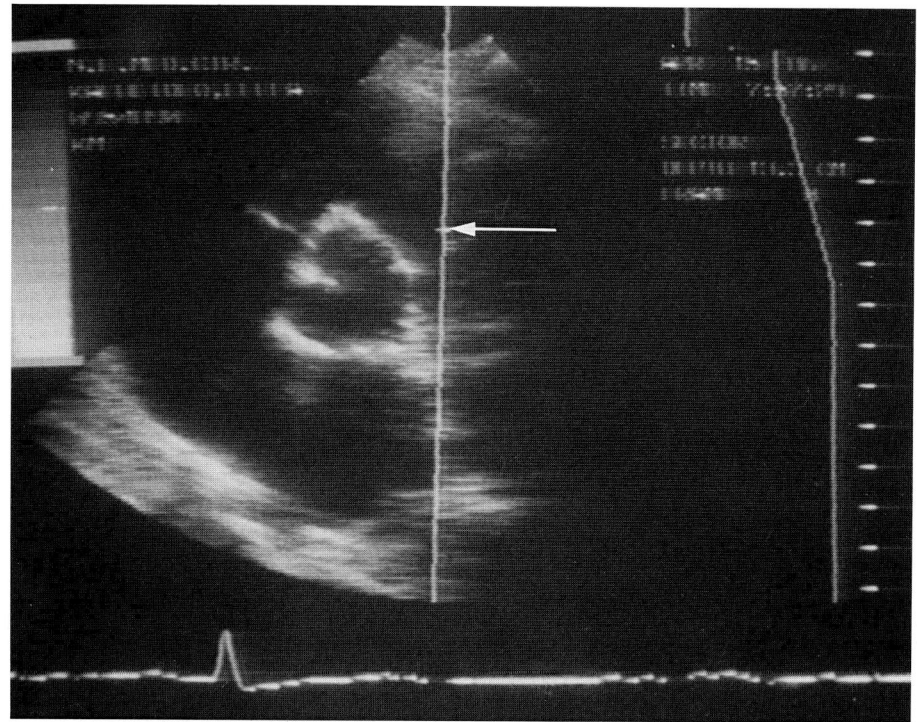

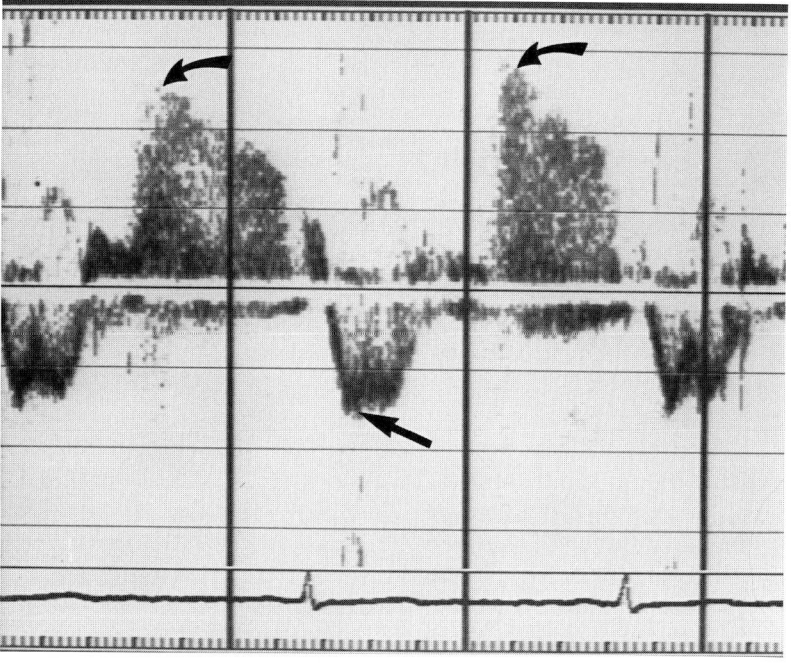

Fig. 3.34A,B. Trace pulmonic insufficiency. In a normal individual, a small amount of pulmonic insufficiency is often seen. **A**. Short axis two-dimensional image with the Doppler sample cursor placed just inside the ventricular side of the closed pulmonic valve leaflets (*long thin white arrow*). **B**. Pulsed-Doppler tracing taken at the site shown in part **A**. Normal systolic negative flow is seen (*straight arrow*) along with positive diastolic flow (*curved arrows*) with a V max of 0.5 m/s representing trace pulmonic insufficiency (calibration marks, 20 cm/s). This finding was not present more than 1 cm below the valve in this healthy individual.

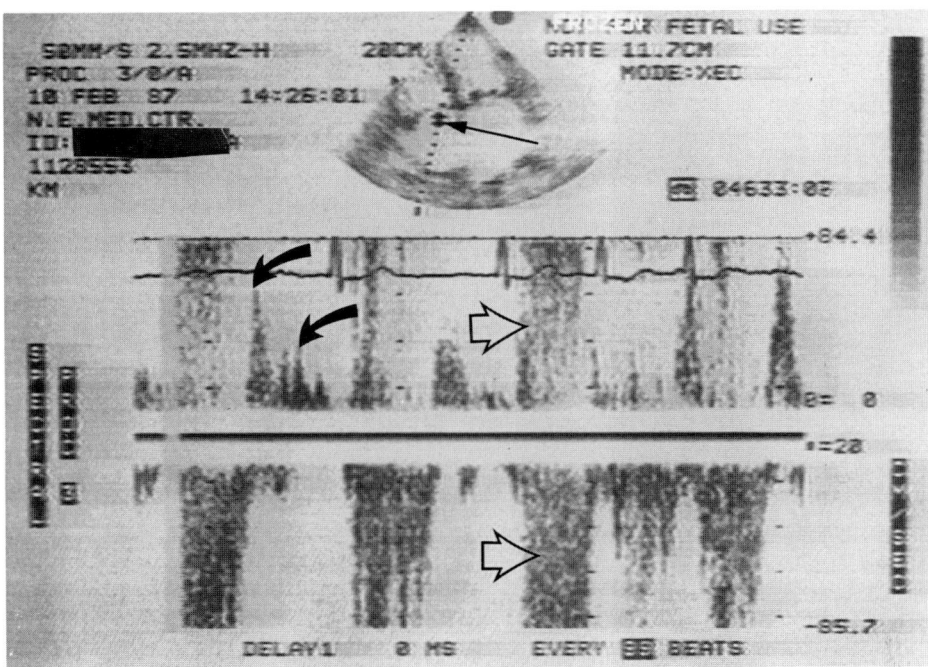

Fig. 3.35. Tricuspid insufficiency with pulsed-Doppler. In the apical four-chamber image of a patient with enlargement of all four cardiac chambers, shown at the top of the illustration, the Doppler sample volume is located about 2 cm inside the right atrium, deep to the tricuspid valve (*long thin arrow*). The regurgitant jet through the tricuspid valve is shown on the pulsed-Doppler tracing at the bottom as severely aliased flow throughout systole at this site (*open broad arrow*). Normal tricuspid inflow with a V max of 0.6 m/s is seen as a positive biphasic wave in diastole (*curved arrows*).

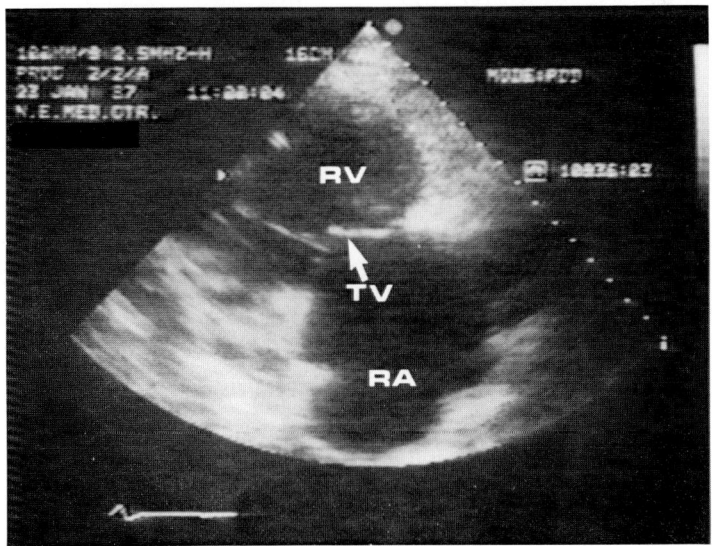

Fig. 3.36A,B. Tricuspid insufficiency. **A.** Black and white parasternal long axis view of the right atrium and right ventricle. Both chambers are enlarged in this patient with severe tricuspid insufficiency (RA, right atrium; RV, right ventricle; TV, tricuspid valve). *(Continued.)*

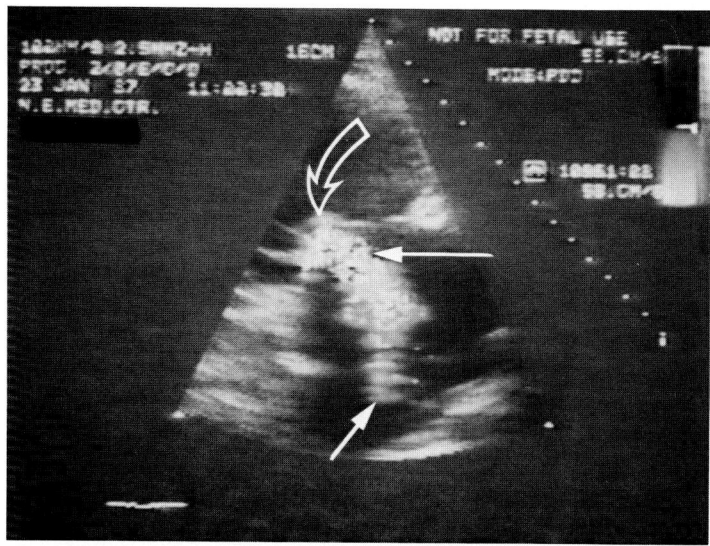

Fig. 3.36B. Color Doppler image in systole, with sector narrowed, showing negative downward high-velocity flow in the right atrium. The blue regurgitant jet (*curved arrow*) through the tricuspid valve reaches the back of the right atrium and is classified as severe. The portion of the jet from the tricuspid valve to the mid-atrial level is displayed as a bright yellow-blue-green mosaic, with some red, indicative of high-velocity aliased flow in this area (*long thin arrow*). Note that the most aliasing and the brightest mosaic pattern is closest to the tricuspid valve. The regurgitant flow slows down to a normal shade of blue as it gets deeper into the right atrium (*short thin arrow*). For a color reproduction of this figure see frontmatter.

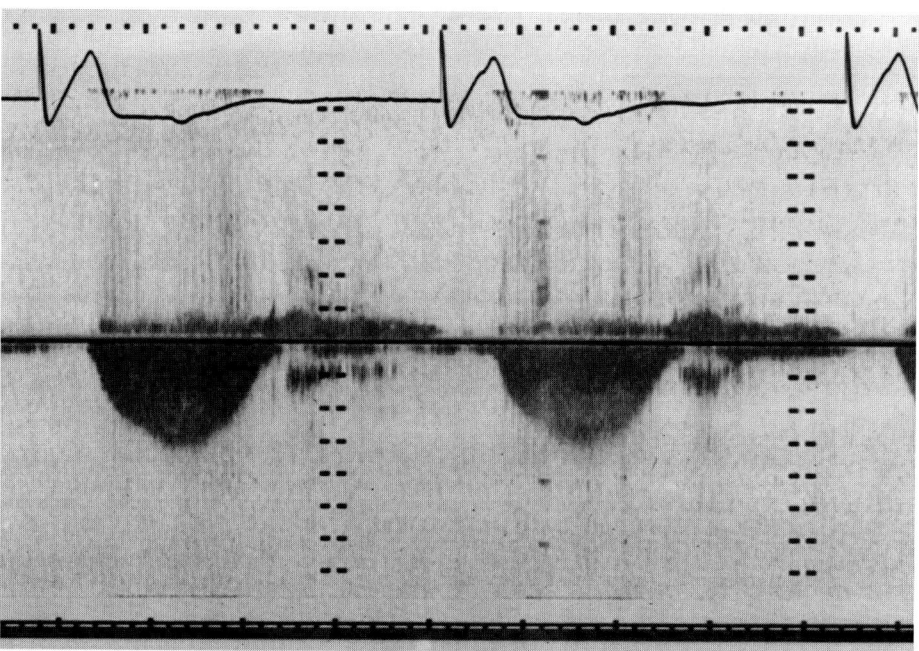

Fig. 3.37. Severe tricuspid insufficiency with continuous-wave Doppler. Because of pulsed-Doppler's inability to measure high flow velocities at the right atrial depth, continuous-wave Doppler is used from an apical approach to demonstrate this high-velocity jet of severe tricuspid regurgitation as a negative ystolic wave with a V max of 3.2 m/s (calibration marks, 1 m/s).

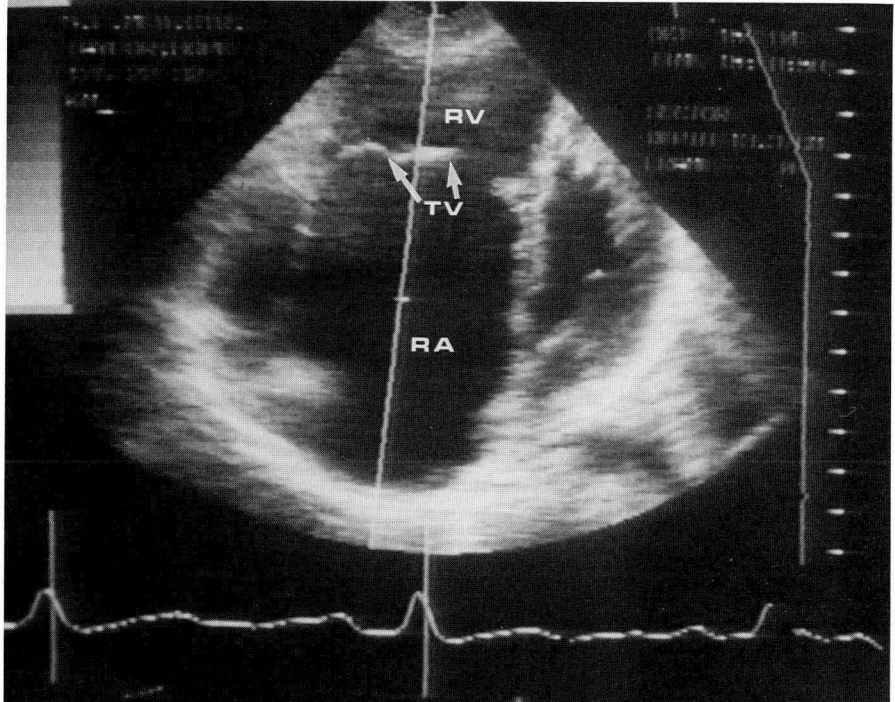

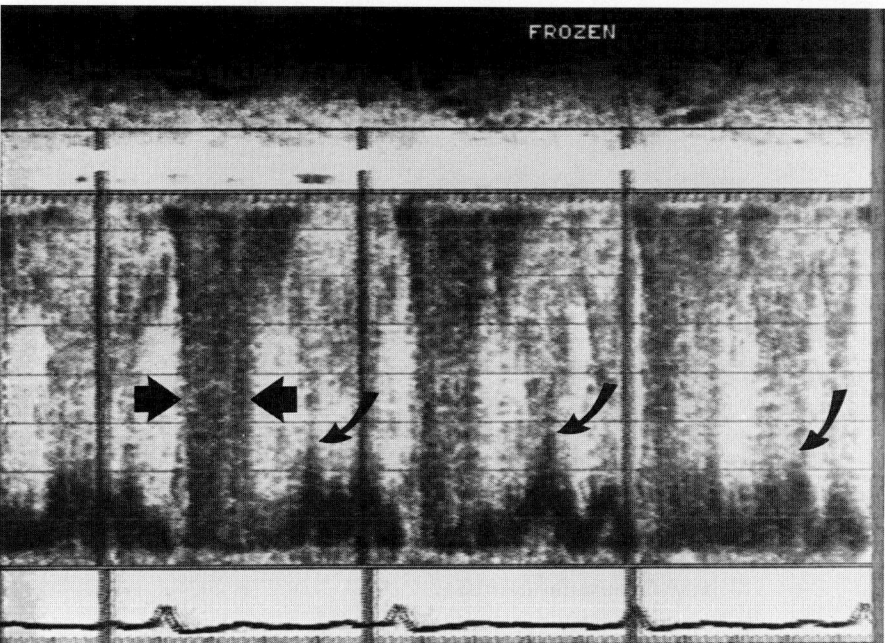

Fig. 3.38A,B. Ebstein's anomaly with pulsed Doppler showing severe tricuspid regurgitation. **A.** Long-axis two-dimensional view from the apex showing a portion of the right ventricle and an enormous right atrium, with the Doppler cursor in the middle of the right atrium, several centimeters deep to the tricuspid valve, which is apically displaced (RV, right ventricle; RA, right atrium; TV, tricuspid valve). **B.** Pulsed-Doppler tracing taken at the site shown in part **A** demonstrating severely aliased flow in systole (*broad closed arrows*) characteristic of severe tricuspid insufficiency. There is also increased positive flow (*curved arrows*) in diastole across the tricuspid valve with a V max of 1.2 m/s also representing the degree of insufficiency with its increased load on the ventricle.

tricuspid regurgitation (Fig. 3.38). Minimal amounts of trisucpid insufficiency close to the valve have been shown to be normal and should be considered physiologic (2, pp 79–82).

By using the modified Bernoulli equation, the pressure drop across regurgitant valves can be measured. In the presence of tricuspid regurgitation, this can be used as a noninvasive way of estimating right ventricular systolic pressure, by adding the jugular venous pressure, which can be estimated at the bedside, to the calculated pressure drop across the regurgitant tricuspid valve (19).

Prosthetic Valves

The noninvasive postoperative evaluation of surgically implanted valvular prostheses is one of the ideal applications of Doppler ultrasound (Fig. 3.39). Before the use of this technique, suspected leaks around a prosthetic valve required confirmation by cardiac catheterization. Again, the combination of all three Doppler techniques is used in a fashion similar to examining native valves. Multiple approaches and multiple sampling sites are used. Pulsed-Doppler is used to localize and map leaks, and continuous-wave Doppler will record the highest velocity of a leak in a parallel fashion if one is found. Pressure gradients can be calculated, and effective valve opening areas of the prostheses can be estimated using the Bernoulli equation and pressure half-time formulas, respectively. Again, here is an ideal situation for the use of color flow mapping.

Both mitral and aortic valve prostheses offer slightly more obstruction to blood flow than native valves. This results in higher maximum flow velocities and higher pressure gradients than in normal valves; a picture similar to mild stenosis is seen. Mild degrees of valvular insufficiency are not uncommon, but moderate or severe regurgitation is always abnormal. For these reasons, it is important to obtain a baseline Doppler ultrasound after cardiac valve replacement to document each valve's individuality in the immediate postoperative period, in order to be ready for comparison with future changes should they develop. In a study of prosthetic aortic and mitral valves by Labovitz and Williams (2, pp 91–92) the following results were obtained (Table 3.2). Orifice size for the mitral prosthesis was calculated using the pressure half-time formula, and pressure gradients across the aortic valve were calculated from the modified Bernoulli equation (20).

Cardiac Output

There has been interest in the possibility of measuring cardiac output noninvasively with Doppler ultrasound, and assessing the relative flows between the left side of the heart and the right. This offers help in the noninvasive evaluation of intracardiac shunts. Goldberg and others (21) have shown that Doppler ultrasound can be used to calculate a shunt ratio by estimating the cardiac output on each side of the heart, as derived from flow velocity recordings made in both the aorta and the pulmonary artery. The volume outputs from both sides of the heart are then compared; in the normal individual, they should be nearly equal. Any ratio of discrepancies between the cardiac outputs estimated for each side of the heart should be indicative of the shunt ratio (21). Determination of cardiac output with Doppler ultrasound has inherent technical difficulties that can be minimized with meticulous technique. Cross-sectional areas of the great vessels leaving the heart must be measured, with two-dimensional echocardiography, to estimate stroke volume.

If, in the heart of a patient with an atrial septal defect (ASD) the cardiac output, as calcu-

Table 3.2. Prosthetic Valves

Type	Orifice Size (cm^2)	Range (cm^2)	Mild Regurgitation (%)
Mitral Valves			
Bjork-Shiley	2.5 (+/− 0.8)	1.8–3.7	11
Starr-Edwards	2.0 (+/− 0.3)	1.2–2.5	19
Porcine	2.1 (+/− 0.7)	1.1–4.0	30

Type	Mean Gradient (mmHg)	Range (mmHg)	Mild Regurgitation (%)
Aortic Valves			
Bjork-Shiley	22 (+/− 10)	5–38	42
Starr-Edwards	29 (+/− 13)	12–50	28
Porcine	23 (+/− 10)	4–36	26

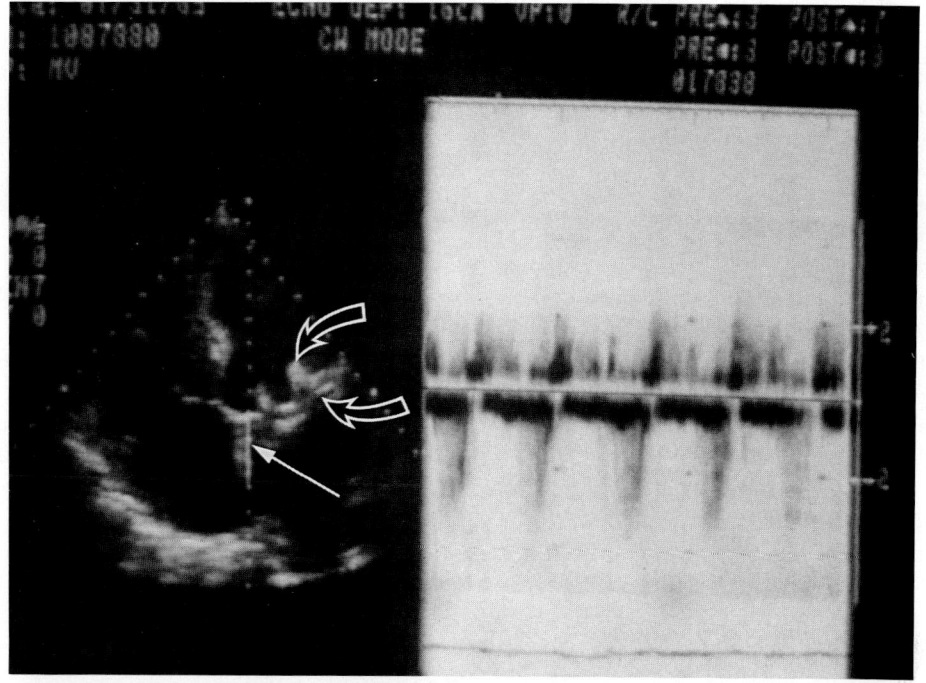

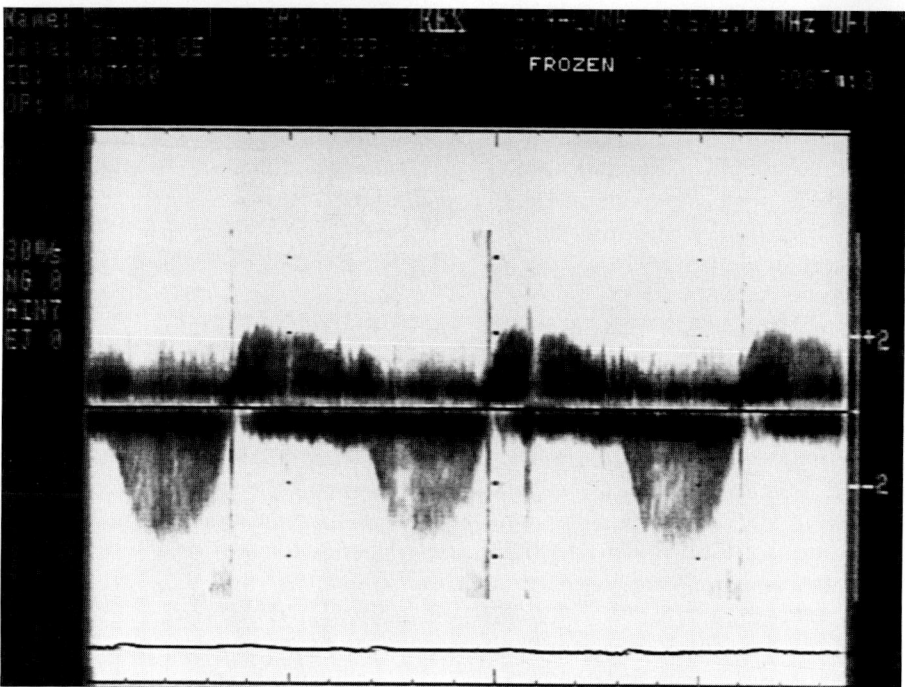

Fig. 3.39A,B. Leaking prosthetic valve. **A.** Apical four-chamber view with the Doppler sample volume (*fine white arrow*) placed close to the atrial septum in the left atrium at a fair distance from the prosthetic mitral valve (*curved open white arrows*). On the right side of this illustration is a pulsed-Doppler recording of poor quality. Nevertheless, a strong jet of mitral insufficiency is detected at this level. **B.** Continuous-wave Doppler tracing in the same patient showing a negative systolic regurgitant jet through the leaking mitral prosthesis with a V max of 3.7 m/s (calibration marks, 2 m/s).

lated from aortic flow velocity measurements, is 3 l/min on the left side, and 6 l/min on the right side, as determined from flow velocity recordings in the pulmonary artery, then the left-to-right shunt ratio in this patient would be 6:3 or 2:1.

The use of Doppler ultrasound in the determination of cardiac output offers appeal in the noninvasive evaluation of cardiac output during therapeutic management with pacemakers, during stress testing, and in estimating regurgitant fractions and calculating intracardiac shunt ratios. When ventricular systolic function is depressed, aortic flow Doppler tracings show prolonged acceleration times and reduced maximal velocity (22). This can be helpful in monitoring therapy in patients with chronic cardiac conditions with reduced ventricular function, such as in cardiomyopathies.

Intracardiac Shunts

Intracardiac shunts make up a considerable amount of the applications of Doppler in the pediatric age group. Whereas it is beyond the scope of this chapter to discuss in detail the vast area of Doppler ultrasound in the evaluation of congenital heart disease, this large and unique topic is thoroughly covered in pediatric textbooks devoted entirely to this one subject.

Nevertheless, certain congenital heart lesions can persist undiscovered into adulthood, such as ventricular septal defect (VSD), atrial septal defect (ASD), and, rarely, patent ductus arteriosus (PDA) and coarctation of the aorta (COA). Not uncommonly, intracardiac shunts develop in adults on an acquired basis. Septal defects can be seen after severe, acute myocardial infarction involving the intraventricular septum, or after rupture of a previously repaired ASD or VSD, and in penetrating cardiac trauma. Left-to-right shunts can be demonstrated after rupture of one of the sinuses of Valsalva into the right side of the heart, either from the bursting of an aneurysm of one of the sinuses, or by extension of an aortic dissection downward into the right ventricle.

Doppler evaluation of intracardiac shunts is similar to flow mapping and velocity measurement in other situations, such as regurgitant and/or stenotic valvular lesions. Doppler ultrasound is used to investigate both the atrial septum (23) and ventricular septum (24) to demonstrate septal defects and the accompanying abnormal turbulent flow through them. The abnormal flow patterns can be mapped, with pulsed-Doppler techniques, throughout the recipient chamber, similar to regurgitant valvular lesions (Fig. 3.40). High velocity flows are measured with continuous-wave Doppler. Increased flow velocities through normal outflow areas often are indicative of the increased volume load in the shunt. The pictorial demonstration of abnormal flow patterns through septal defects again is beautifully represented in color flow mapping. As mentioned in the preceding section on cardiac output, cardiac outputs can be determined from Doppler recordings in the aorta and pulmonary artery, and shunt ratios can be estimated.

With ventricular septal defects, high-velocity jets are seen in systole within the right ventricle, usually associated with increased velocity and turbulence of blood flow in the pulmonary artery (25).

In atrial septal defects, which, along with ventricular septal defects, are often best seen in short-axis or subcostal views, mildly increased flows are seen across the atrial septal defect throughout the cardiac cycle, along with associated evidence of elevated pulmonic flow secondary to the overload.

Coarctation of the aorta is rarely an adult diagnosis; however, it is easily evaluated by Doppler imaging similar to the evaluation of other obstructing lesions. The lesion is best approached from the suprasternal region where the Doppler path can be lined up in a direction parallel to aortic blood flow beyond the aortic arch. Maximum velocity recordings are obtained from samples recorded above and below the lesion, and pressure gradients can be calculated with the Bernoulli equation. Increased flow velocities in the descending aorta, distal to the coarctation, are characteristically found.

Patent ductus arteriosus is, like aortic coarctation, rarely diagnosed in the adult. The Doppler examination is usually done in the pulmonary artery, and two findings characteristic of a patent ductus are found. The first is increased systolic flow velocities in the pulmonary artery; the second is prominent diastolic flow in the pulmonary artery, which is not seen in the right ventricular outflow tract, below the pulmonic valve (26).

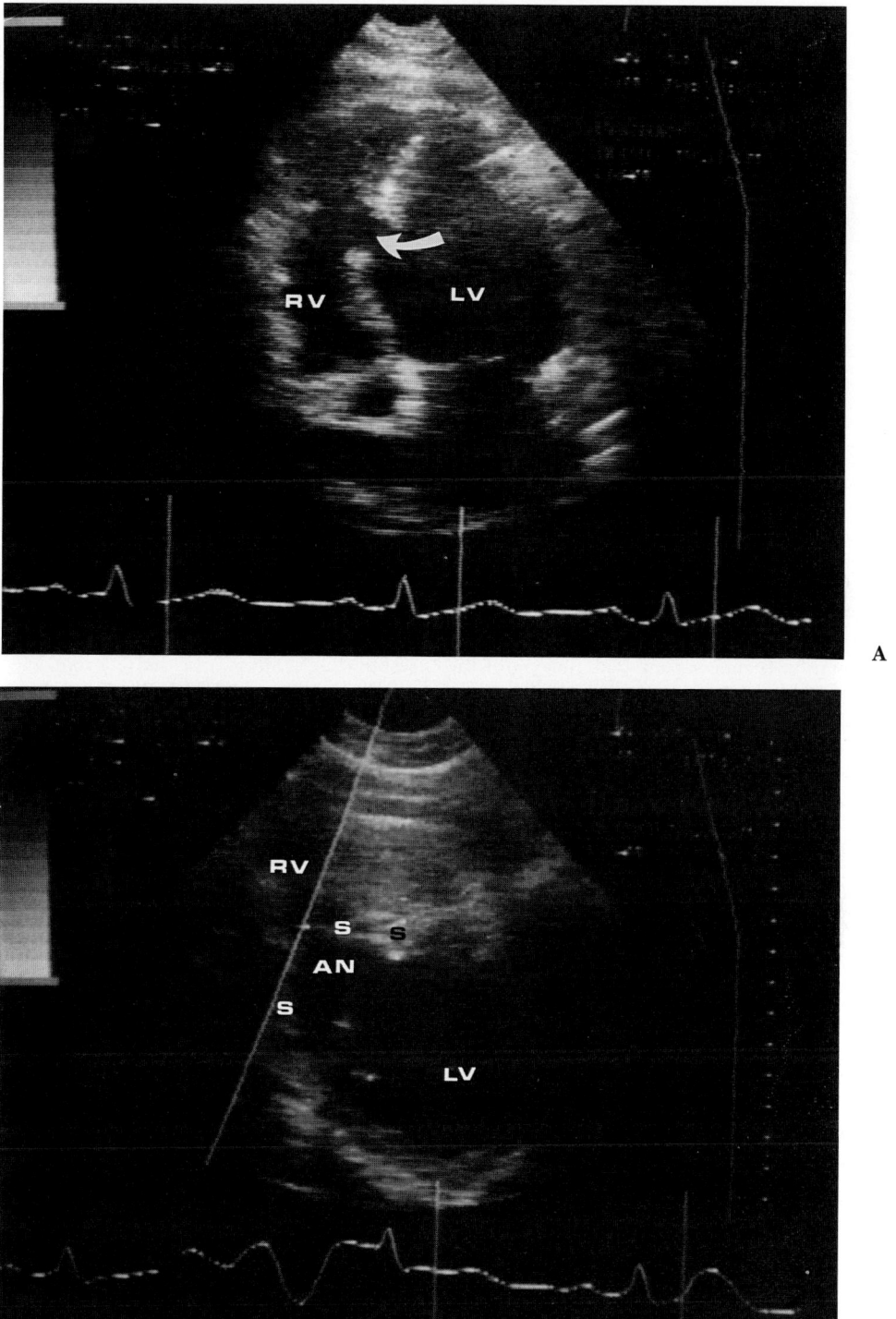

Fig. 3.40A–C. Ventricular septal defect after myocardial infarction. **A.** Apical four-chamber view showing a large defect in the ventricular septum (*closed curved white arrow*) (RV, right ventricle; LV, left ventricle). **B.** Short axis view with the Doppler cursor placed within the septal defect that resulted from the rupture of a large ventricular septal aneurysm after a myocardial infarction (LV, left ventricle; AN, septal aneurysm; S, ventricular septum; RV, right ventricle). *(Continued)*

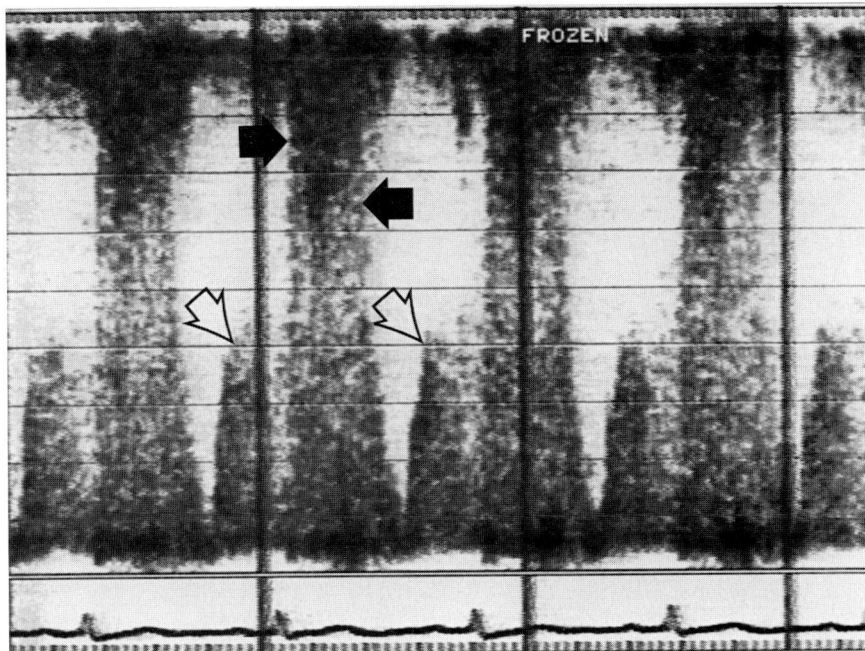

Fig. 3.40C. Pulsed-Doppler tracing obtained at the site inside the VSD showing marked aliasing of the systolic flow (*broad closed arrows*) and some left-to-right flow through the VSD in later diastole as well as in a positive direction with a V max of 0.9 m/s, corresponding to flow into the left ventricle after left atrial contraction (*broad open arrows*) (calibration marks, 20 cm/s).

Miscellaneous Cardiac Lesions

As was seen with the evaluation of prosthetic heart valves, the use of Doppler techniques can be tailored to specific situations. This usually requires only a simple extrapolation and reapplication of methods already discussed.

Hypertrophic Cardiomyopathy

The restriction to the left ventricular outflow tract seen in patients with idiopathic hypertrophic subaortic stenosis (IHSS) can be evaluated with Doppler ultrasound from the apex, in a fashion similar to the interrogation of stenotic aortic valves. The flow velocity disturbances around the obstruction are sampled at multiple sites with pulsed-Doppler guided by a two-dimensional image for mapping the lesion. With continuous-wave Doppler, the maximum velocity is determined, and the pressure gradient across the obstructing muscle mass in the intraventricular septum is calculated with the modified Bernoulli equation (Fig. 3.41) (27). The Doppler tracings obtained in patients with IHSS show a characteristic concave appearance to the high-velocity flow profile due to the late systolic peak of the high-velocity intraventricular jet, after the obstruction has been overcome by the ventricular squeeze. The demonstration of obstruction to the outflow of left ventricular blood flow velocity in patients with IHSS is dramatically pictured with color flow mapping.

Left Atrial Myxoma

Patients with left atrial myxoma have characteristic diagnostic two-dimensional echocardiograms, where there is no significant extra information that Doppler ultrasound need apply. Nevertheless, these patients are encountered in clinical practice, and although the two-dimensional images are diagnostic, the Doppler findings (Fig. 3.42) that are seen with both pulsed-Doppler and continuous-wave Doppler are virtually identical to what is seen in mitral

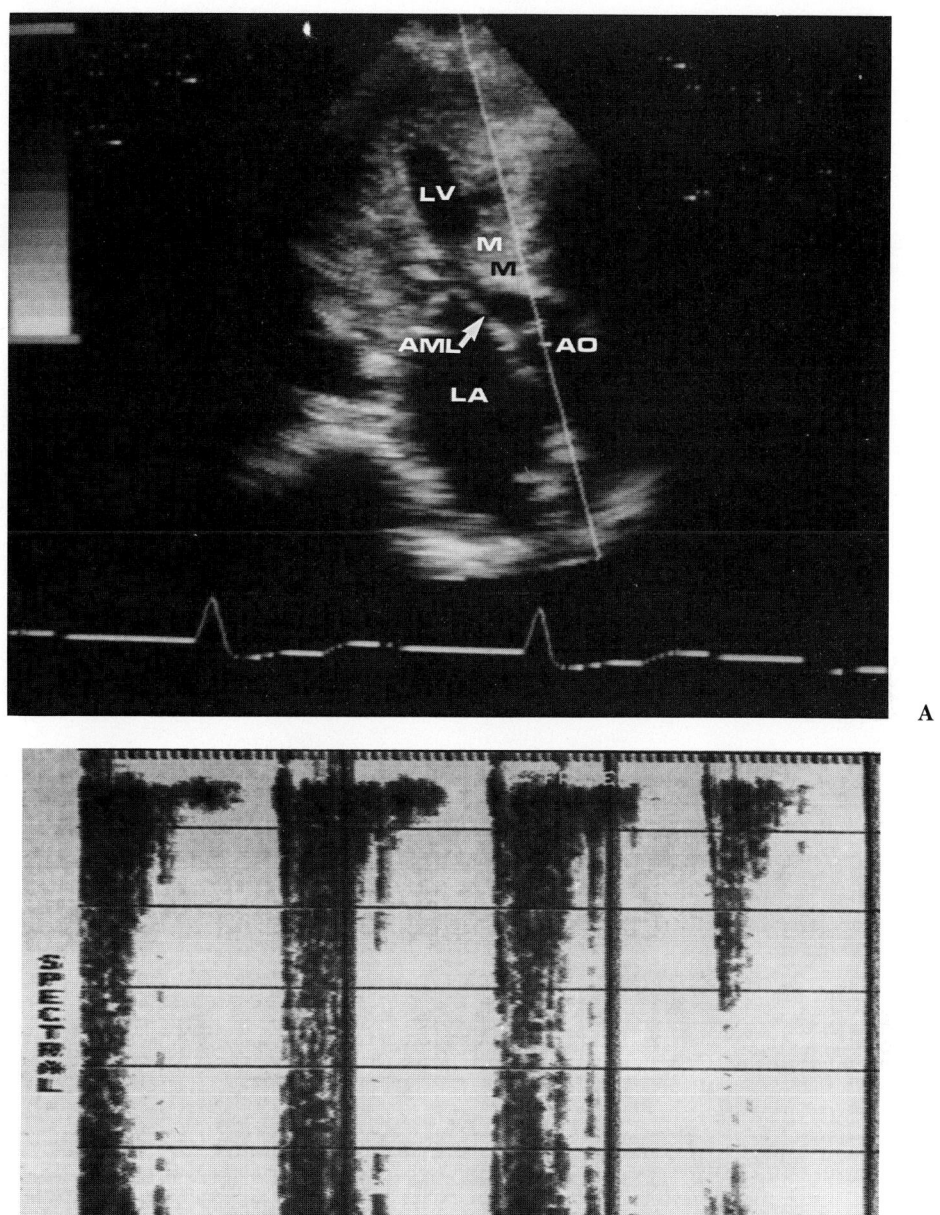

Fig. 3.41A–E. IHSS—Idiopathic hypertrophic subaortic stenosis. Pulsed- and continuous-wave Doppler. **A.** Long axis two-dimensional view from the apex with the Doppler cursor placed in the ascending aorta, just distal to the aortic valve in a patient with IHSS. The hypertrophied muscle mass, which causes left ventricular outflow tract obstruction, is seen projecting from the upper septum into the left ventricle adjacent to the anterior mitral valve leaflet in the subaortic region. There is also left ventricular hypertrophy as well in this patient (LV, left ventricle; LA, left atrium; M, hypertrophied upper septum; AO, aorta; AML, anterior leaflet of mitral valve). **B.** Pulsed-Doppler tracing at the site shown in part **A** with aliased high-velocity flow in systole (calibration marks, 20 cm/s). *(Continued.)*

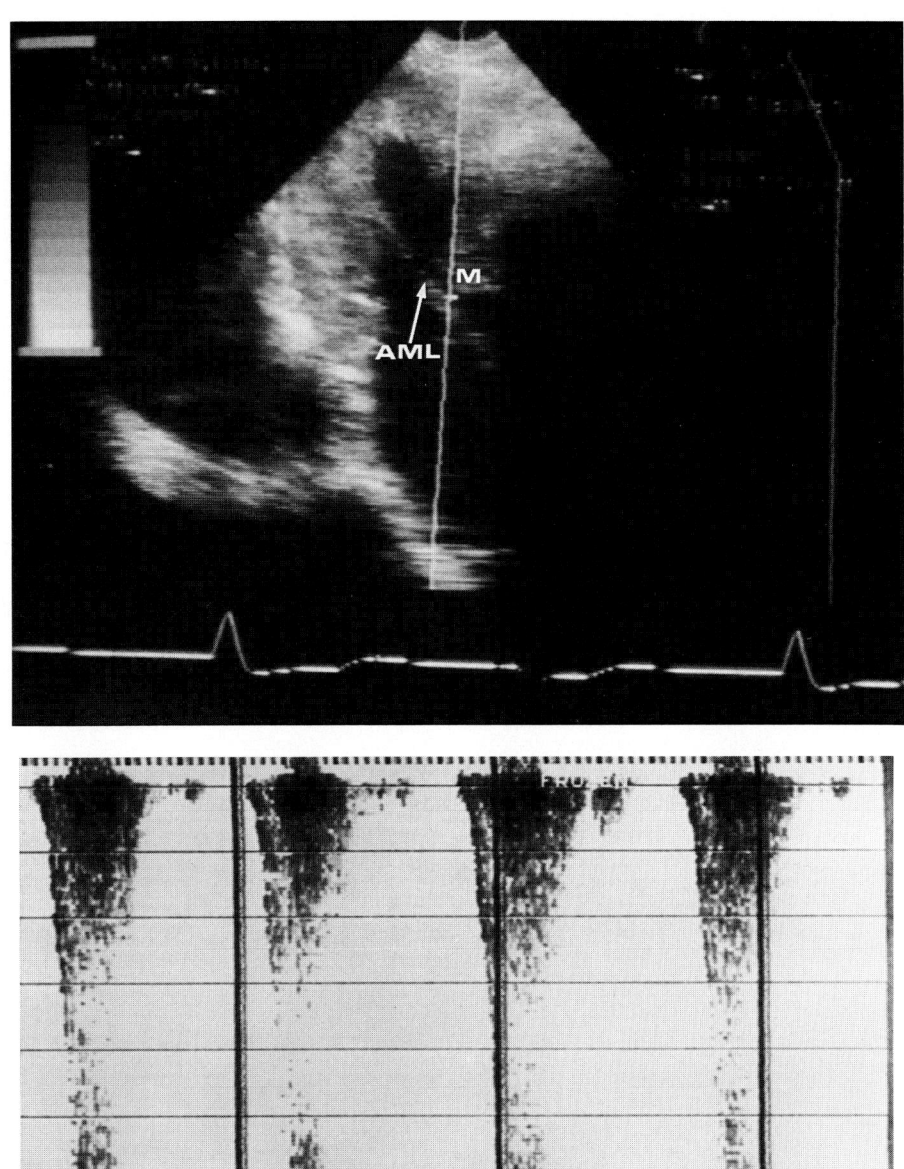

Fig. 3.41C. Long axis apical view with Doppler cursor placed at the site of obstruction between the hypertrophied septum and the anterior mitral leaflet (AML, anterior mitral valve leaflet; M, hypertrophied upper septum). **D.** Pulsed-Doppler in high PRF mode at the site shown in part **C**. Again, aliased flow is seen in systole, which cannot be measured. **E.** Continuous-wave Doppler tracing obtained in the subaortic region, with a linear tracing of the Doppler profile, showing a negative systolic flow of 5.8 m/s (*curved solid arrow*) which represent a pressure gradient of 101 mm Hg (*curved open arrows*) as derived from the modified Bernoulli equation.

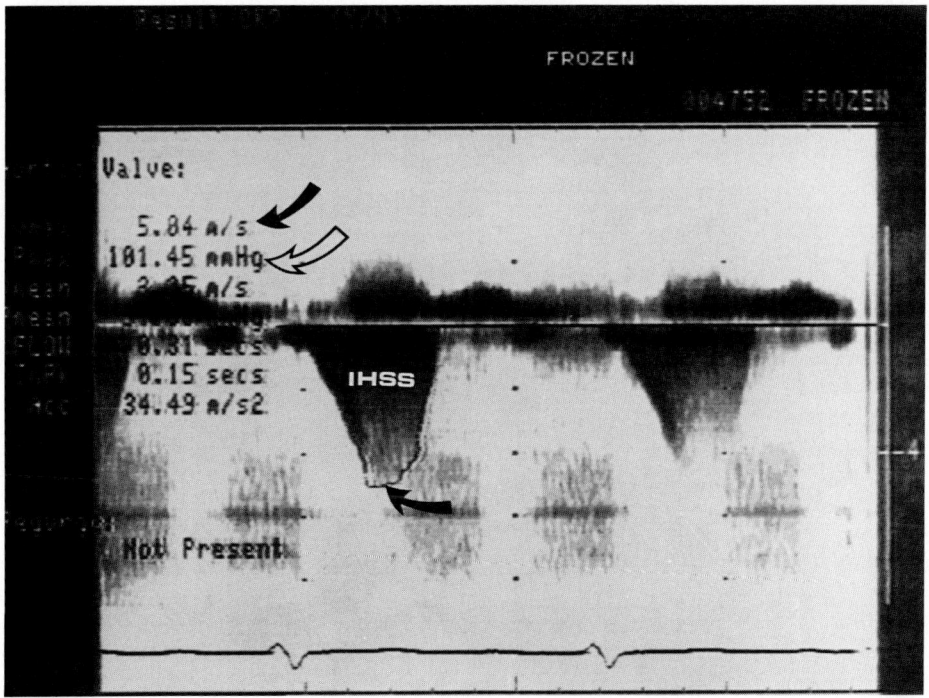

Fig. 3.41.

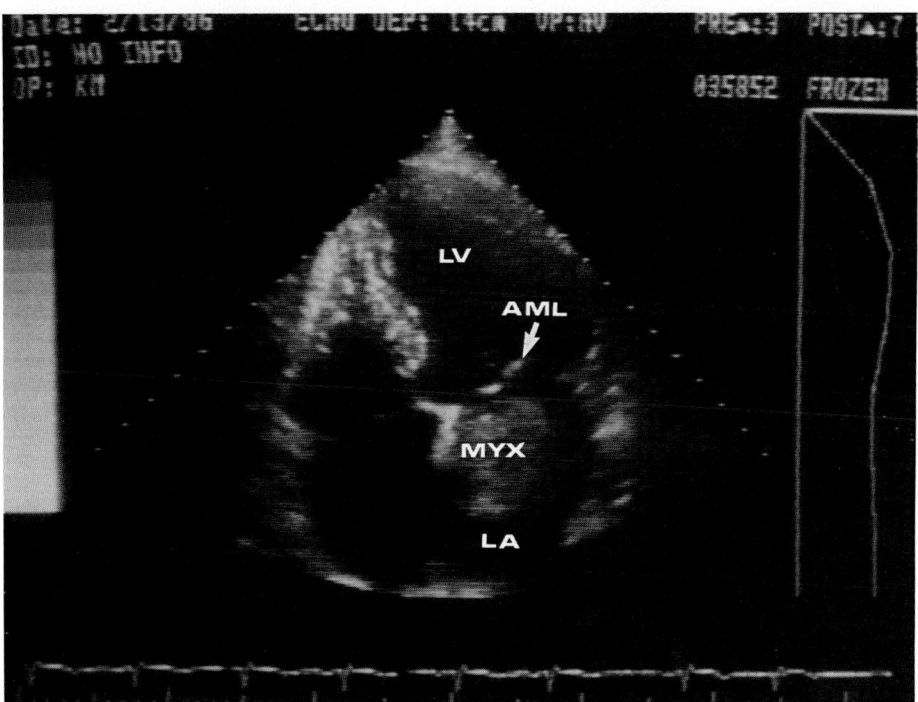

Fig. 3.42A–D. Left atrial myxoma. **A.** Apical four-chamber view in systole. The mitral leaflets are closed, and the myxoma, which is attached to the atrium and atrial side of the anterior mitral leaflet, resides in the left atrium (LV, left ventricle; AML, anterior mitral valve leaflet; LA, left atrium; MYX, myxoma). *(Continued.)*

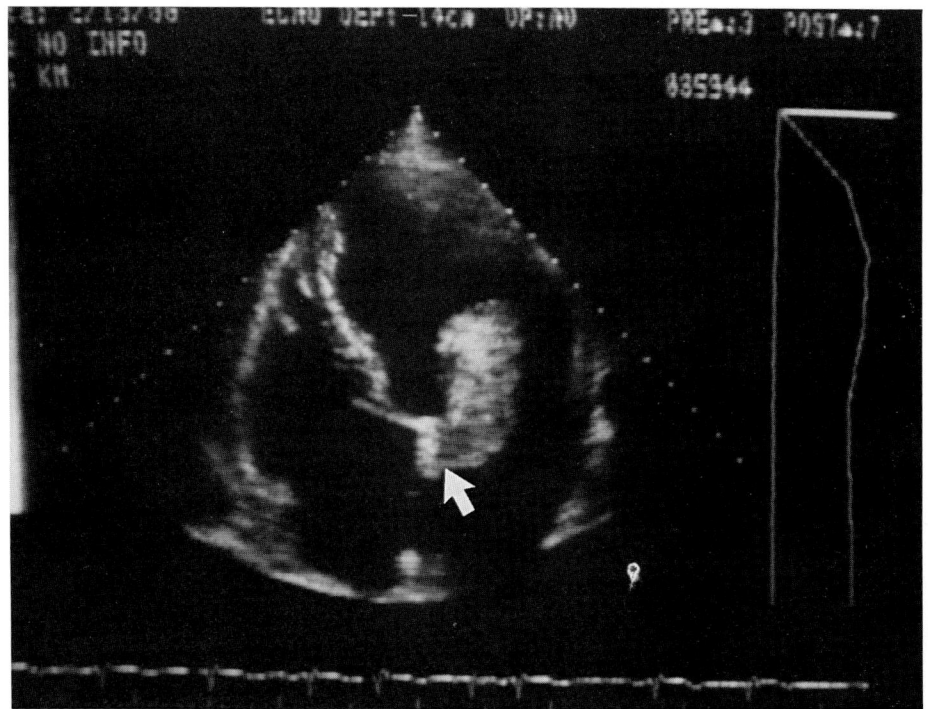

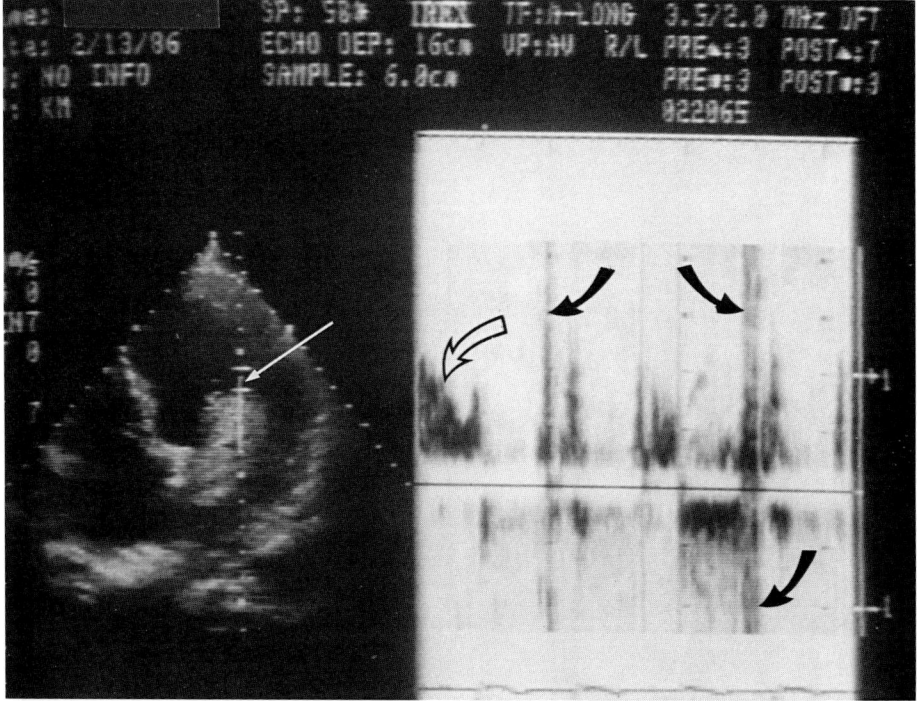

Fig. 3.42B. Apical four-chamber view in diastole. The mitral leaflets have opened, and the myxoma prolapses from the left atrium through the mitral orifice into the left ventricle. Its septal attachment is clearly seen (*arrow*). **C.** Pulsed-Doppler tracing in the right half of the illustration, showing the pattern obtained using the image at left for guidance, with the Doppler cursor placed in the left ventricular inflow area (*long thin white arrow*). Tumor motion (*curved solid arrows*), as well as flow information similar to mitral stenosis is seen (*curved open arrow*). This is better shown in part **D**. *(Continued.)*

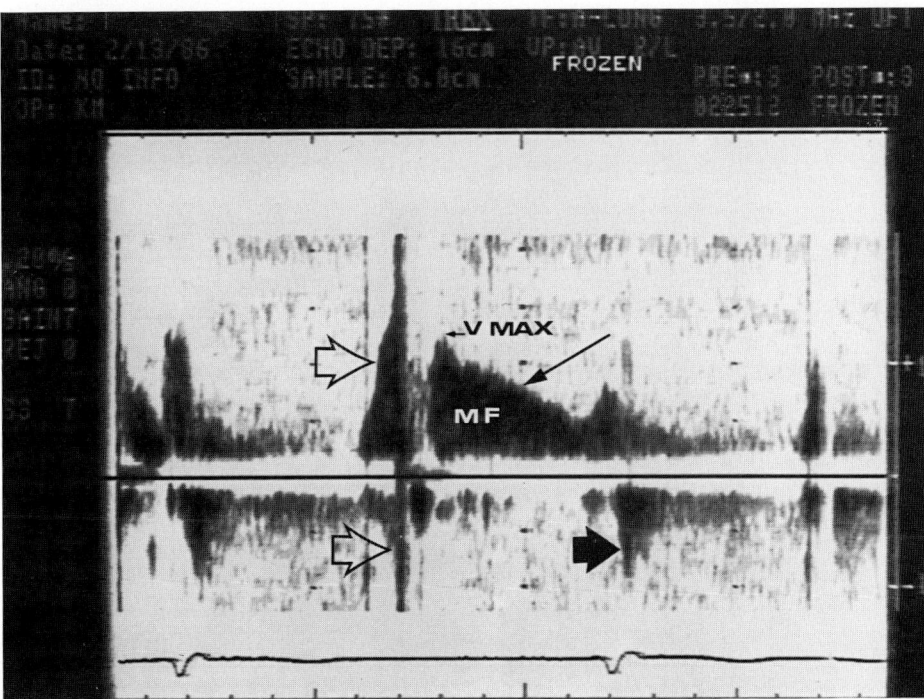

Fig. 3.42D. Continuous-wave tracing of left ventricular inflow. High-amplitude spikes in early diastole (*broad open arrows*) and at systole (*broad closed arrow*) represent tumor movement into and out of the left ventricle. These movements precede and follow the positive diastolic mitral flow velocity profile (MF), which resembles the pattern of mitral stenosis, slightly elevated mitral flow velocity of 1.5 m/s and a slow deceleration curve after V max, indicating a prolonged mitral pressure half-time and physiologic mitral stenosis (*long thin black arrow*).

stenosis (1, p 88). Dramatic pictures of the abnormal flow associated with myxomas can be shown with color flow mapping.

Conclusion

As can be seen, Doppler ultrasound now plays a significant role in the noninvasive evaluation of the heart in suspected cardiac disorders. An invaluable amount of quantifiable information about intracardiac flow dynamics is now available with Doppler techniques to supplement the high-resolution anatomic detail already available in echocardiography. The combination of echocargiographic imaging techniques along with the flexible use of pulsed- and continuous-wave Doppler techniques, together with color flow mapping, offers a rapidly increasing wealth of reliable and important dynamic information about the heart that is available through no other single technique.

It has been the attempt of this chapter to organize the Doppler approach to the heart in as clear a fashion as possible, without entering into too much detail as to make this complex subject more difficult. Doppler echocardiography is not a casual examination, and the importance of the skill and experience on the part of those who perform these sophisticated examinations cannot be underemphasized. Unique information is now available that was never before seen. The explosion in Doppler echocardiographic capability puts us at the advent of the opportunity to further our understanding of circulatory problems.

References

1. Hatle L, Angelsen B: Doppler Ultrasound in Cardiology (2nd ed). Philadelphia, Lea & Febiger, 1985.
2. Labovitz AJ, Williams GA: Doppler Echocardiography—Quantitative Methods of Pulsed and

Continuous Wave Cardiac Doppler. Philadelphia, Lea & Febiger, 1985.
3. Miyatake K, Okamoto M, Kinoshita N, et al: Clinical applications of a new type of real-time two-dimensional Doppler flow imaging system. Am J Cardiol 54:857, 1984.
4. Sahn DJ: Real-time two-dimensional Doppler echocardiographic flow mapping. Circulation 71:849, 1985.
5. Demaria AN, Smith MD, Kwan OL: Doppler flow imaging: Another step in the evolution of ultrasound. *In* Echocardiography—A Review of Cardiovascular Ultrasound, Vol. 2. pp 495–500, 1985. *Editor in Chief*, Vincent E. Friedwald, Jr.; *Associate Editors*, Anthony DeMaria, Navin C. Nanda, Pravin M. Shah, Arthur E. Weyman, Futura Publishing Co., Inc., 295 Main St. P.O. Box 330, Mount Kisco, N.Y. 10549.
6. Libanoffal AJ, Rodbard MD: Evaluating the severity of mitral stenosis and regurgitation. Circulation 33:218, 1966.
7. Libanoffal AJ, Rodbard MD: Atrioventricular pressure half time. Measurement of mitral valve orifice area. Circulation 38:144, 1968.
8. Hatle L, Angelsen B, Tromsdale A: Noninvasive assessment of atrioventricular pressure half time by Doppler ultrasound. Circulation 60:1096, 1979.
9. Hatle L, Angelsen B, Tromsdale A: Noninvasive assessment of aortic stenosis by Doppler ultrasound. Br Heart J 43:284, 1980.
10. Requarth JA, Goldberg SJ, Vasko SD, et al: In vitro verification of Doppler prediction of transvalve pressure gradient and orifice area in stenosis. Am J Cardiol 53:1369, 1984.
11. Currie PJ, Seward JB, Reeder GS, et al: Continuous wave Doppler echocardiographic assessment of severity of calcific aortic stenosis: A simultaneous Doppler-catheter correlative study in 100 adult patients. Circulation 71:1162, 1985.
12. Williams GA, Labovitz AJ, Nelson JG, et al: Value of multiple echocardiographic views in the evaluation of aortic stenosis in adults by continuous wave Doppler. Am J Cardiol 55:445, 1985.
13. Ciobanu M, Abassi AS, Allen NW, et al: Pulsed Doppler echocardiography in the diagnosis and estimation of severity of aortic insufficiency. Am J Cardiol 49:339, 1982.
14. Pearlman AS, Acoblioko DP, Saal AK: Assessment of valvular heart disease by Doppler echocardiography. Clin Cardiol 6:573, 1983.
15. Abassi AS, Allen NW, Decristofaro D, et al: Detection and estimation of the degree of mitral regurgitation by range gated pulse Doppler echocardiography. Circulation 61:143, 1980.
16. Kitabatake A, Inove M, Adao M, et al: Noninvasive evaluation of pulmonary hypertension by a pulsed Doppler technique. Circulation 68:1096, 1983.
17. Skjaerpe T, Hatle L: Diagnosis and assessment of tricuspid regurgitation with Doppler ultrasound. *In* Rijsterborgh H (ed): Echocardiography. The Hague, Holland, Martinus Nijhoff, 1981.
18. Pennestri F, Loperfido F, Salvatori MP, et al: Assessment of tricuspid regurgitation by pulsed Doppler ultrasonography of the hepatic veins. Am J Cardiol 54:363, 1984.
19. Yock PG, Popp RL: Noninvasive estimation of right ventricular systolic pressure by Doppler ultrasound in patients with tricuspid regurgitation. Circulation 70:657, 1984.
20. Williams GA, Labovitz AJ: Doppler hemodynamic evaluation of prosthetic (Starr Edwards and Bjork-Shiley) and bioprosthetic (Hancock and Carpentier-Edwards) cardiac valves. Am J Cardiol 56:325, 1985.
21. Goldberg SJ, Sahn DJ, Allen HD, et al: Evaluation of pulmonary and systemic blood flow by two-dimensional Doppler echocardiography using fast fourier transform spectral analysis. Am J Cardiol 50:1394, 1982.
22. Pearlman AS: Evaluation of ventricular function using Doppler echocardiography. Am J Cardiol 49:1324, 1982.
23. Minagoe S, Tei C, Kisanuki A, et al: Noninvasive pulsed Doppler echocardiographic detection of the direction of shunt flow in patients with atrial septal defect: Usefulness of the right parasternal approach. Circulation 71:745, 1985.
24. Stevenson JG, Kawabori I, Guntheroth WG: Differentiation of ventricular septal defects from mitral regurgitation by pulsed Doppler echocardiography. Circulation 56:14, 1977.
25. Stevenson JG, Kawabori I, Dooley T, et al: Diagnosis of ventricular septal defect by pulsed Doppler echocardiography—sensitivity, specificity, and limitations. Circulation 58:322, 1978.
26. Stevenson JG, Kawabori I, Guntheroth WG: Noninvasive detection of pulmonary hypertension in patent ductus arteriosus by pulsed Doppler echocardiography. Circulation 60:355, 1979.
27. Hatle L: Noninvasive assessment and differentiation of left ventricular outflow obstruction with Doppler ultrasound. Circulation 64:381, 1981.

4
Duplex Sonography of the Abdomen

E. MAUREEN WHITE and PETER L. CHOYKE

Duplex sonography, which integrates real-time imaging with pulsed-Doppler analysis, has greatly expanded the diagnostic capabilities of conventional ultrasound examinations. Within the abdomen, several applications have been established and, through clinical research, new indications are being defined. Information regarding blood flow is obtained by placing a sample volume within a desired location and detecting the backscattered sound beam (1). After processing of the Doppler shift signals, the data is then available both as an audible output and as a graphical display, with Doppler frequency shift (or velocity) on the vertical axis versus time on the horizontal axis. The configuration of the waveform reflects the status of the proximal circulation as well as the receiving vascular bed. Specific parameters that determine waveform shape include cardiac contractility, vascular wall compliance, luminal diameter, velocity of blood flow, presence or absence of turbulence, and downstream vascular resistance (2). These, in turn, are affected by other factors such as the individual's physiologic status. Notable examples include altered circulatory impedance of the distal aorta and lower extremities between resting and postexercise states, as well as variation in superior mesenteric arterial flow between fasting and postprandial states.

Both quantitative and qualitative information may be obtained with Doppler analysis (3,4). To date, most abdominal applications have been qualitative in nature. One of the most frequent uses involves the determination of vascular patency. On real-time ultrasound imaging, low-level echoes may be demonstrated in patent vessels, with an appearance indistinguishable from thrombus. Causes for this finding include high instrument gain settings as well as echogenic blood flow, whether laminar or turbulent in nature (5–8). When this appearance is visualized on real-time sonograms, demonstration of normal intraluminal Doppler signals will confirm vascular patency. Duplex ultrasound may also help in defining abnormal structures as being vascular or nonvascular in origin. In addition, dentification of blood flow directionality is possible through analysis of the spectral display. A normal waveform is deflected above baseline when blood is flowing toward the transducer and below baseline when blood is flowing away from the transducer. Use of Doppler also allows for the identification of turbulent blood flow. Turbulence produces an increased spectrum of blood flow velocities, which may be displayed on the waveform by "filling in" under the systolic peak. This finding is termed spectral broadening. With severe degrees of turbulence, distortion of the waveform shape often accompanies spectral broadening.

More quantitative information is acquired with duplex ultrasound by calculation of various indexes from waveform data (9). One of the most commonly used is the pulsatility index (PI). This is defined as the peak-to-peak (sytolic-to-diastolic) amplitude of the spectral display, divided by the mean amplitude. This provides an indication of downstream impedance to blood flow, with a high PI suggesting increased peripheral vascular resistance (10). In general, blood vessels with increased resistance have diminished or absent flow in diastole, whereas with low downstream resistance, flow continues throughout the entire cardiac cycle.

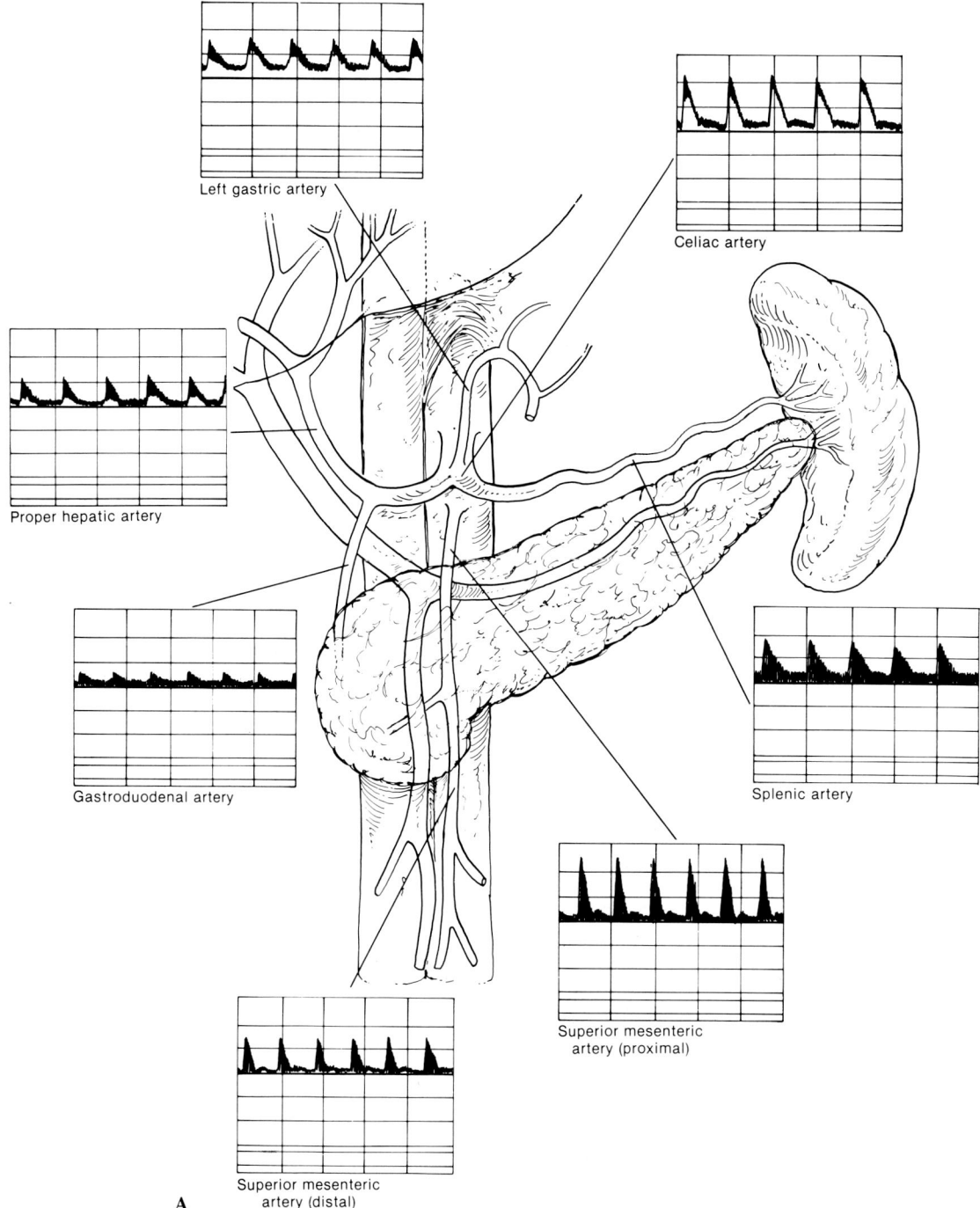

Fig. 4.1A,B. Duplex sonography may be used to evaluate several vascular structures within the upper abdomen. These are depicted on these diagrams, with the corresponding normal waveform displays.

4. Duplex Sonography of the Abdomen

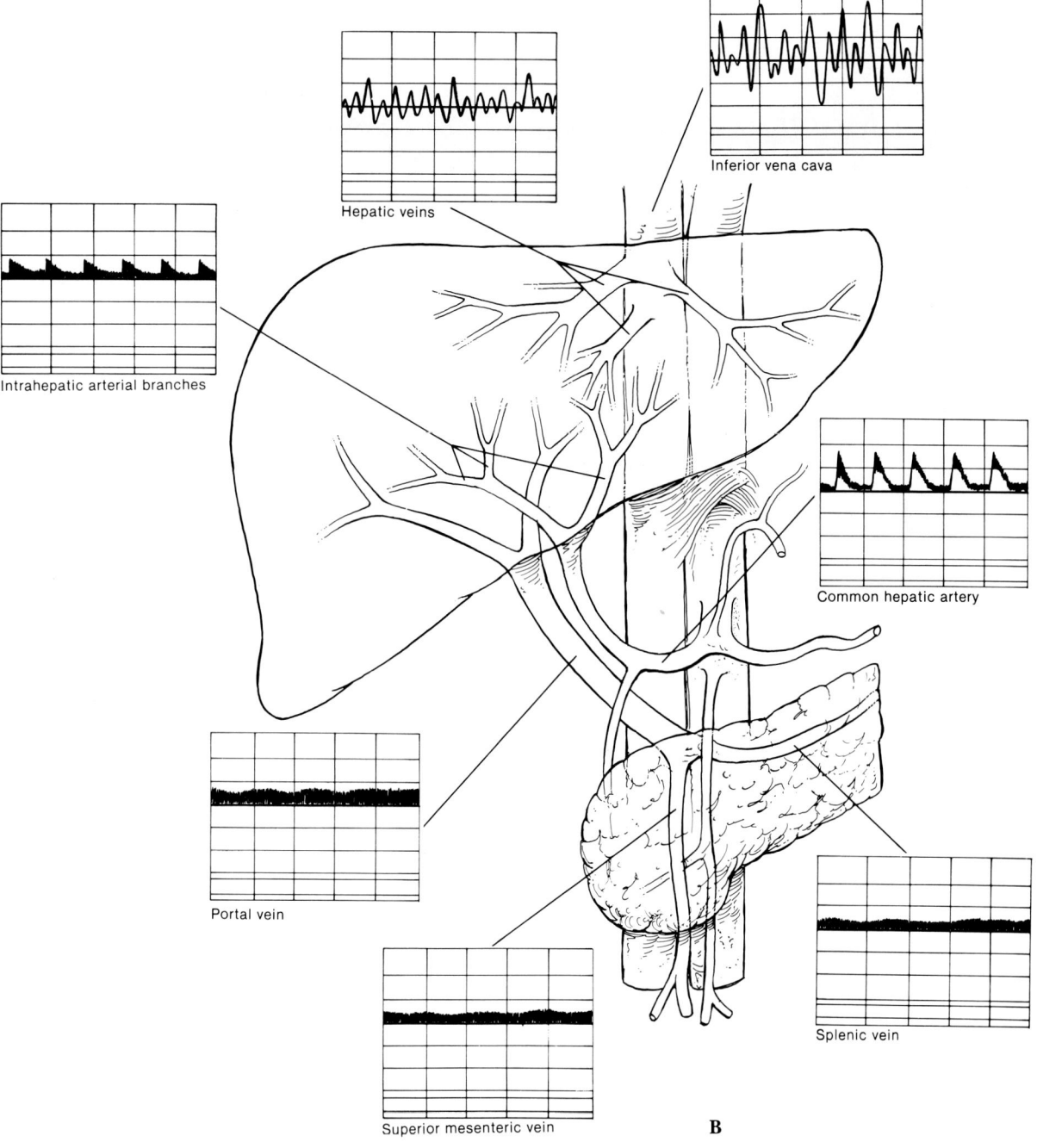

Fig. 4.1.

Proper interpretation of duplex abdominal studies requires familiarity with the normal vascular waveforms. In this chapter, several abdominal vessels are examined by duplex sonography. Normal time-velocity spectra, which are often relatively characteristic for specific blood vessels, are described and illustrated (Figs. 4.1 and 4.2). These findings are then compared with waveforms obtained in various disease states.

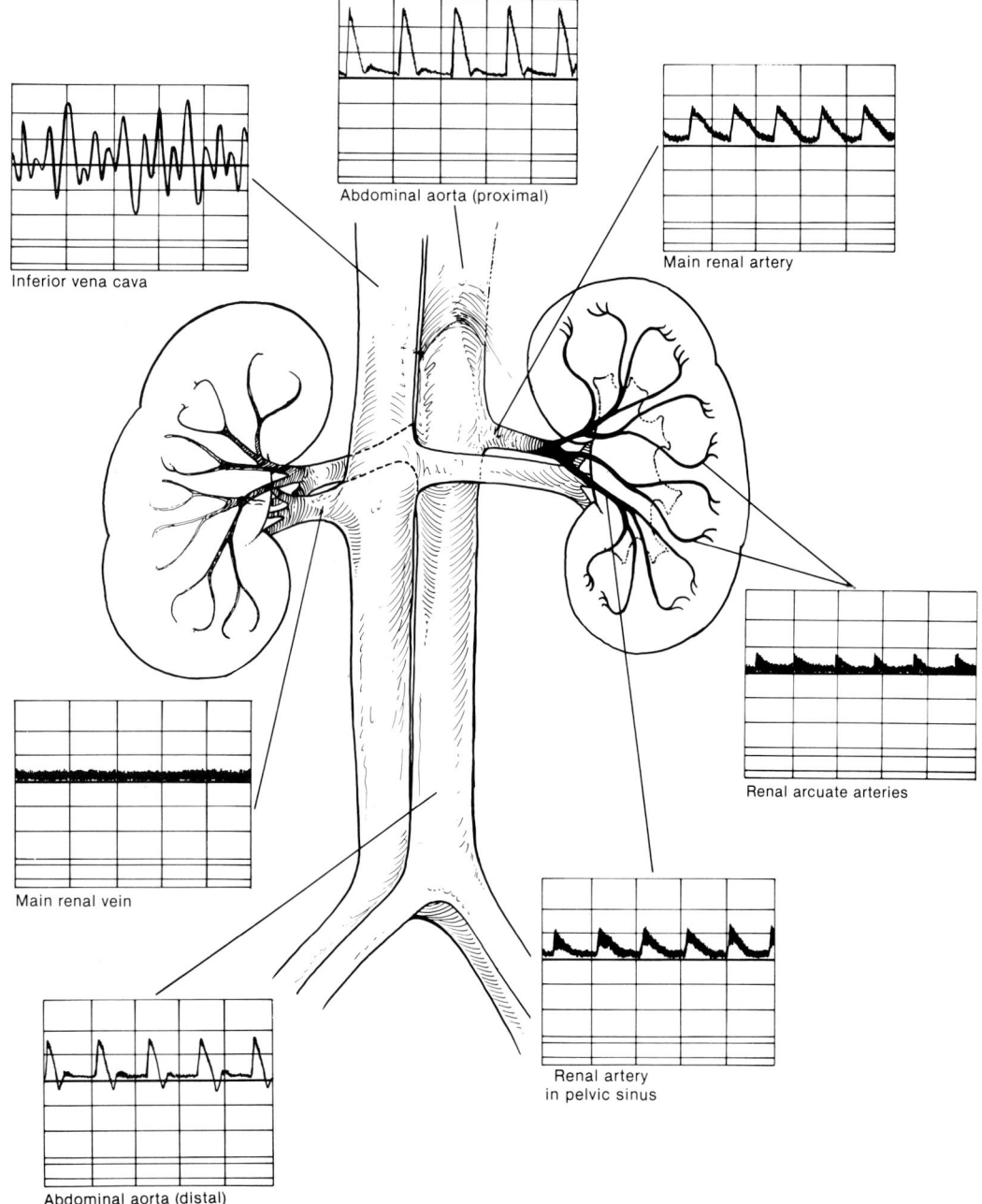

Fig. 4.2. Schematic illustration of the normal Doppler waveforms in the renal vasculature.

Duplex Ultrasound of the Normal Abdomen

Abdominal Aorta

A typical waveform display from the abdominal aorta shows a sharp systolic peak, which rapidly returns toward baseline during diastole. The relatively uniform velocity of flowing red blood cells within the upper abdominal aorta is represented on the Doppler spectrum as a clear "window" under the systolic peak. Uniformity in the systolic blood flow velocity is maintained more inferiorly within the abdominal aorta. The diastolic portion of the waveform, however, normally changes at progressively more distal sites in the aorta. Absence or even reversal of flow develops during diastole (Fig. 4.3). Graphi-

Fig. 4.3A,B. Normal abdominal aorta (Ao). **A.** Sagittal ultrasound image of a normal abdominal aorta (*arrows*). **B.** Doppler spectral display from the aorta demonstrates a clear window under the systolic peak and reversal of flow in diastole.

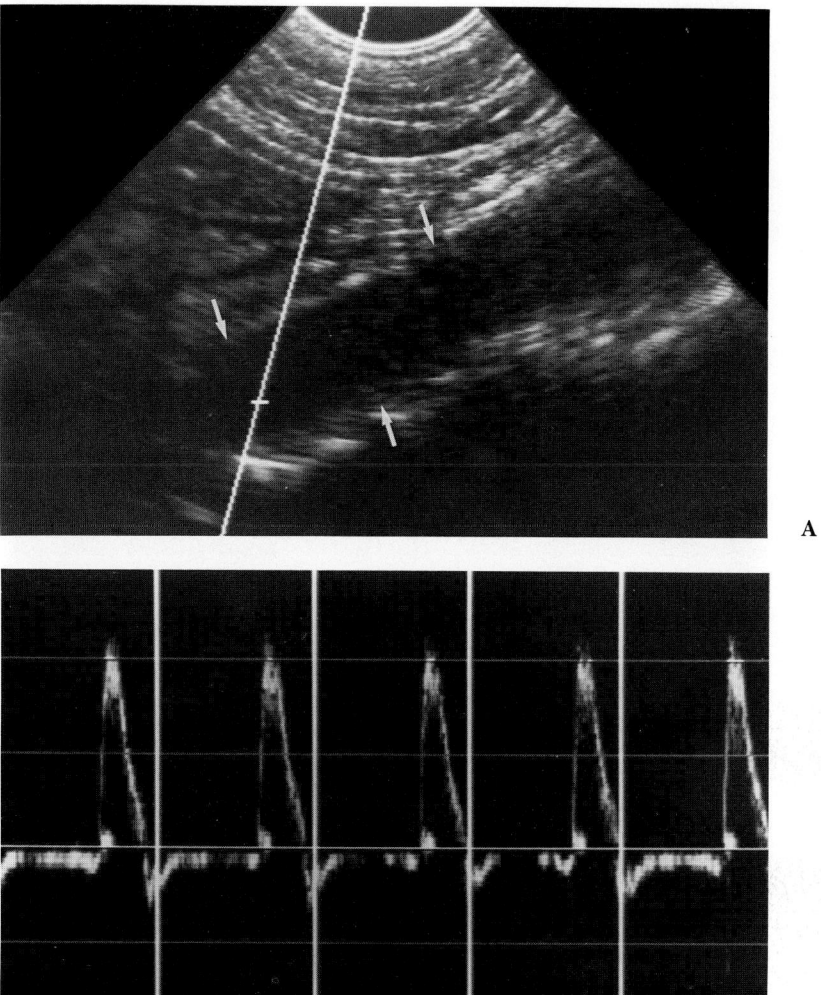

cally, this is depicted as a small peak projecting on the opposite side of the baseline from the systolic wave. Transient diastolic reversal of blood flow in the lower abdominal aorta results from the high resistance in the receiving vascular bed of the lower extremity musculature. This is most prominent at rest and is gradually abolished with exercise, due to reactive hyperemia and decreased peripheral resistance in the lower extremities. An important consequence of the high resting impedance within the lower aorta is to optimize renal artery blood flow during diastole.

Celiac Artery and Branches

The normal Doppler spectrum of the celiac artery demonstrates a systolic peak with mild spectral broadening (Fig. 4.4). The latter finding results from an increased distribution in the velocities of flowing red blood cells. Blood flow continues throughout diastole, due to the low impedance of the receiving circulatory beds, particularly to the liver. Similar waveform configurations are found in the common, proper, and main right hepatic arteries, which are sonographically visualized in approximately 92, 75, and 73% of patient examinations, respectively (11) (Fig. 4.5). As progressively smaller and more distal hepatic arterial branches are sampled, the peak velocities gradually diminish and the velocity profiles demonstrate a greater spectrum of Doppler shift frequencies; consequently, spectral broadening increases. The gastroduodenal artery (GDA) is demonstrated to course along the ventral aspect of the pancreatic head, inferior to its origin from the com-

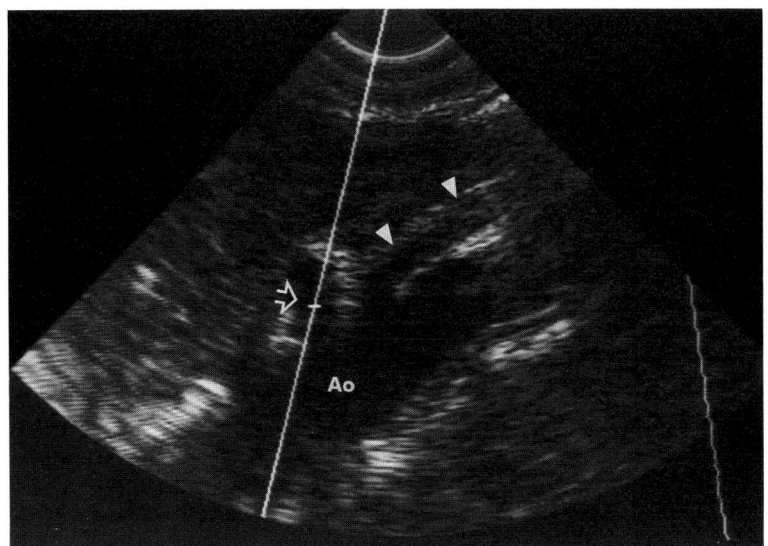
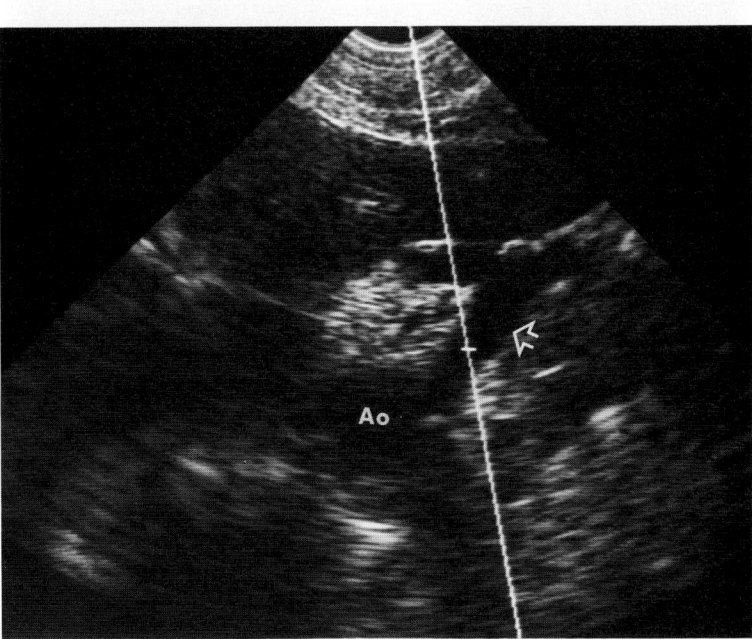

Fig. 4.4A–C. Normal celiac artery. **A.** Sagittal scan of the abdominal aorta (Ao), celiac artery (*open arrow*), and SMA (*arrowheads*). The Doppler sample volume is located within the celiac artery. **B.** Celiac artery imaged transversely (*open arrow*). The Doppler cursor is positioned centrally in the vascular lumen. **C.** The normal celiac arterial tracing demonstrates mild spectral broadening and continuous flow in diastole.

Fig. 4.5A–C. Normal hepatic artery. **A.** Transverse sonogram of the celiac trifurcation, with the cursor positioned in the common hepatic artery (*solid arrow*). **B.** Ultrasound image of the porta hepatis. The Doppler sample volume is located in the hepatic artery (*arrowheads*). **C.** Spectral display obtained from image 5B. This demonstrates spectral broadening and continuous diastolic flow in the hepatic artery.

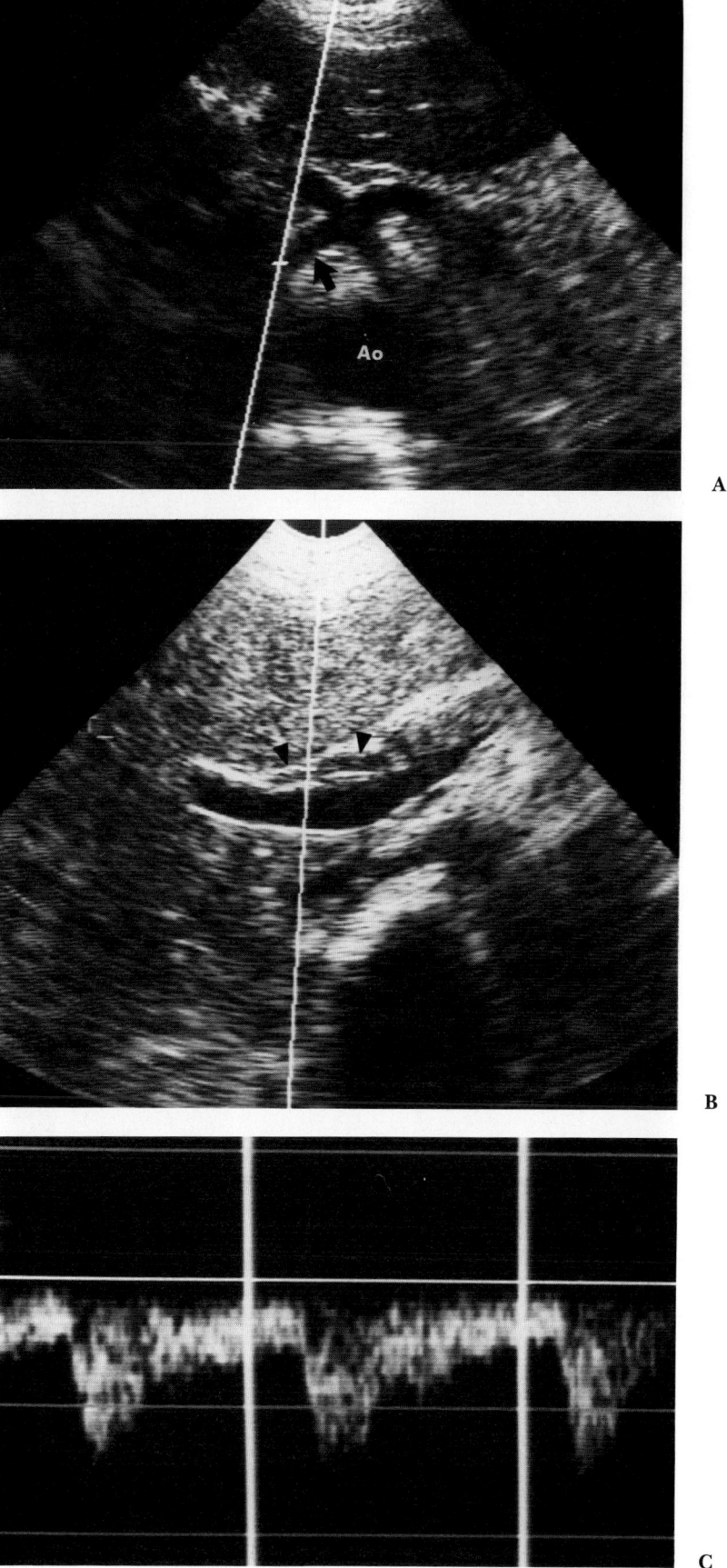

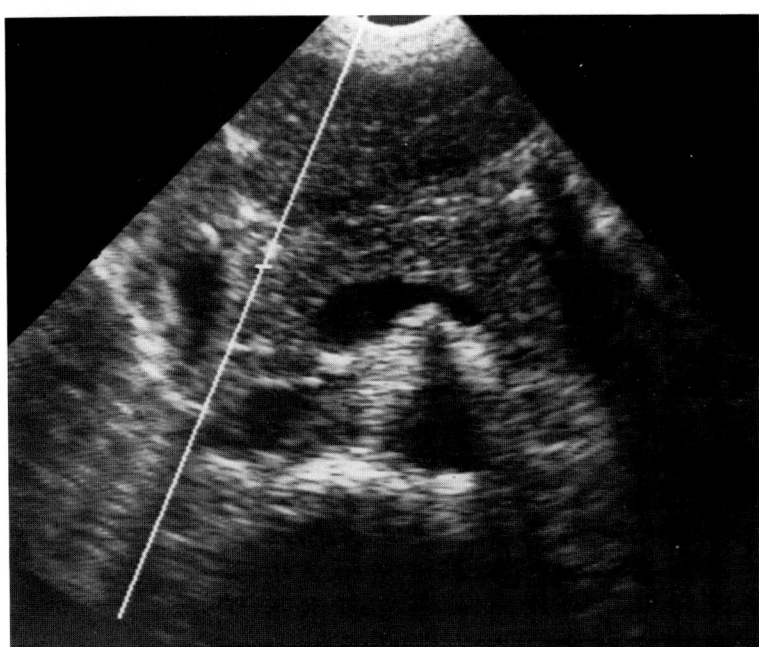

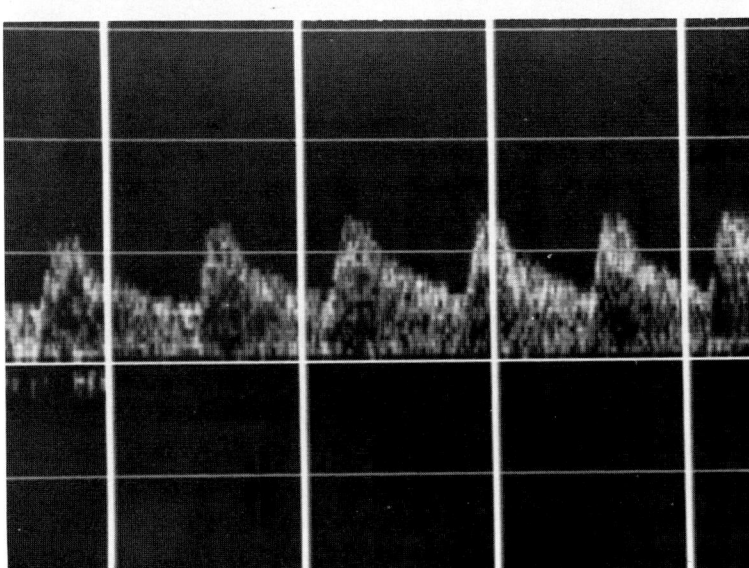

Fig. 4.6A,B. Normal gastroduodenal artery (GDA). **A.** Transverse image at the level of the pancreas. The cursor is located in the GDA, which courses ventral to the pancreatic head. **B.** Normal Doppler waveform in the GDA, with spectral broadening under the systolic peak.

mon hepatic artery, in approximately 30% of abdominal sonograms (11) (Fig. 4.6). The spectral display within this vessel often shows low-flow velocities, with spectral broadening.

Just beyond the celiac trifurcation, the proximal portions of the left gastric (Fig. 4.7) and splenic (Fig. 4.8) arteries are often visualized with ultrasound. Doppler waveforms in these vessels are similar to the main hepatic artery. Findings include a systolic peak with variable degrees of spectral broadening, followed by persistent diastolic flow. Due to the frequent tortuosity of the splenic artery, more turbulence may be demonstrated in this vessel than in the other celiac branches. This may be manifest by significant spectral broadening.

Superior Mesenteric Artery

The superior mesenteric artery (SMA), which supplies blood to much of the duodenum, the

Fig. 4.7A,B. Normal left gastric artery. **A.** Transverse sonogram of the celiac trifurcation, with Doppler sampling near the origin of the left gastric artery (*arrow*). **B.** Turbulent flow, manifest by the degree of spectral broadening, is demonstrated in the proximal portion of this vessel.

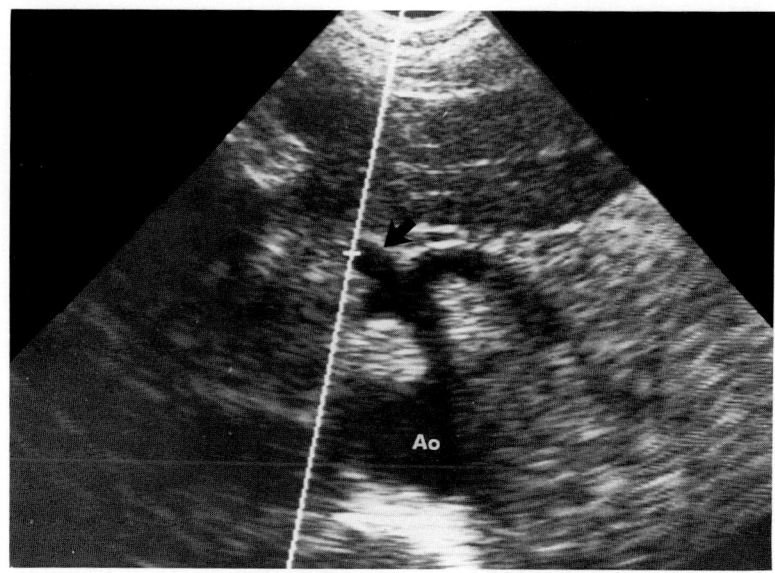

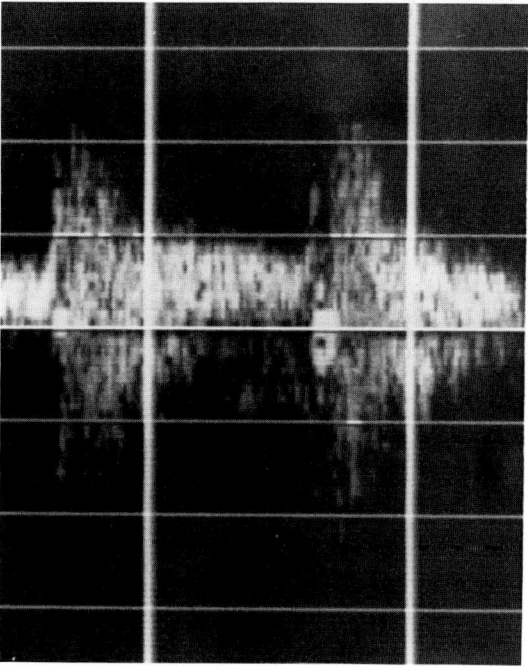

entire small bowel, and the right half of the colon is often sonographically imaged over a distance of several centimeters from its origin, just inferior to the celiac artery. The waveform display shows a relatively high velocity profile and variable degrees of spectral broadening (12) (Fig. 4.9). The latter finding is due to turbulence, which normally exists within the proximal portion of this vessel. Blood flow becomes more orderly when sampling at sites progressively further into the SMA. This is manifest by a lower peak velocity and often a clearer window under the systolic peak.

In the normal fasting state, high impedance exists within the superior mesenteric arterial circulation. This produces little or no diastolic flow and sometimes even transient flow reversal. When the latter occurs, a triphasic waveform is displayed, similar to spectra seen in peripheral arteries and in the external carotid arteries. The normal postprandial response in the SMA is decreased vascular resistance, caused by dilatation of the splanchnic circulation. Blood flow within the SMA has been shown to more than double within 15 minutes of a meal (13). Lowering of the vascular impedance within the SMA enhances diastolic flow, with loss of the reverse component on the Doppler waveform display.

Quantitation of the normal SMA Doppler signal may be undertaken using the pulsatility index (PI). It has been shown that the PI in the SMA is not influenced by either age or sex (2). The mean resting PI in fasting individuals has been reported as 3.57 (+0.11), with a range between 1.83 to 6.78 (2). This presumably results from physiologic variation in splanchnic blood flow, a finding documented in both humans and animals. Within 5 minutes after the completion of a meal, the PI may diminish by as much as 46% (2). This reduction is due to a

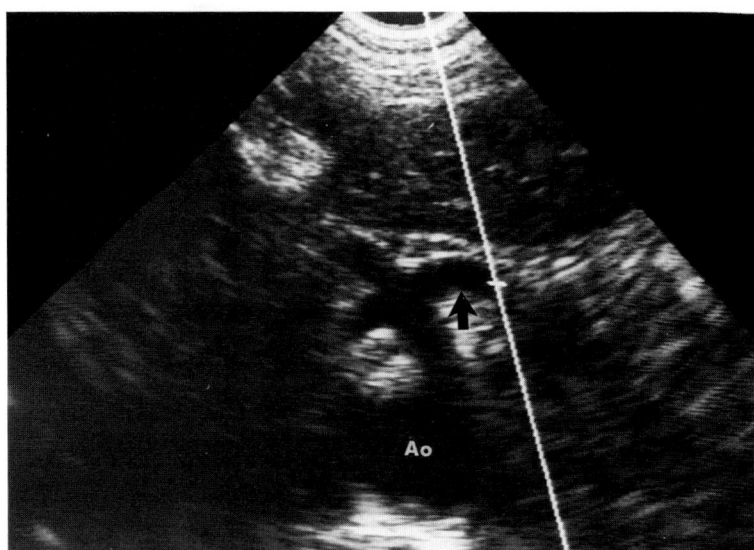

Fig. 4.8A,B. Normal splenic artery. **A.** Transverse imaging of the celiac trifurcation demonstrates the Doppler cursor within the splenic artery (*arrow*). **B.** Marked turbulence in the splenic arterial waveform display is a common finding, primarily due to the normally tortuous course of this vessel.

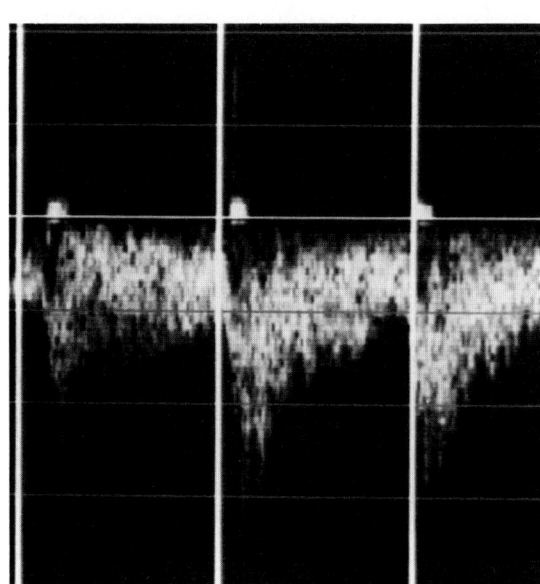

postprandial decrease in mesenteric resistance and has been shown to persist for more than 2 hours (2).

Renal Arteries and Veins

The main renal arteries, which arise from the lateral aspects of the midabdomen aorta, are often difficult to sonographically image due to overlying bowel gas. The proximal portions of these vessels are usually best demonstrated on transverse imaging through the anterior abdomen (Fig. 4.10*A*). Occasionally, on sagittal scans obtained through the flank, the main right renal artery is detected as it crosses posterior to the inferior vena cava (Fig. 4.10*B,C*). Waveforms from the renal parenchymal arteries are almost invariably detected when studying the kidney through a translumbar or (lateral) transabdominal approach. The spectral display from the main renal arteries characteristically shows a moderately high frequency systolic phase, followed by a continuous diastolic flow component. Waveforms that are obtained from the renal sinus region, as well as from the corticomedullary junction (arcuate arteries), have a similar appearance except for gradual diminution in the systolic peak amplitude and greater spectral broadening.

The main renal veins may also be interrogated with duplex ultrasound, when overlying bowel gas does not preclude adequate study (Fig. 4.11). The normal spectra from these systemic veins is characterized as a low-velocity tracing, with continuous flow and mild amplitude variation resulting from respiratory and cardiac motion. Not infrequently, Doppler tracings obtained at various sites within the renal parenchyma will simultaneously display both arterial and venous waveforms, being detected within the same sample volume (Fig. 4.12).

Fig. 4.9A–E. Normal superior mesenteric artery (SMA). **A.** Transverse and **B.** Sagittal images of the proximal SMA (*arrowheads*). **C.** The corresponding Doppler tracing reveals a relatively high-velocity profile and spectral broadening in the proximal SMA. *(Continued.)*

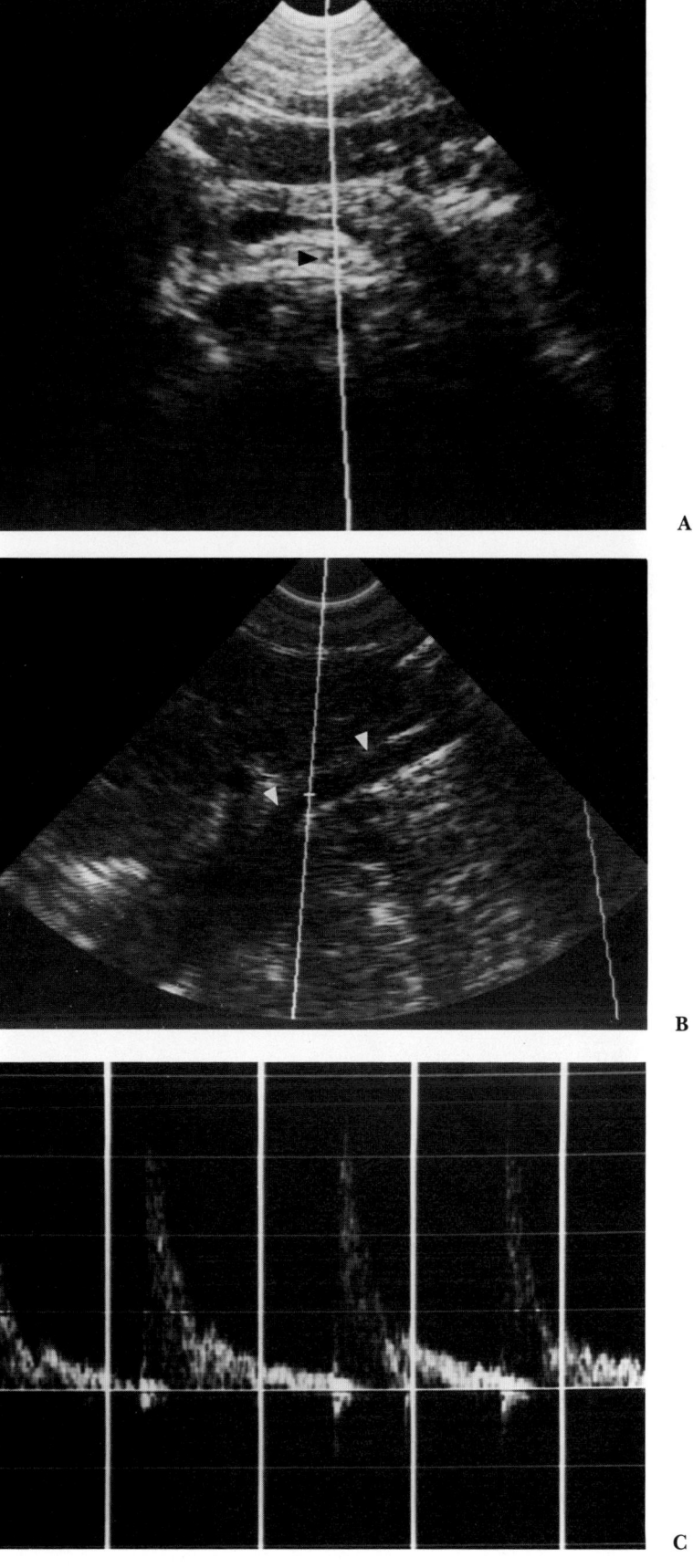

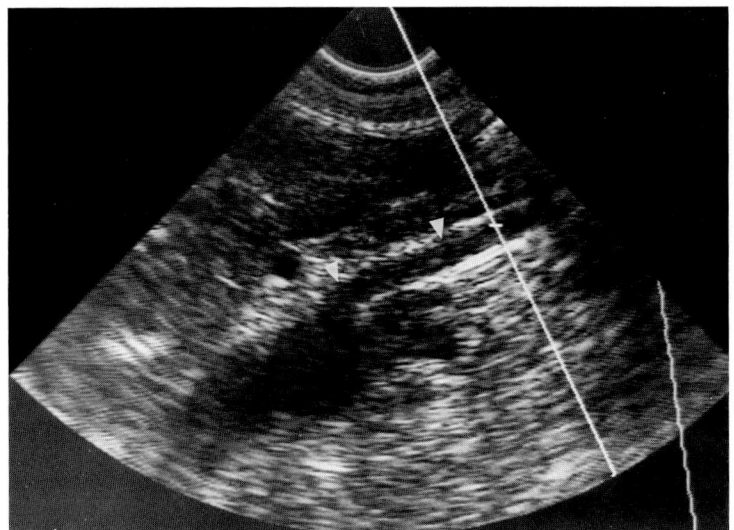

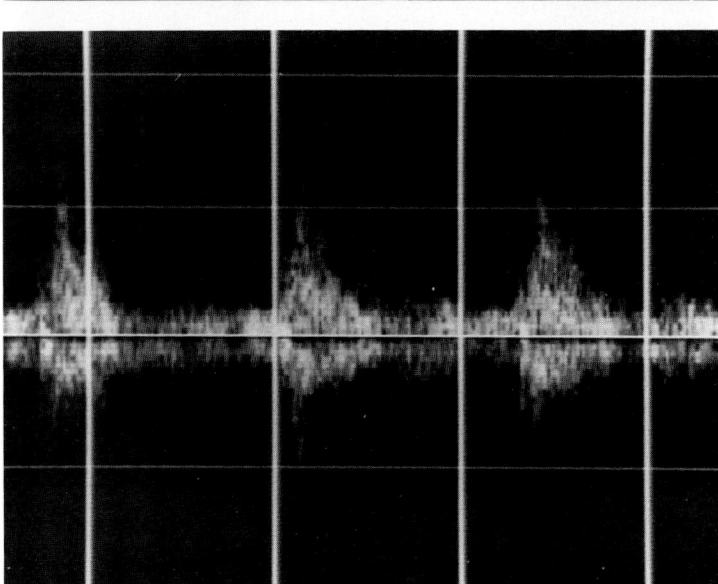

Fig. 4.9D. Sagittal image with Doppler sampling in the distal SMA (*arrowheads*). **E.** Decrease in the amplitude of the frequency shift (velocity) is often observed at progressively more distal sites in the SMA.

Hepatic Veins and Inferior Vena Cava

Significant variation in both blood flow velocity and directionality are demonstrated within the hepatic veins and inferior vena cava (IVC) (Fig. 4.13). These changes depend in large part on the phase of respiration and on cardiac activity. Normally, there is free reflux of blood from the right atrium during systole. This, combined with changes in flow due to respiratory excursions, results in a complex bidirectional spectral display with portions of the waveform both above and below the baseline. In instances where these structures are difficult to visualize, performance of a Valsalva maneuver may help to distend the veins and facilitate Doppler sampling.

Splenoportal Venous System

Almost invariably, the normal central intrahepatic portal venous branches are adequately visualized for pulsed-Doppler analysis. The extrahepatic portal vein is sonographically demonstrated in more than 90% of individuals studied, the splenic vein in approximately 85%, and the superior mesenteric vein in about 75%

Fig. 4.10A–C. Normal renal artery. **A.** Transverse sonogram shows the origin of the right renal artery (*open arrows*) from the aorta (Ao), ventral to the spine (Sp). **B.** Sagittal abdomen ultrasound demonstrates the cursor within the right renal artery (*curved black arrow*) as it crosses posterior to the IVC (*white arrows*). **C.** Typical renal artery Doppler waveform, with a systolic peak and continuous diastolic flow.

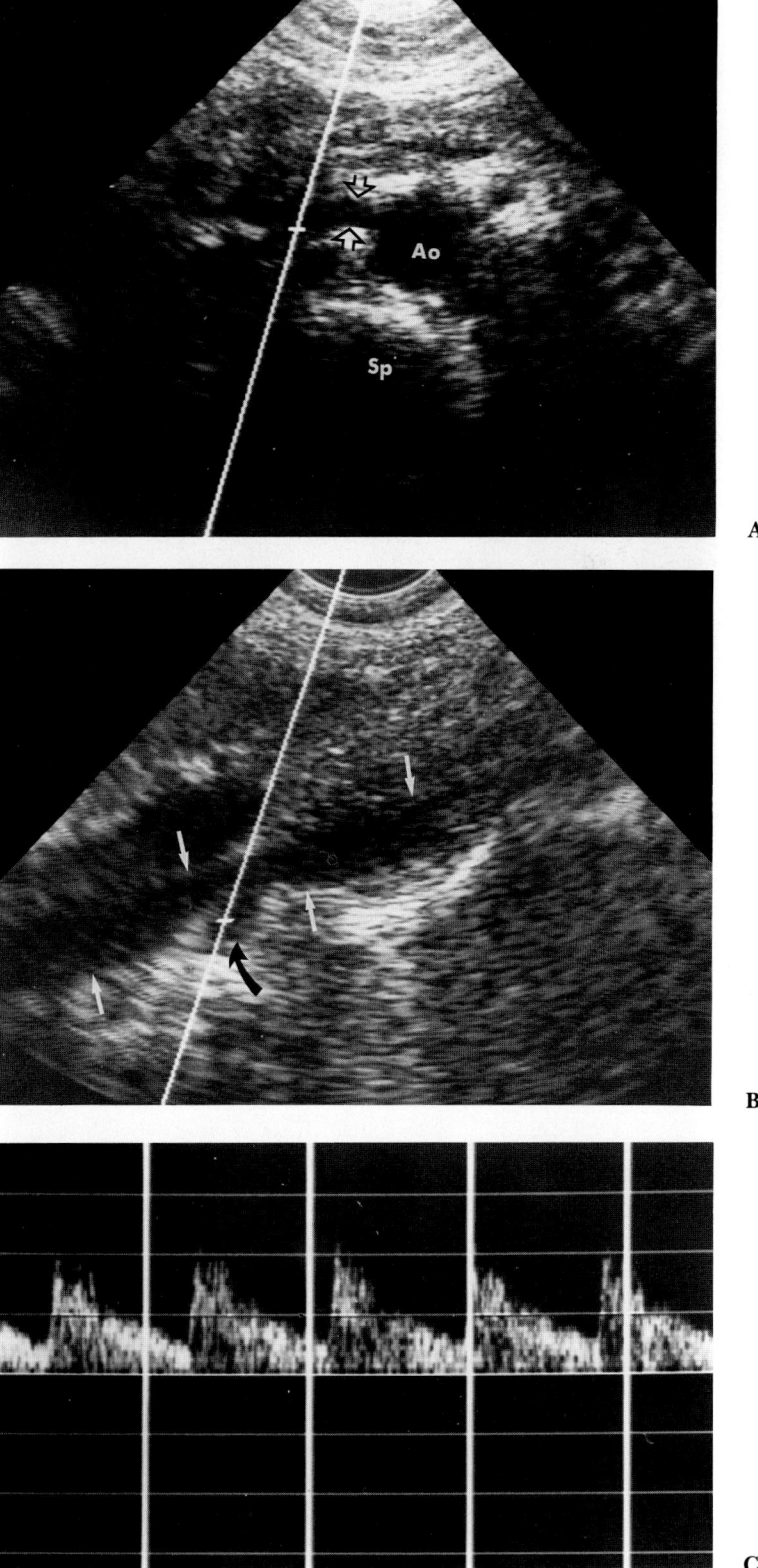

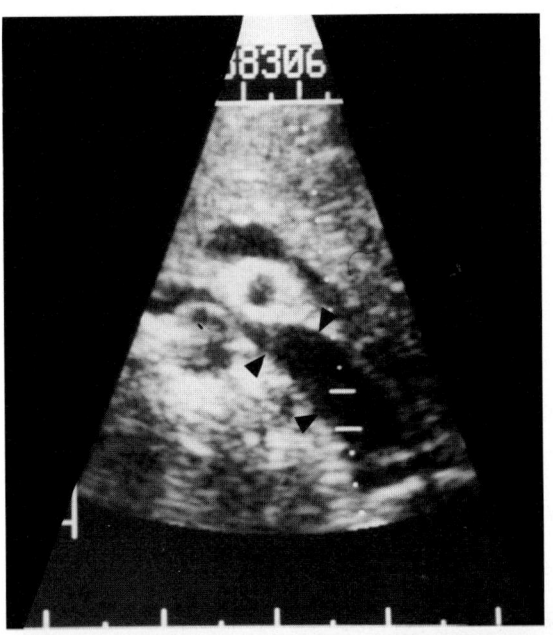

Fig. 4.11A,B. Normal renal vein. **A.** The normal left renal vein (*arrowheads*) is imaged transversely, as it courses between the aorta and SMA to drain into the IVC. **B.** A low-velocity, continuous venous flow is typically observed within this vessel.

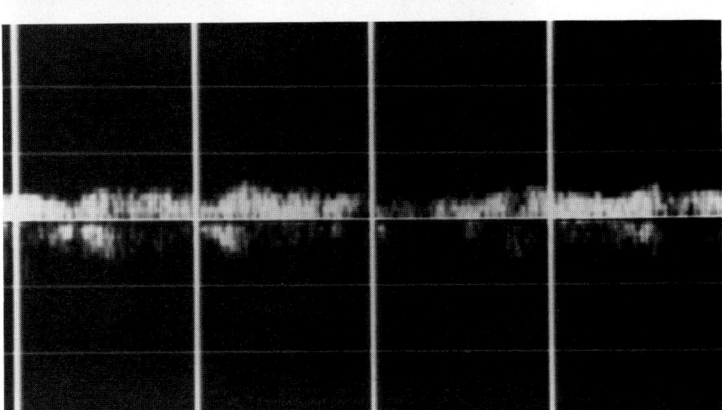

of cases (14). Inability to visualize these vessels with ultrasound usually results from overlying bowel gas.

The normal spectra within the portal, splenic, and superior mesenteric veins differs significantly from both the systemic arterial and venous systems. The unique splenoportal waveform results from the location of this vascular system between two capillary beds, the mesenteric and hepatic circulations. This buffering effect leads to a continuous, low-velocity blood flow that is directed hepatopetally (Fig. 4.14). Normally, there is mild respiratory variation in waveform amplitude, with increased flow during inspiration. In addition, slight flow turbulence may be present in the splenoportal systems, appearing as "roughness" in the spectral waveform. The audible output from these vessels typically resembles a low-pitched rumble.

Duplex Analysis of Diseases Affecting Abdominal Blood Flow

Abdominal Aorta

Pulsed-Doppler analysis provides a useful adjunct to conventional real-time ultrasound imaging in the evaluation of abdominal aortic pathology. In the adult population, one of the

Fig. 4.12A,B. Normal intrarenal vessels. **A.** Sagittal scan of the kidney obtained during duplex examination within the renal parenchyma. **B.** The spectral waveforms present within the renal cortex frequently demonstrate both arterial and venous tracings, simultaneously detected within the sample volume.

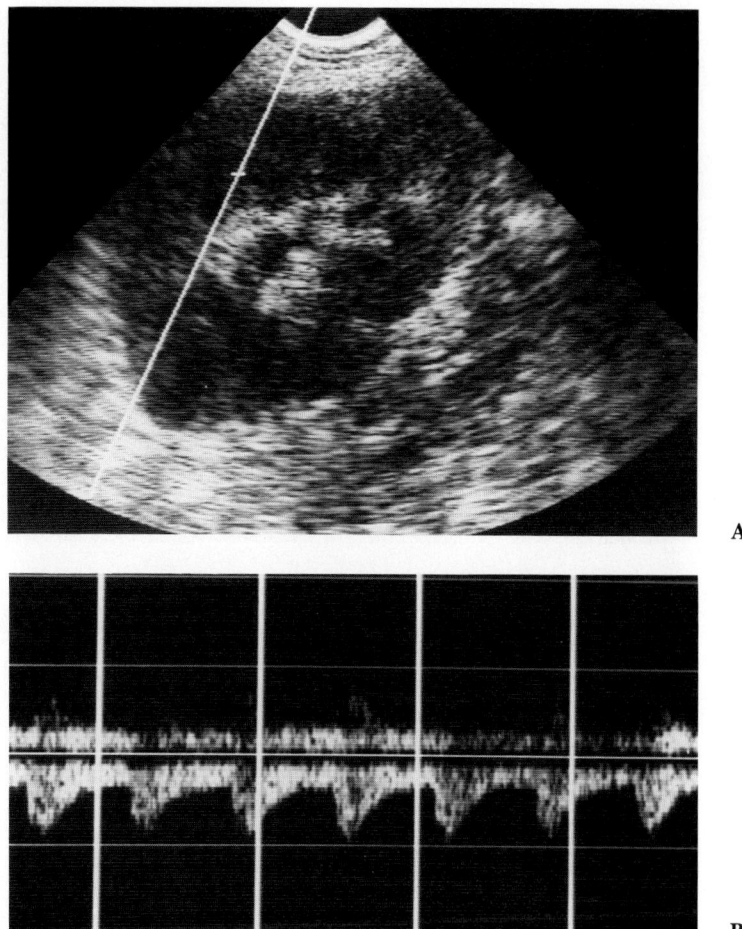

most common diseases to affect the aorta is atherosclerosis. Identification of atherosclerotic plaque, whether calcified or noncalcified, is easily accomplished by real-time sonography. Doppler may be used to demonstrate regions secondarily affected by turbulent blood flow. On the waveform display, this appears as spectral broadening and, with significant luminal narrowing, an increased Doppler frequency shift in the stenotic area. With more severe turbulence, the waveform becomes further distorted.

Aneurysms represent another common abnormality of the abdominal aorta. Dimensions of an aneurysm may be established by real-time imaging. The location of the aneurysm and involvement of major aortic branches, particularly the renal arteries, are other important factors to define for appropriate surgical planning. Doppler analysis provides additional information regarding blood flow alteration within the aneurysm. Different waveform displays have been demonstrated in aortic aneurysms. Spectral broadening caused by turbulent blood flow is frequently present. Turbulence results from eddies and vortexes that form as blood suddenly passes from the normal caliber aorta into the dilated segment (Fig. 4.15). With severe turbulence, bidirectional blood flow may develop, manifest by a waveform variably deflected above and below the baseline. In addition, the amplitude of the velocity profile usually diminishes within an aneurysm. The degree of damping in blood flow velocity depends on several factors, such as the severity of luminal aortic dilation. For example, large aneurysms, particularly those with little organized thrombus along the walls, often have

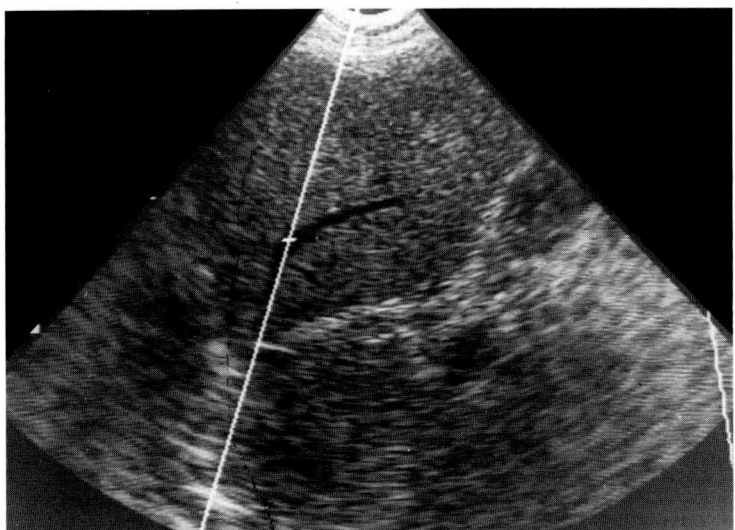
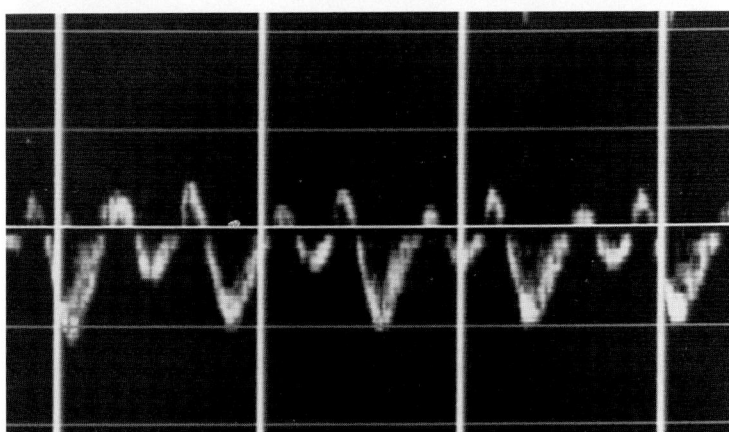

Fig. 4.13A,B. Normal hepatic veins. **A.** Doppler analysis of a normal hepatic vein on this sagittal scan of the liver. **B.** The normal spectra within the hepatic veins and IVC demonstrates a complex, bidirectional waveform, deflected on both sides of the baseline. This is due in large part to the free reflux of blood from the right atrium during systole.

marked blood flow turbulence. Finally in the case of aortic dissection, duplex sonography may be helpful in confirming two lumens. This modality may also allow for identification of the true and false lumens (Figs. 4.16 and 4.17).

Inferior Vena Cava

Within the upper abdomen, the inferior vena cava is usually well visualized sonographically using the liver as an acoustic window. However, low-level echoes may be present within the vascular lumen (Fig. 4.18). This is frequently caused either by high gain settings necessary for adequate imaging or by echogenic laminar blood flow. The appearance may simulate luminal occlusion from thrombus or tumor. In this situation, Doppler analysis is extremely useful for establishing vascular patency. When thrombus is documented, Doppler sampling may help to identify a residual lumen or recanalized channel (Figs. 4.19 and 4.20). Duplex sonography has also been used as a noninvasive technique to study patients with inferior vena cava filters (15). Not only may the filter position within the IVC be confirmed by real-time imaging, but blood flow information may also be acquired through use of duplex ultrasound. For instance, the extent of intracaval thrombus may be better clarified with Doppler analysis than by real-time imaging alone. Furthermore, patency of vessels which supply the IVC, such as the renal and hepatic veins, may be documented.

Fig. 4.14A–C. Normal splenoportal venous system. **A**. Transverse image of the liver, with the sample volume positioned in the portal venous lumen. **B**. Transverse sonogram of the pancreas, with the Doppler cursor located in the splenic vein. **C**. Typical waveform display in the splenoportal venous system. This is characterized by continuous, low-velocity flow and mild amplitude variation with respiration.

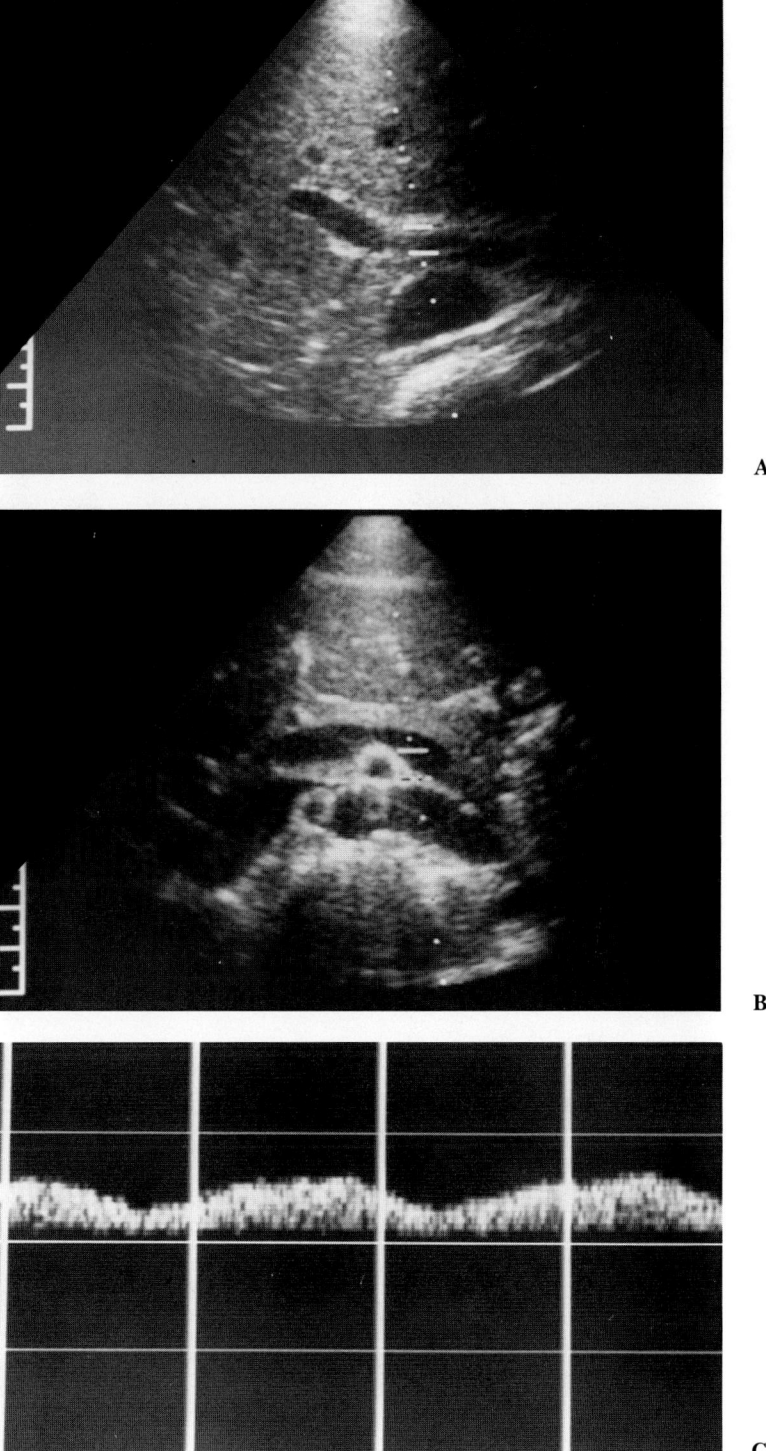

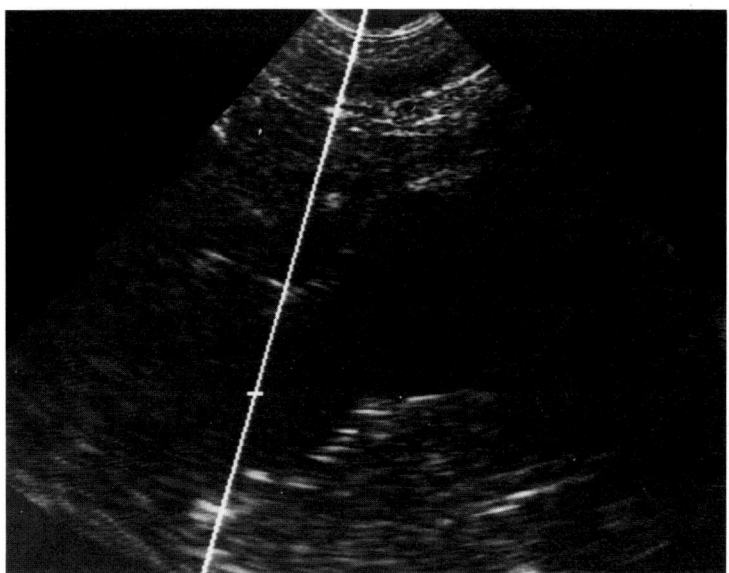

Fig. 4.15A–D. Abdominal aortic aneurysm. **A.** Sagittal image of the midabdominal aorta. The sample volume is placed proximal to the aneurysm. **B.** The corresponding waveform (to 15**A**) demonstrates a relatively normal aortic waveform. **C.** A sagittal scan obtained more inferiorly shows the cursor within the central portion of the aneurysm. **D.** The correlative tracing (to 15**C**) reveals a turbulent blood flow pattern often demonstrated within these aneurysms. The spectra appears as a low-velocity, complex, bidirectional waveform.

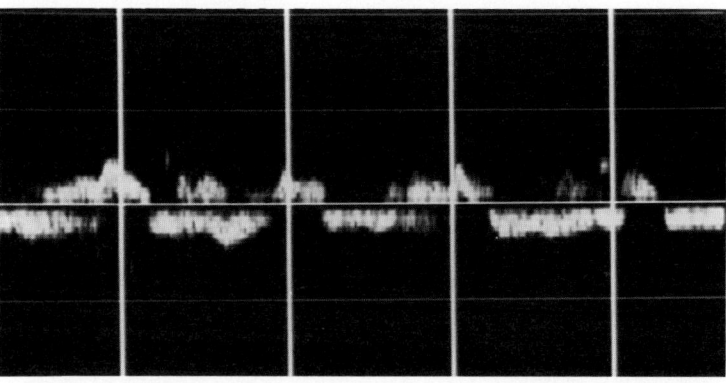

Fig. 4.15.

When the IVC is markedly displaced by large retroperitoneal masses, duplex ultrasound may allow for verification of patency within the compressed lumen (Fig. 4.21).

Duplex sonography also provides a noninvasive means to diagnose congenital anomalies of the IVC. Doppler sampling within the aberrantly located vessel confirms a central systemic venous waveform and may help in following its intraabdominal course. Some developmental defects of the IVC that can be diagnosed by duplex ultrasound include interruption of the IVC with azygous-hemiazygous continuation, transposition of the IVC, and duplication of the IVC. With interruption of the IVC, the cava has a normal course from the common iliac venous bifurcation to the level of the renal veins. The intrahepatic portion of the IVC is absent, with hepatic veins draining directly into the right atrium (16). Enlargement of the azygous-hemiazygous veins may be identified in the retrocrural space, on either side of the aorta. Although infrahepatic interruption of the IVC occurs as an isolated anomaly, it is often associated with other developmental defects, including cyanotic and acyanotic congenital heart disease as well as abnormalities in cardiac orientation and abdominal situs (17). It is frequently found in polysplenia and asplenia, and other findings of these syndromes should be sought for during the ultrasound examination (17). In transposition of the IVC, duplex sonography may demonstrate the cava as it crosses from an aberrant left-sided position to the normal right-sided location, at the level of the renal veins. Finally, duplication of the IVC may be identified by demonstrating systemic venous flow in two vascular channels on either side of the lower abdominal aorta. These structures ascend to the level of the renal veins. At this site, the left-sided cava joins the right side through a small vascular channel. Doppler sampling at selected locations in the abdomen may be extremely helpful in clarifying this anatomy.

Hepatic Circulation

Many applications of duplex ultrasound have been described to evaluate the liver. These are considered separately under hepatic arterial or portal venous inflow to the liver, or under hepatic venous drainage of this organ.

Hepatic Artery

Both aneurysms and pseudoaneurysms may develop in the hepatic arterial system. The hepatic artery represents the fourth most frequent location for abdominal aneurysms, followed by the infrarenal aorta, iliac arteries, and splenic artery (18). Approximately 75% develop extrahepatically, and the remaining 25% occur intrahepatically (19). The most common etiologies, in order of frequency, include atherosclerotic disease, infection, and trauma (20). The primary concern regarding hepatic artery aneurysms is catastrophic rupture, which occurs in up to 80% of cases (18). As with the abdominal aorta, aneurysms are identified and

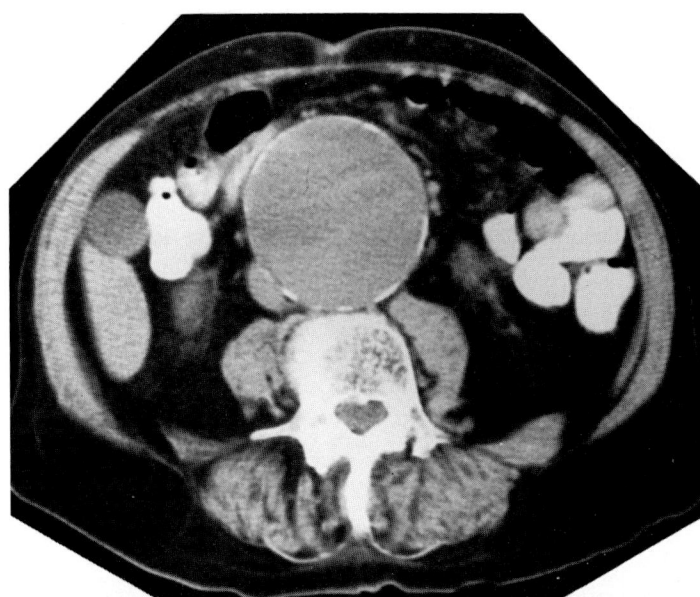

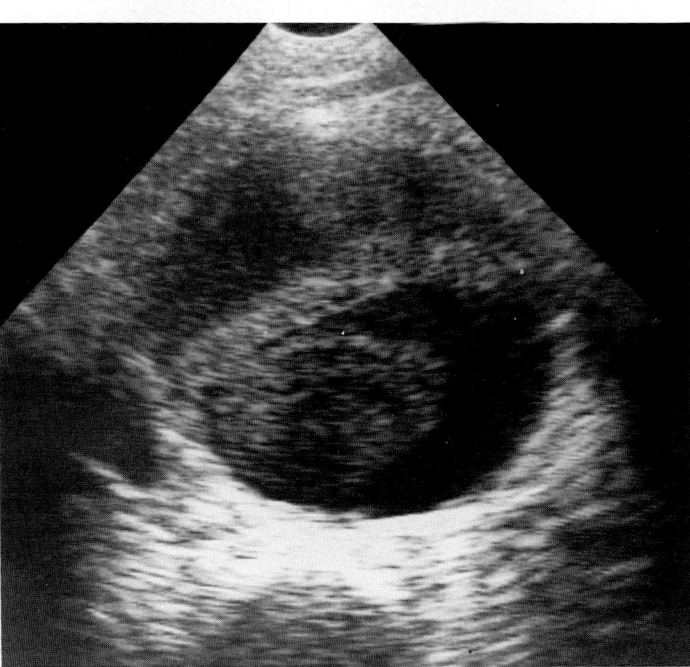

Fig. 4.16A–H. Abdominal aortic dissection. **A.** A non-contrast-enhanced CT scan of the abdomen demonstrates marked dilatation of the aorta. **B.** Transverse sonogram reveals two lumens within the aorta, separated by a thick echogenic band. Swirling blood was visualized in the posterior lumen on real-time imaging. **C.** Sagittal image with the Doppler cursor placed proximal to the aneurysm. **D.** The waveform display obtained at 16**C** shows a normal aortic tracing. **E.** Duplex analysis of the posterior (true) lumen. *(Continued.)*

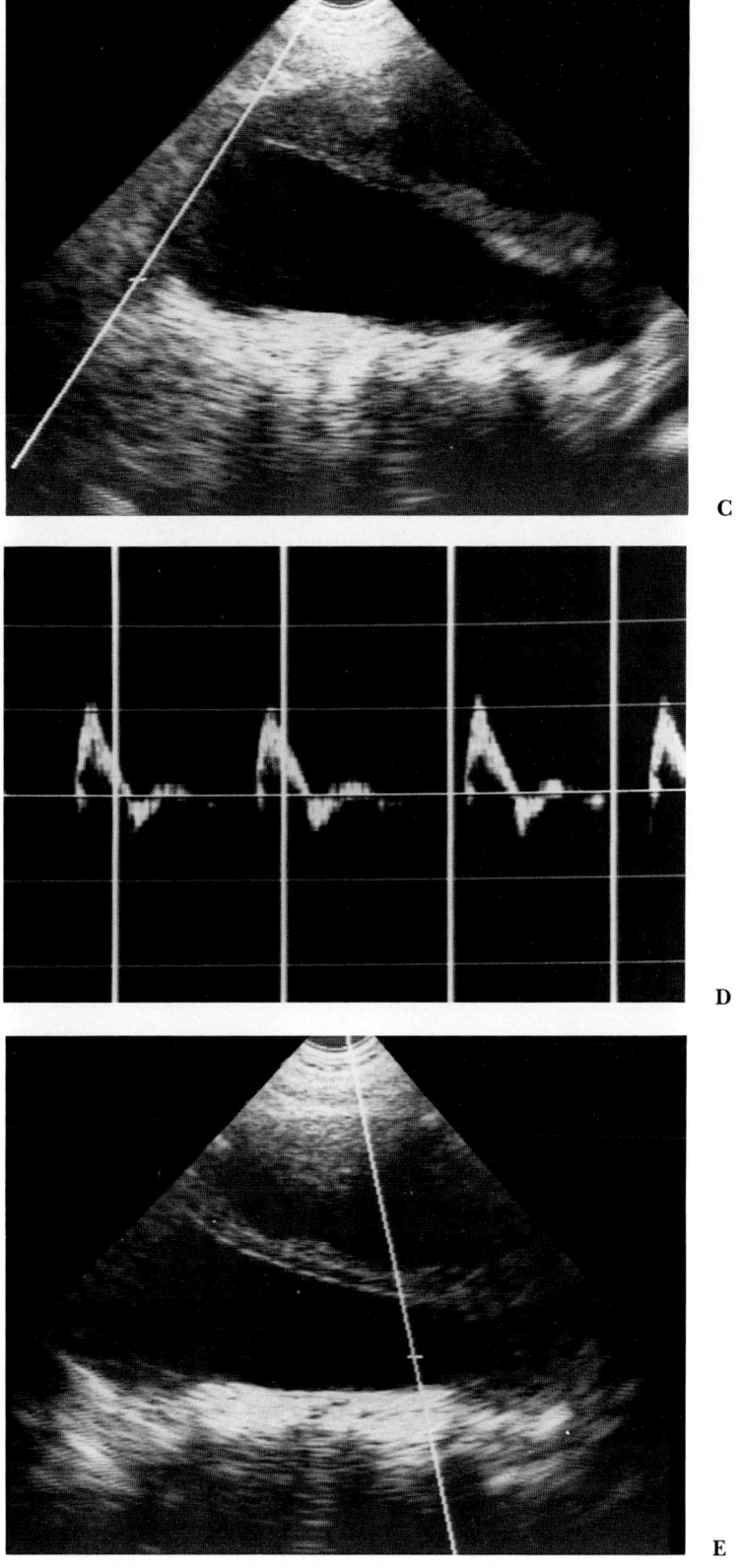

Fig. 4.16.

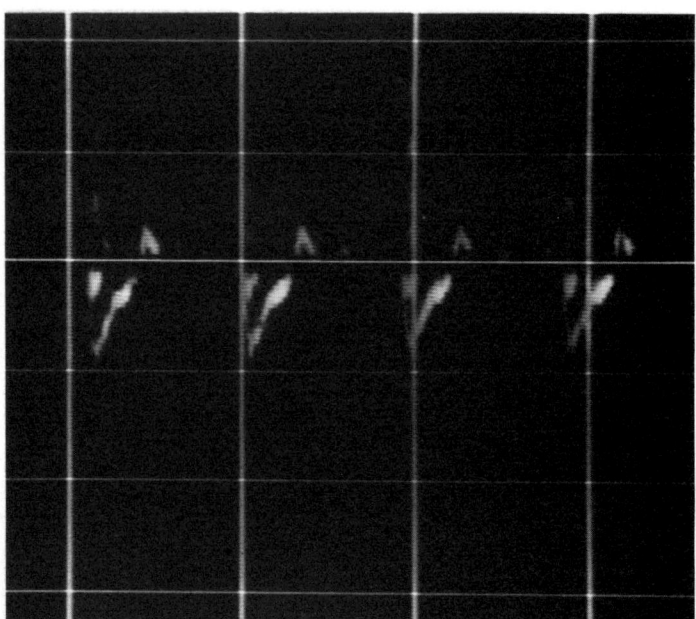

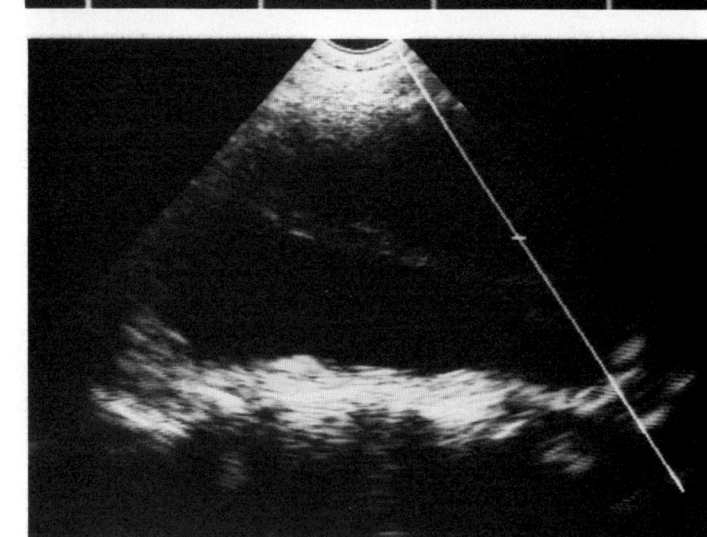

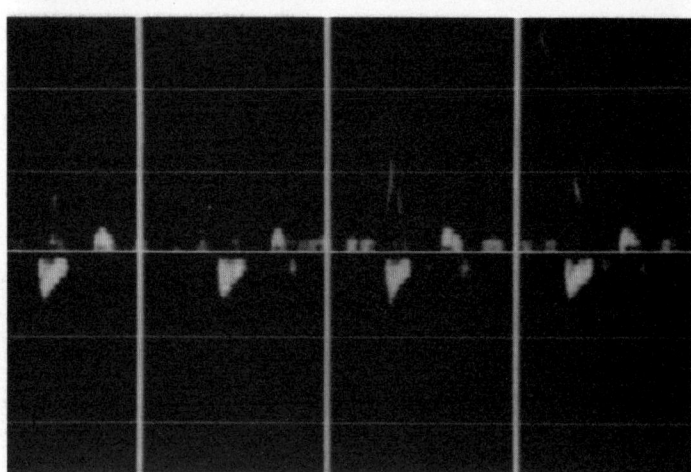

Fig. 4.16F. The waveform obtained at 16**E** resembles that seen in the proximal, normal aorta. **G.** Doppler sampling in the anterior (false) lumen. The spectral display obtained at 4.16**G** shows decreased signal amplitude compared with the normal aorta, proximally. There is also evidence of a turbulent, bidirectional component in blood flow.

Fig. 4.17A–H. Abdominal aortic dissection. **A.** Sagittal scan in the abdominal aorta, which has two vascular lumens. The anterior lumen is being sampled on this tracing. **B.** The waveform display obtained from 4.17A appears normal. *(Continued.)*

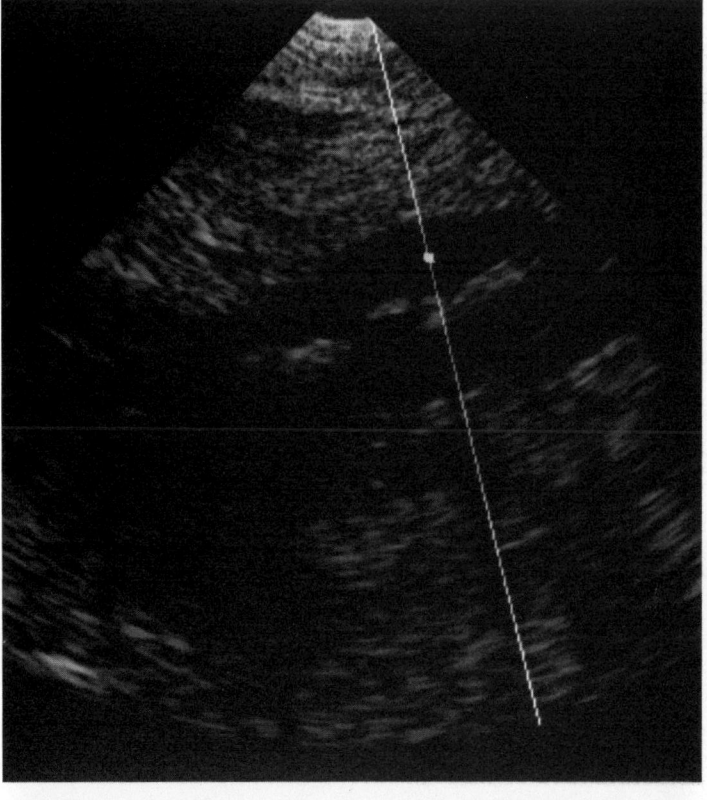

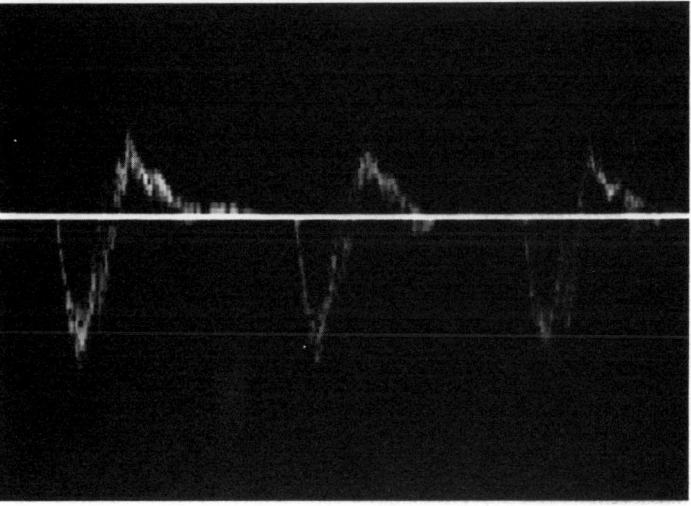

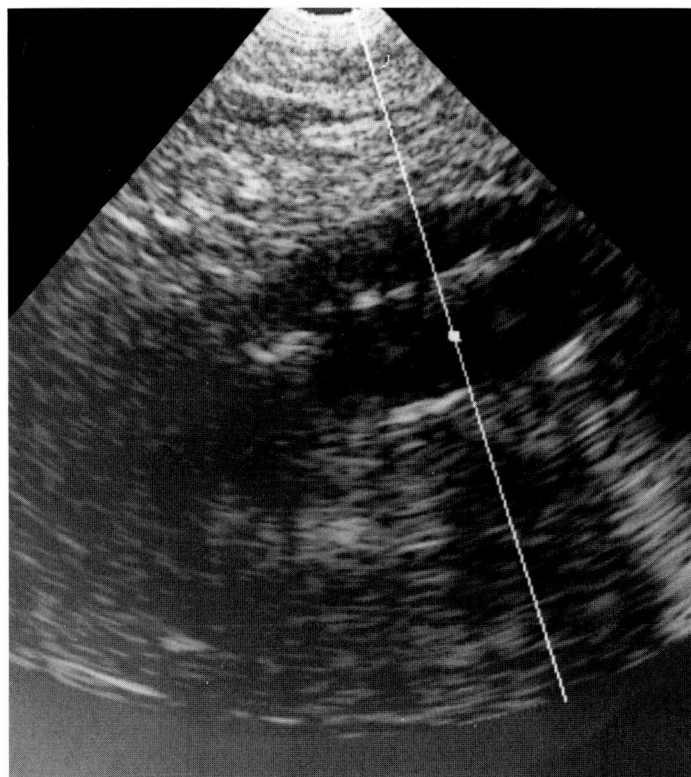

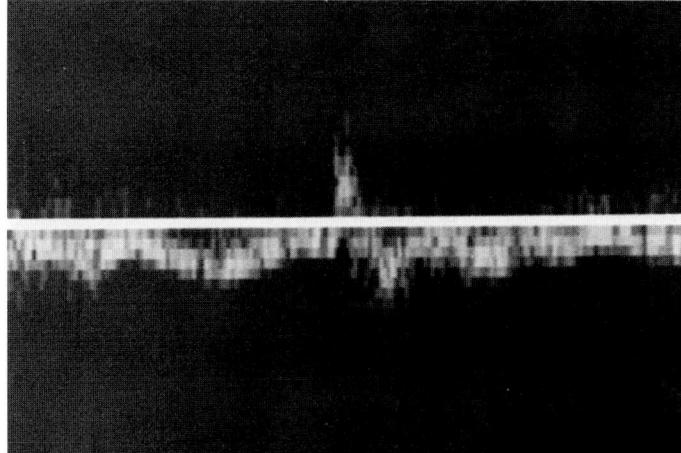

Fig. 4.17C. Duplex examination of the posterior lumen of this aortic dissection. **D.** A continuous flow pattern is demonstrated, with occasional small peaks resulting from transient velocity acceleration. **E,F.** Lateral views from an abdominal aortogram. Note two catheters in place, one within the anterior (true) lumen and the other within the posterior (false) lumen. On initial contrast injection, the true lumen opacifies. *(Continued.)*

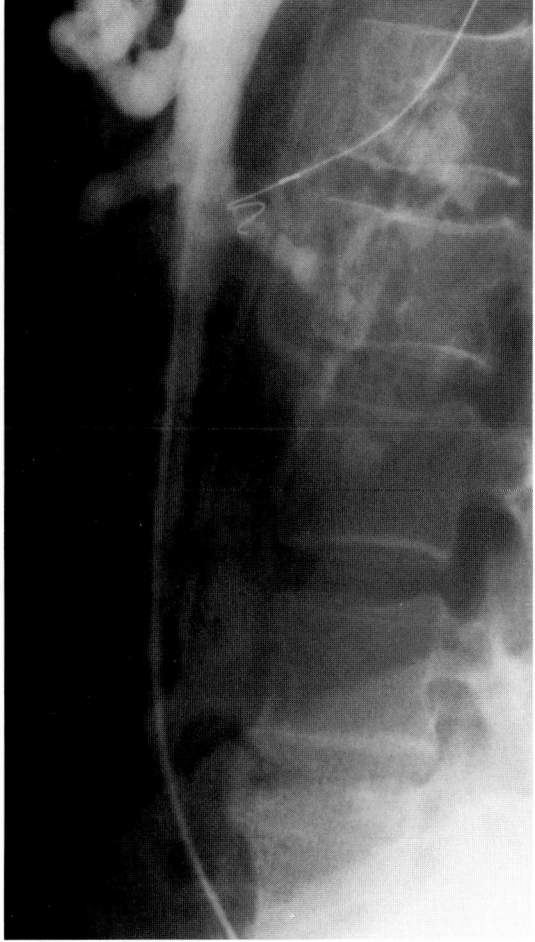 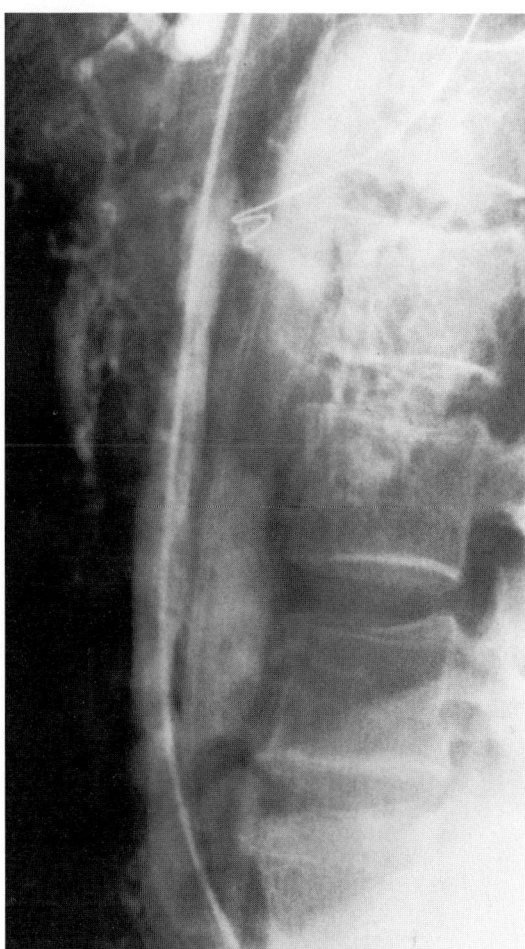

E F

Fig. 4.17.

dimensions measured by real-time imaging. In one report describing sonographic findings of five hepatic artery aneurysms, the four intrahepatic lesions appeared as primarily anechoic, well-circumscribed masses that were nonpulsatile, although flow was demonstrated in one case (21). The single extrahepatic aneurysm in this series presented as a lobulated, anechoic, pulsatile mass (21). When such findings are demonstrated on real-time scans, duplex sonography may be used as an adjunct to confirm an arterial tracing and to assess the degree of turbulent blood flow. Large aneurysms often demonstrate more severe turbulence and greater waveform damping than in small aneurysms. Sampling distal to hepatic arterial aneurysms will usually demonstrate at least partial reconstitution of a more normal hepatic arterial waveform.

Pseudoaneurysms of the hepatic artery also may present as nonpulsatile, circumscribed, sonolucent masses (22). These usually develop in patients with a history of chronic pancreatitis. The inflammatory process may affect any of the peripancreatic arteries, with pseudoaneurysm formation complicating 10% of cases (23). When the lesion is nonpulsatile, the sonographic appearance may be indistinguishable from a pseudocyst. Use of Doppler analysis within the pseudoaneurysm, however, will confirm turbulent arterial flow (Fig. 4.22). With larger pseudoaneurysms, the waveform may become markedly distorted, with damping and

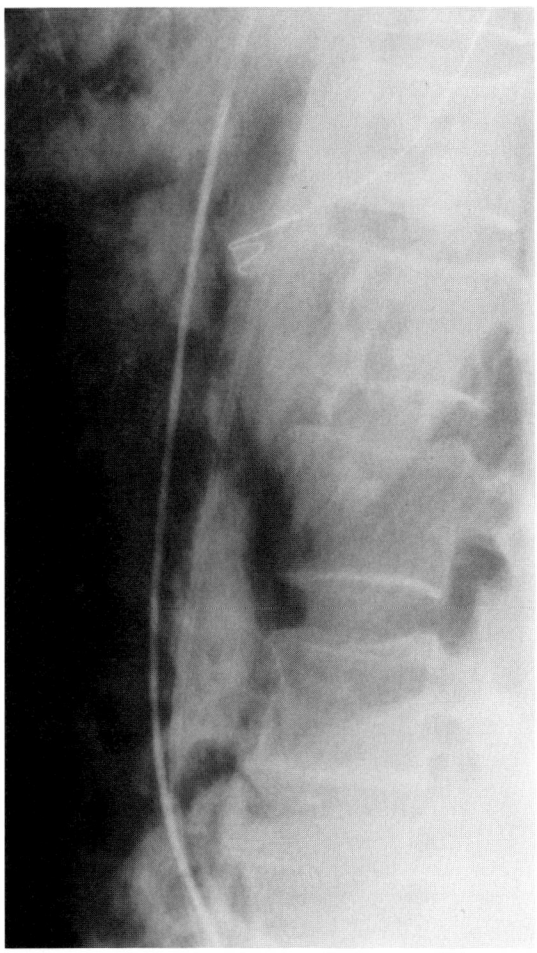

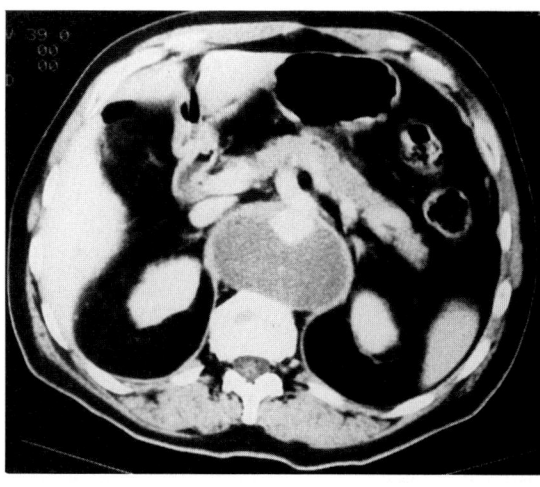

Fig. 4.17G. During progressively later phases of the injection, the posterior false lumen becomes better visualized. **H.** A few months later, this contrast-enhanced CT examination shows enlargement of the posterior false lumen of this dissection.

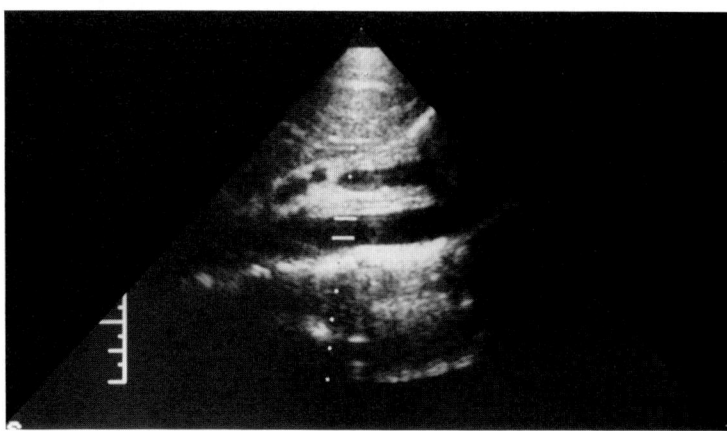

Fig. 4.18A,B. Inferior vena cava—Intraluminal echoes. **A.** Sagittal image of the IVC demonstrating low-level internal echoes. On occasion, this may be confused with intraluminal disease. **B.** The Doppler waveform confirms vascular patency by demonstrating a normal IVC tracing.

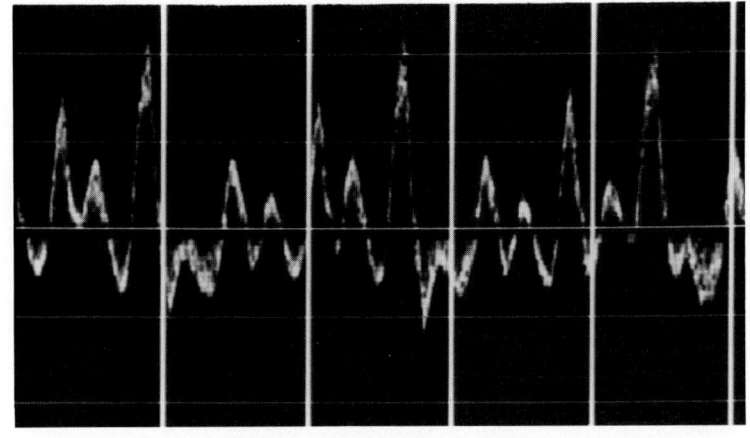

Fig. 4.18.

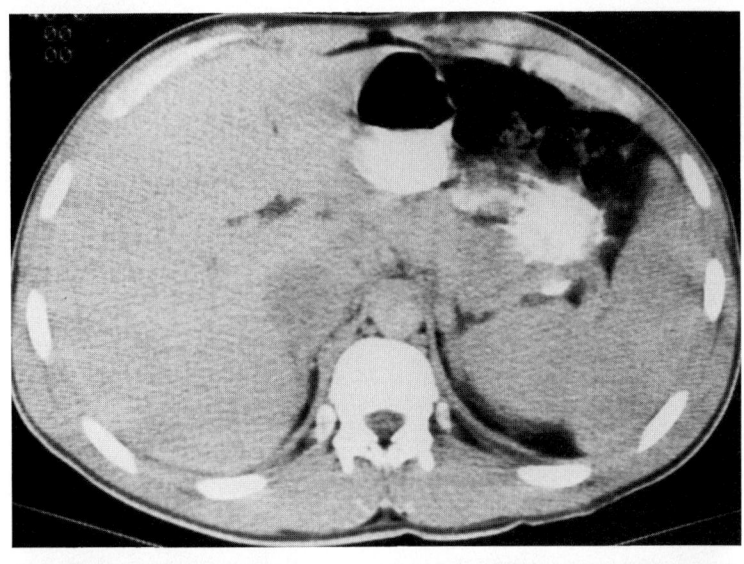

Fig. 4.19A,B. IVC thrombus. **A.** Non-enhanced CT image obtained through the upper abdomen demonstrates a large IVC. Without intravenous contrast (contraindicated due to allergy), the presence of thrombus cannot be determined on this examination. **B.** Sagittal ultrasound image of the IVC shows a large thrombus. This completely occludes the lumen inferiorly (*solid arrows*), but is patent superiorly (*open arrow*).

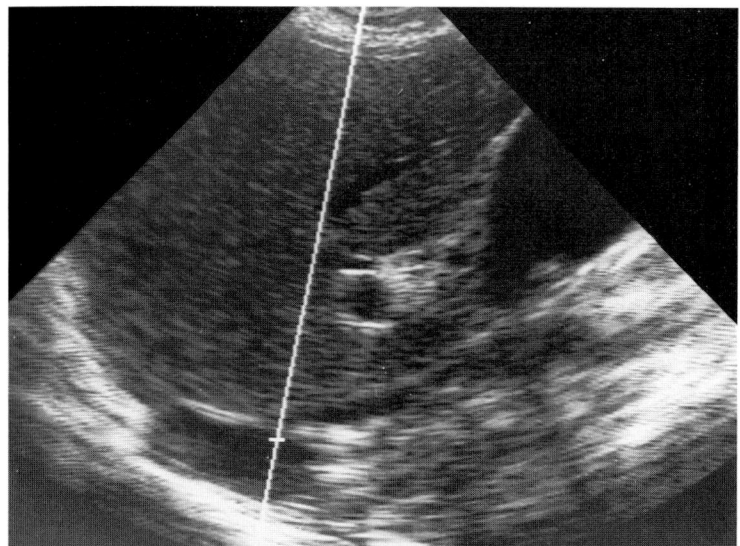

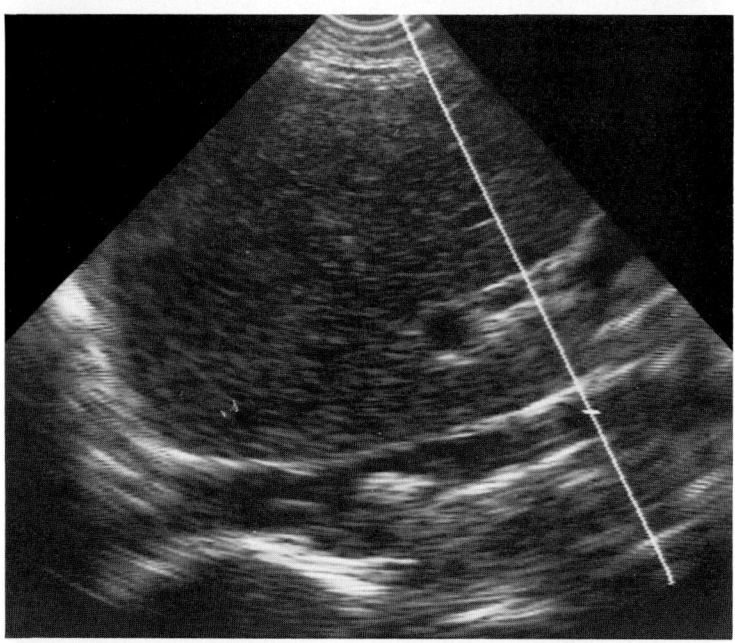

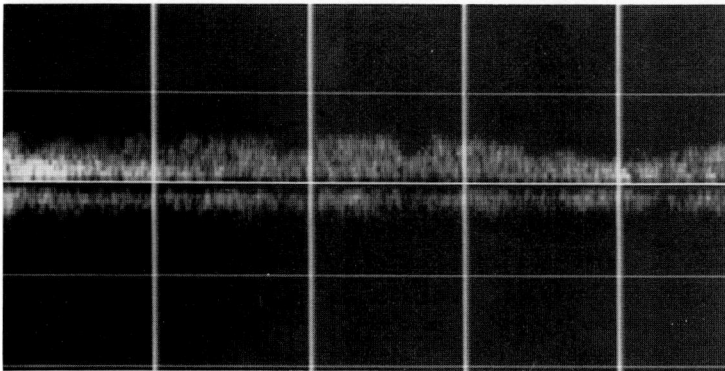

Fig. 4.20A–D. IVC thrombus. **A,B.** Doppler cursor placement at different sites within the IVC. Note the partial intraluminal thrombus. **C.** Spectral display demonstrates venous flow around the thrombus. **D.** Inferior vena cavogram shows thrombus extending along a portion of the IVC lumen (*arrows*).

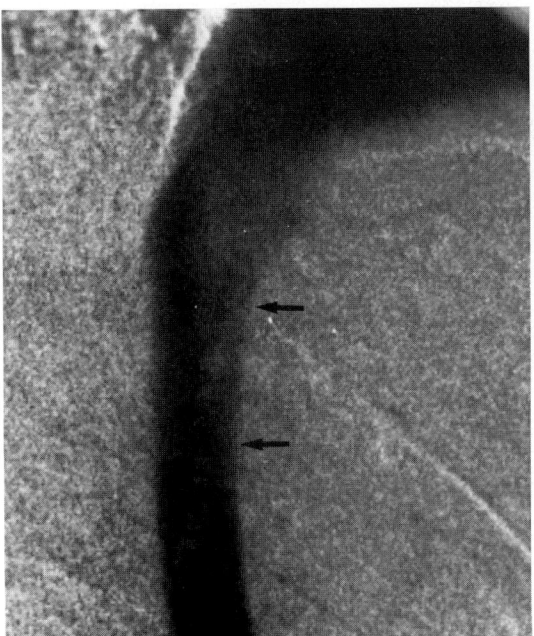

D

Fig. 4.20.

severe turbulence. Difficulty occasionally arises in differentiating true from false aneurysms by real-time imaging alone. Furthermore, many of the Doppler features are indistinguishable. One finding that we have observed in a few pseudoaneurysms is a "jet," or sudden systolic velocity acceleration, at a peripheral site within the abnormal vascular structure. This finding suggests identification of the pseudoaneurysm neck. The "jet effect" is caused by a high volume of blood flowing rapidly across a relatively narrow orifice. The result is an abrupt increase in the Doppler frequency shift of the arterial waveform, usually associated with marked spectral broadening. Sampling within the pseudoaneurysm at more distant sites from the neck demonstrates progressive damping in velocity. This constellation of findings may prove helpful in diagnosing pseudoaneurysms and perhaps also in distinguishing true and false aneurysms.

Within the porta hepatis, duplex scanning has been used to defined structures comprising the portal triad, which include the hepatic artery, portal vein, and bile duct. At the hilum of the liver, the hepatic artery and bile duct have a variable relationship. In one study, 85% of sonograms that adequately visualized the porta hepatis demonstrated the right hepatic artery to course between the dorsally located portal vein and the ventrally situated bile duct (24). In the remaining 15% of cases, the right hepatic artery was positioned ventral to the bile duct (24). These anatomic variations, combined with frequent inability to trace structures to known landmarks, often make it difficult to define the components of the portal triad by real-time imaging alone. Duplex ultrasound may readily identify the hepatic artery and portal vein by their different Doppler waveforms. The bile duct is then recognized as the remaining tubular structure with absence of Doppler signal. Definition of this anatomy is particularly important among patients with enlarged hepatic arteries, which may simulate a dilated biliary ductal system (Fig. 4.23). In one study of eight patients with histories of alcoholism and/or cirrhosis, duplex ultrasound allowed for correct identification of enlarged hepatic arteries, which resembled dilated bile ducts (25). This distinction, which is critical for appropriate patient management, may not be possible with real-time imaging alone.

The hepatic artery may occasionally become thrombosed. This is often traumatic or iatrogenic in origin, for instance from dissection which may complicate angiographic catheter placement into the hepatic artery. After liver transplantation, hepatic arterial occlusion has been found to occur in 7% of individuals. This reportedly increases to as high as 23% among patients with complex arterial reconstructions (26). In these patients, duplex ultrasound is extremely useful as a means to noninvasively confirm hepatic arterial flow (26). Another indication for hepatic artery evaluation in liver transplants involves waveform alterations, which frequently accompany rejection. In the rejecting transplant, increased vascular impedance often develops. On the spectral display this may become manifest by loss of hepatic arterial flow in diastole (26). However, this finding is not invariably present in all individuals with liver transplant rejection, possibly due to the dual blood supply to the liver.

Finally, documentation of hepatic arterial patency should be undertaken in all patients with partial or complete portal vein occlusion to verify adequate liver perfusion. Frequently, patients with portal vein occlusion will show

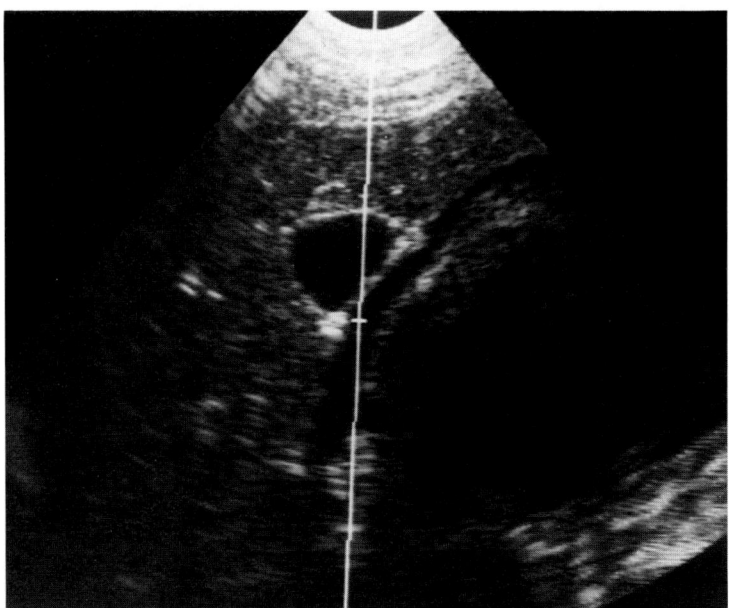

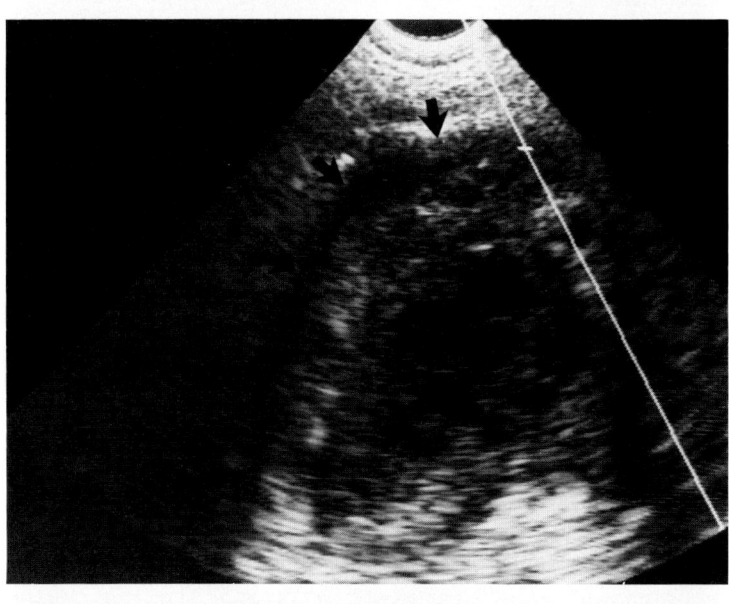

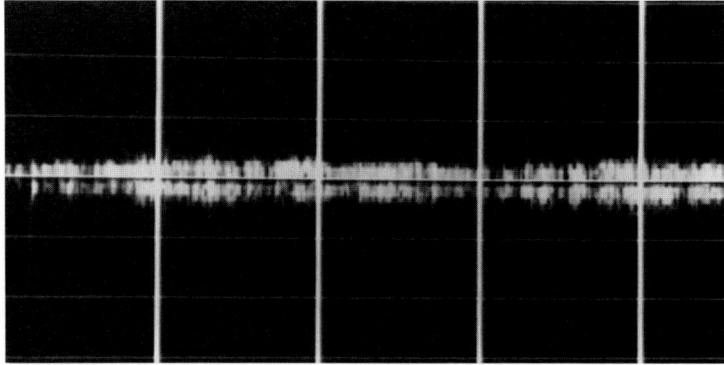

Fig. 4.21A–C. IVC displacement/compression by extrinsic mass. **A.** Transverse image at the level of the junction between the renal veins and IVC. There is marked anterior displacement of these vessels by a large mass of malignant retroperitoneal lymph nodes. The Doppler sample volume is in the right renal vein. **B.** Sagittal image of the ventrally displaced and compressed IVC (*arrows*). **C.** The use of Doppler ultrasound allowed for confirmation of luminal patency throughout the entire course of the IVC.

Fig. 4.22A–F. Hepatic artery pseudoaneurysm. **A.** Non-enhanced CT image of the abdomen demonstrates a large mass adjacent to the pancreas. **B.** Sagittal ultrasound scan of this mass, which has an anechoic central region and thick, echogenic walls. *(Continued.)*

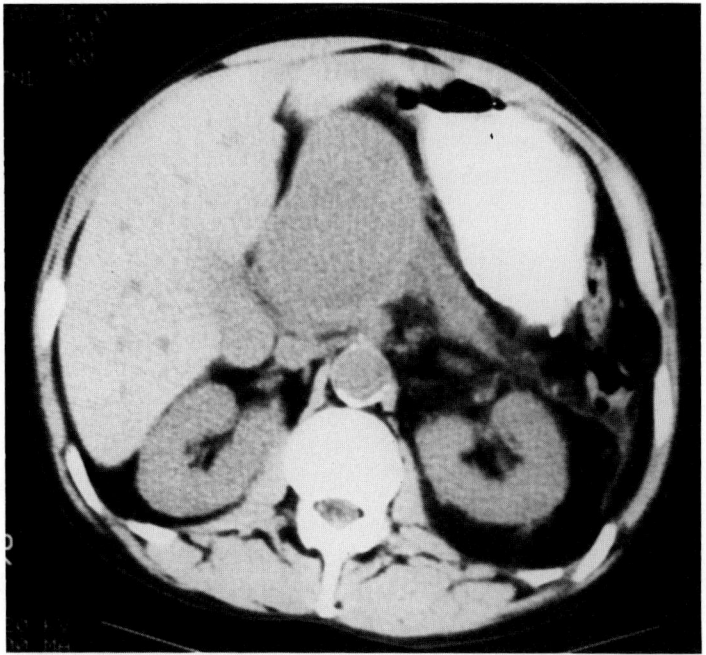

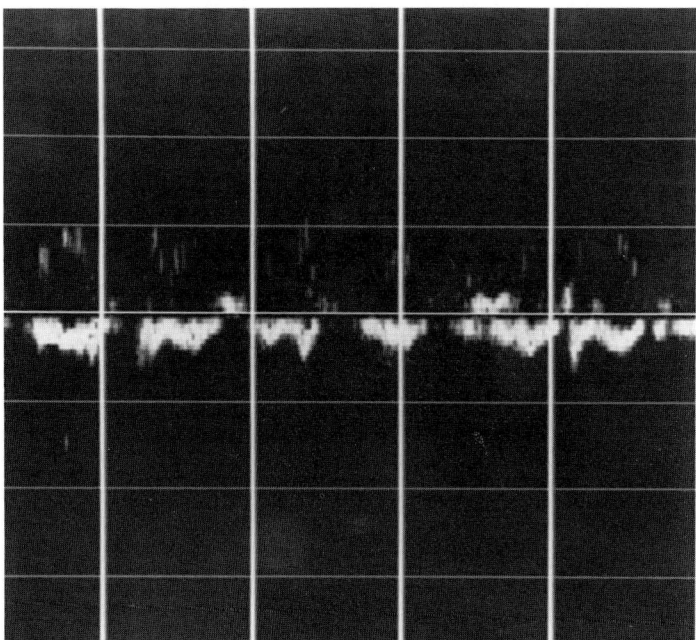

Fig. 4.22C. Doppler sampling within the center of this mass, as shown in **B**, reveals a low-amplitude, disorganized blood flow pattern. **D.** Transverse sonogram along the superior margin of the mass demonstrates a communication with the hepatic artery, in the region of the Doppler cursor. **E.** The waveform obtained at **D** shows a high-frequency shift with turbulence. This results from the rapid flow of blood through the neck of this pseudoaneurysm. **F.** Hepatic anteriogram confirms this mass to represent a large pseudoaneurysm.

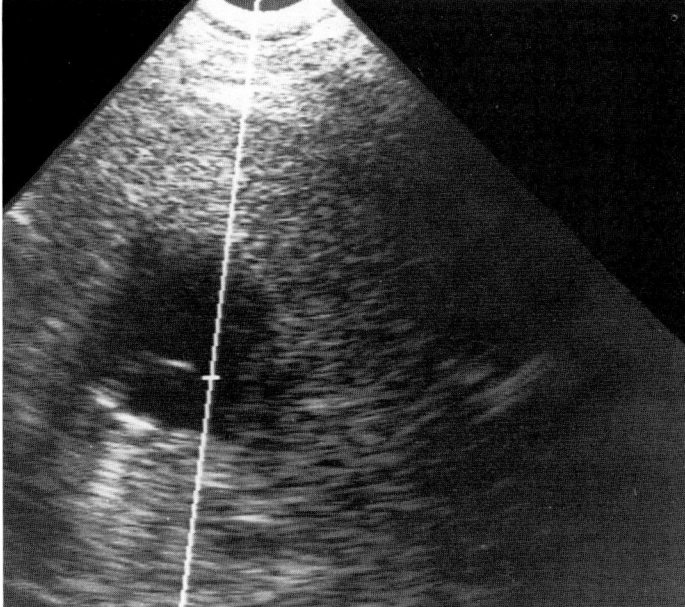

4. Duplex Sonography of the Abdomen

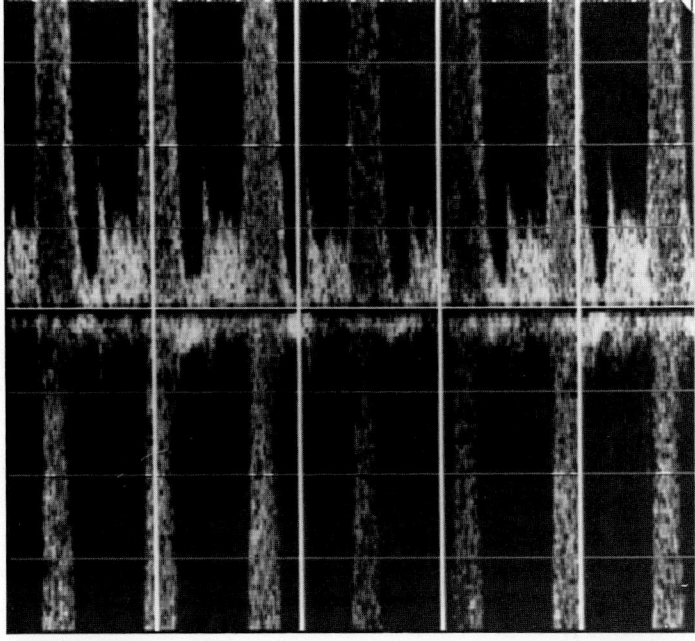

Fig. 4.22.

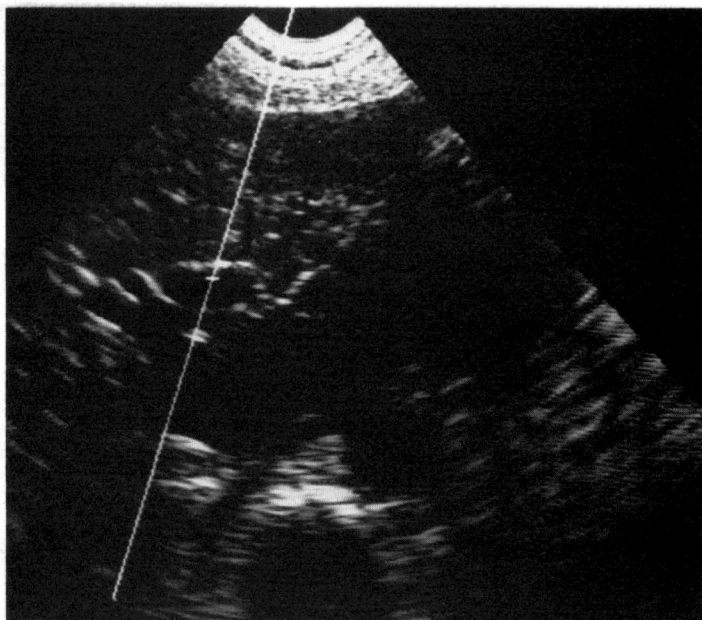
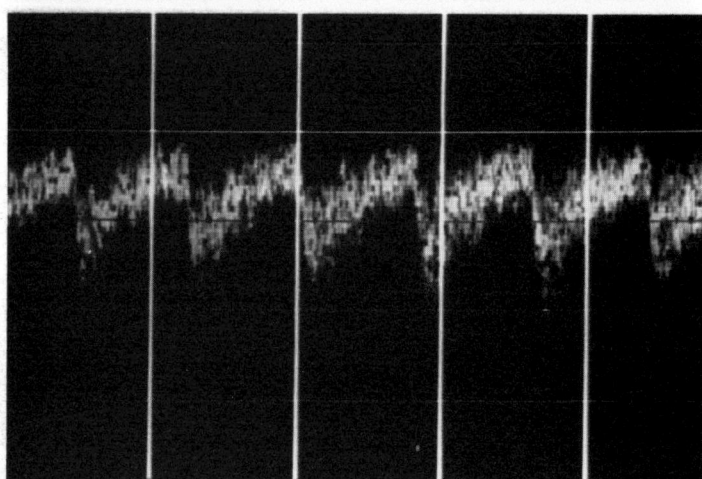

Fig. 4.23A,B. Enlarged hepatic artery. **A.** Sonogram of the porta hepatis that demonstrates a large tubular structure ventral to the portal vein (*arrows*). This could not be traced to known structures (which might have enabled distinction of an large hepatic artery from a dilated bile duct). **B.** Doppler sampling confirms this structure to represent the hepatic artery.

high hepatic arterial flow on Doppler spectral analysis.

Portal Venous System

Occlusion of the portal vein is not uncommon and numerous underlying etiologies have been identified. The most frequent causative factors are cirrhosis, neoplastic invasion (eg, hepatocellular carcinoma, metastatic liver disease, cholangiocarcinoma), inflammatory abdominal disease (eg, appendicitis, colonic diverticulitis, pancreatitis, peritonitis), abdominal trauma, and, finally, blood dyscrasias. In 20 to 50% of cases, the cause remains idiopathic (27). Using real-time imaging, several manifestations of portal vein thrombosis have been described. These include: (1) presence of echogenic material within the portal venous lumen; (2) inability to visualize the main portal vein, with an echogenic appearance in the expected location of this vessel; and (3) dilatation of the superior mesenteric and splenic veins proximal to the occlusion (27). When findings from real-time sonography are ambiguous, Doppler

Fig. 4.24A–C. Portal vein thrombosis in advanced cirrhosis. **A.** Sagittal ultrasound of the liver demonstrates low level echoes within the portal vein. **B.** No blood flow is detected in the portal vein on Doppler sampling. **C.** Splenoportogram verifies absence of portal venous blood flow. *(Continued.)*

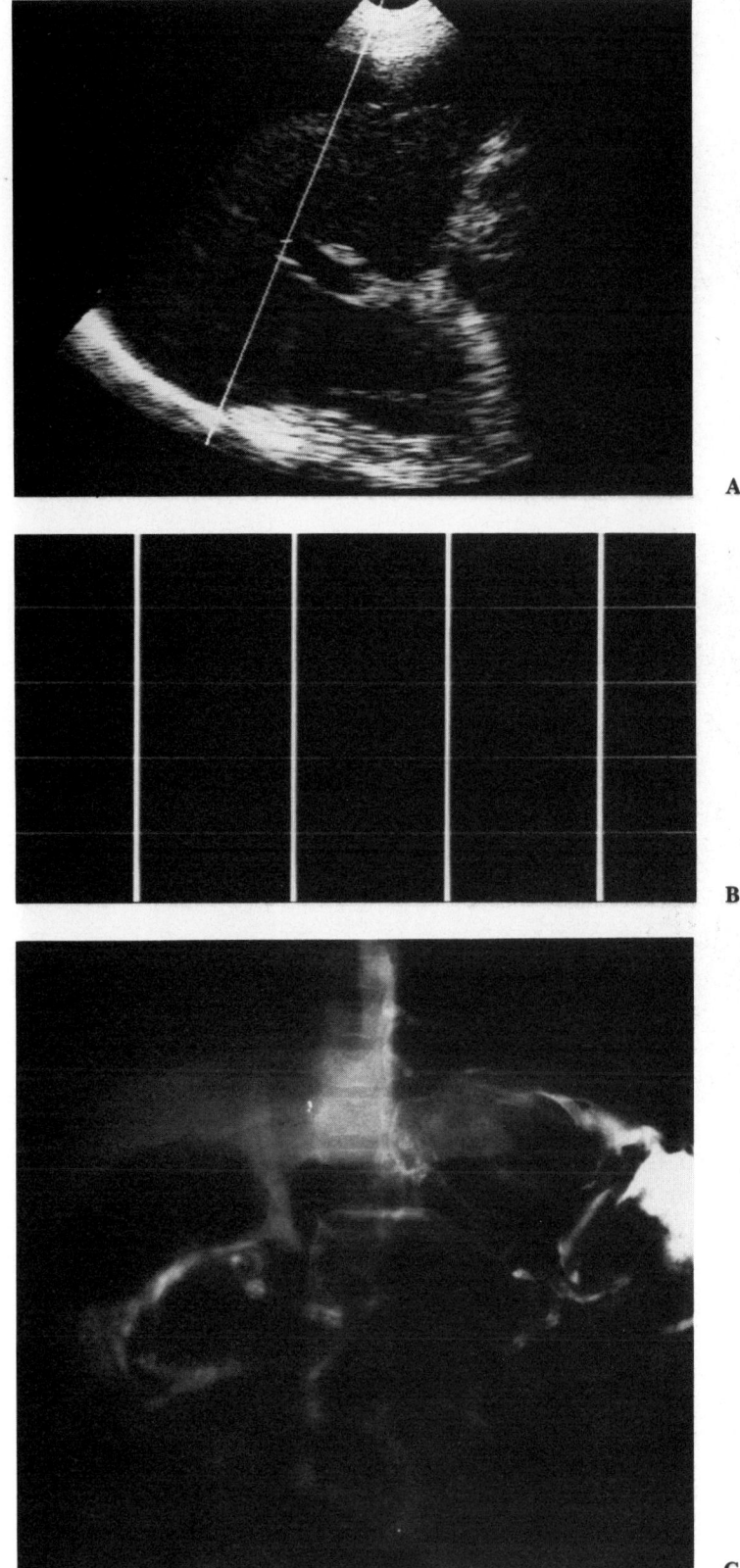

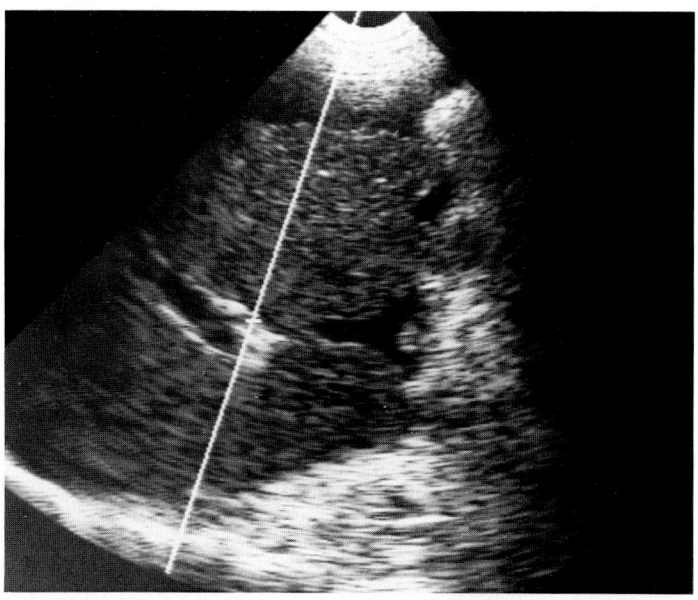

Fig. 4.24D,E. Duplex examination of the hepatic artery in this patient demonstrates a higher frequency than is normally seen. In addition, diastolic blood flow is signficantly diminished. This is attributed to markedly increased resistance in the capillary bed in this patient with severe cirrhosis.

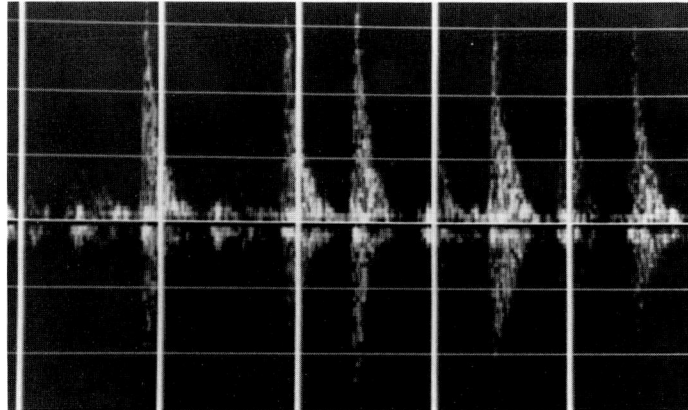

analysis may be used to noninvasively examine for portal venous patency (28) (Fig. 4.24). This is particularly important in patients being evaluated for liver transplantation, both pre- and postoperatively. In one prospective study correlating duplex sonography and angiography of the porta hepatis, Doppler was found to accurately identify total portal vein thrombus, but was less reliable in recognizing partial thrombus (29). It may be that with partial portal thrombosis, Doppler color flow mapping will facilitate diagnosis. This seems particularly applicable to instances in which the clot has a hypoechoic appearance or when only certain branches are occluded. Finally, multiple serpiginous structures are occasionally demonstrated to surround a thrombosed main portal vein. When Doppler analysis demonstrates hepatopetal venous flow within these small vessels, the diagnosis of cavernous transformation of the portal vein may be established (30).

After documentation of portal venous patency by duplex sonography, directionality of blood flow should be assessed. Normally, blood flowing toward the transducer should appear above the baseline of the waveform display. Conversely, blood flowing away from the transducer should be deflected below the baseline. Portal venous blood flow is normally hepatopetal and becomes retrograde or hepatofugal with advanced portal hypertension. Abnormal portal venous flow directional-

Fig. 4.25A–D. Pulsatile portal venous blood flow—secondary to cardiac disease. **A.** Sagittal ultrasound of the liver shows the Doppler sample volume in the portal vein. This patient has moderate-to-severe tricuspid regurgitation. **B.** Instead of the normal continuous antegrade portal venous waveform, the spectra in this patient shows a sinusoidal configuration on the display. This pattern reflects transmission of the right heart pressures into the portal circulation. **C.** Duplex examination of the hepatic vein in this patient. *(Continued.)*

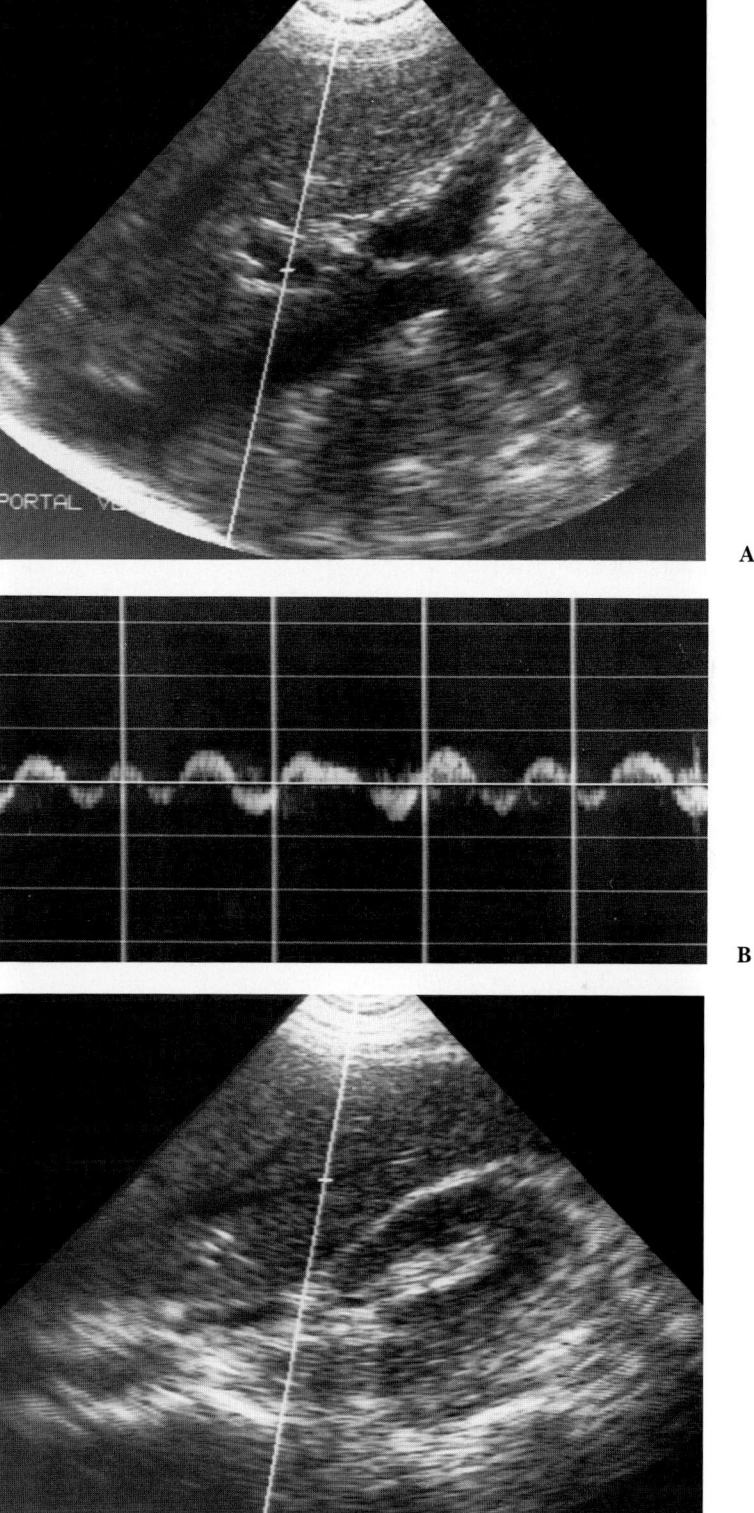

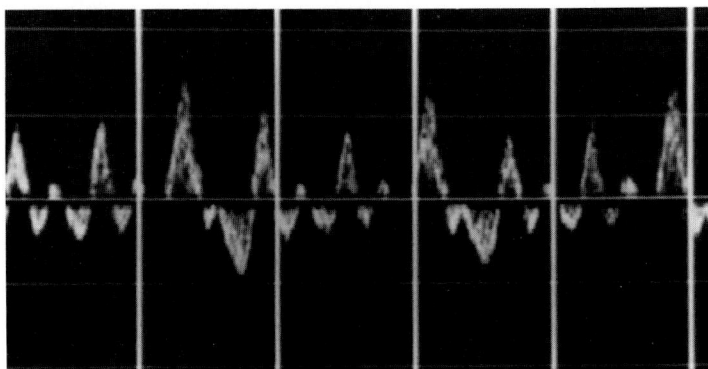

Fig. 4.25D. A normal waveform is obtained from the hepatic vein. Note the similar bidirectional spectral displays in the patient's hepatic and portal veins.

ity is also demonstrated in patients with spontaneous or surgically created portosystemic shunts. Confirmation of shunt patency and flow direction is extremely important, as will be discussed in a later section.

The spectral display of the patent portal venous system is relatively unaltered by various disease states that affect the liver. This is due to the buffering effect of the hepatic and mesenteric capillary beds. One exception to this occurs in patients with moderate-to-severe right heart failure. In these individuals, the elevated systemic venous pressures may be transmitted through the hepatic sinusoids and into the splenoportal venous system. Instead of the continuous, low-velocity waveform display of the normal portal vein, the spectral tracing assumes a pulsatile quality resembling that in the hepatic veins (Fig. 4.25). The periodic waveform may be unidirectional, returning to baseline, or in more severe cases, may be bidirectional, with deflection of the wave both above and below baseline in a sinusoidal manner. The latter pattern more closely resembles spectra from the hepatic veins and IVC.

Portal hypertension, which usually represents a complication of diffuse intrahepatic disease or extrahepatic portal venous obstruction, is often clinically silent, at least in the early stages of disease. When symptoms develop, the most frequent manifestations are gastrointestinal bleeding and ascites. Various modalities have been used as noninvasive screening techniques to evaluate for portal hypertension. Real-time ultrasound findings that have been described in portal hypertension include: (1) a main portal vein greater than 13 mm in diameter (sensitivity around 50%); (2) attenuation of the normal inspiratory increase in the portal vein (sensitivity around 80%); and, finally, (3) detection of enlarged venous collaterals, such as coronary, gastroesophageal, umbilical, duodenal, gastrorenal, and splenorenal varices (31,32). On ultrasound examination, varices generally appear as tubular, serpiginous, sonolucent structures, which may occasionally resemble other disease processes such as lymphadenopathy. The appropriate diagnosis can be easily established when Doppler sampling in these areas yields a venous waveform (33) (Fig. 4.26).

Quantitative data regarding the portal venous system may be obtained with duplex sonography by calculating the "congestion index" (CI). This has been suggested to represent a means for identifying pathophysiologic hemodynamics in the portal venous system. This index is the ratio between the cross-sectional area of the vessel (cm^2) and the blood flow velocity (cm/s) in the portal vein. Criteria have been established for normal individuals and for patients with various forms of liver disease (eg, chronic hepatitis, cirrhosis, and idiopathic portal hypertension). A statistically significant difference was found between patients with cirrhosis and idiopathic portal hypertension, the latter who had CI values 2.5 times higher than normal subjects. Although the absolute numbers appear to vary with such factors as the specific equipment used, standardization and larger patient studies may ultimately prove this to represent a useful tool for noninvasively identifying portal hypertension.

Fig. 4.26A–E. Portal hypertension. **A,B**. Contrast-enhanced CT scans of the upper abdomen in a patient with known portal hypertension. *(Continued.)*

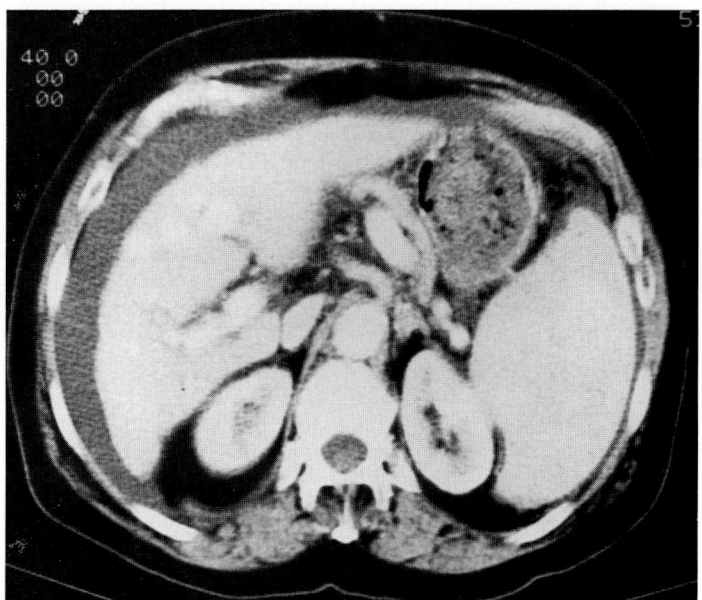

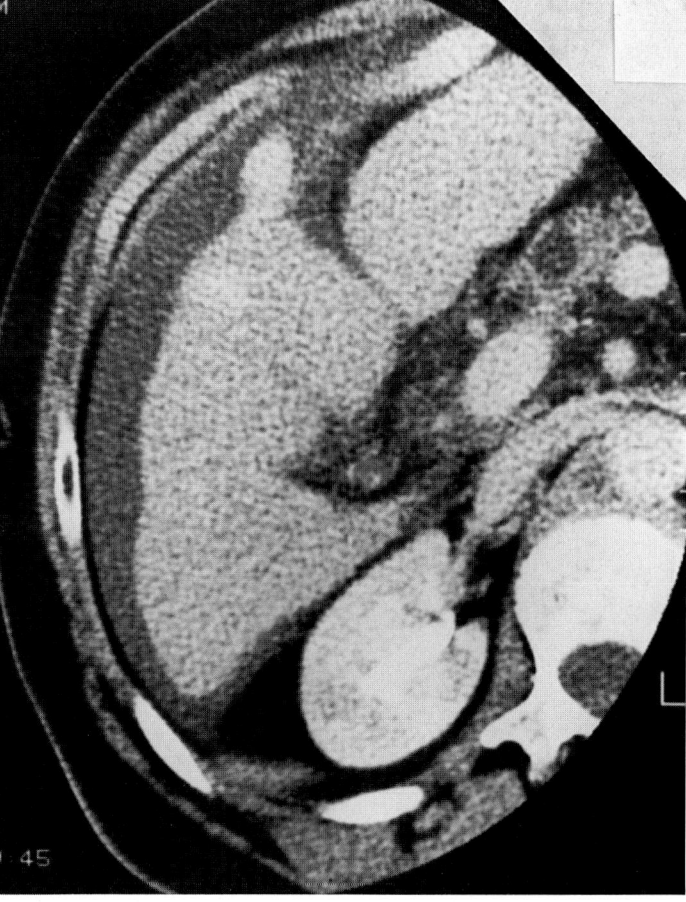

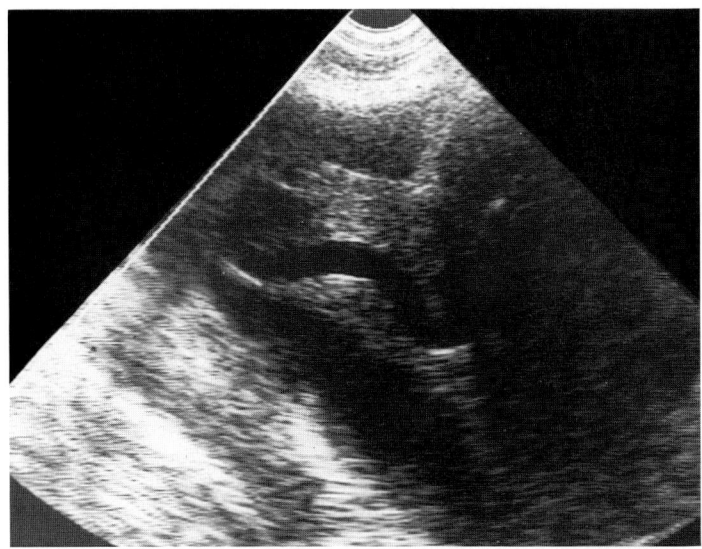

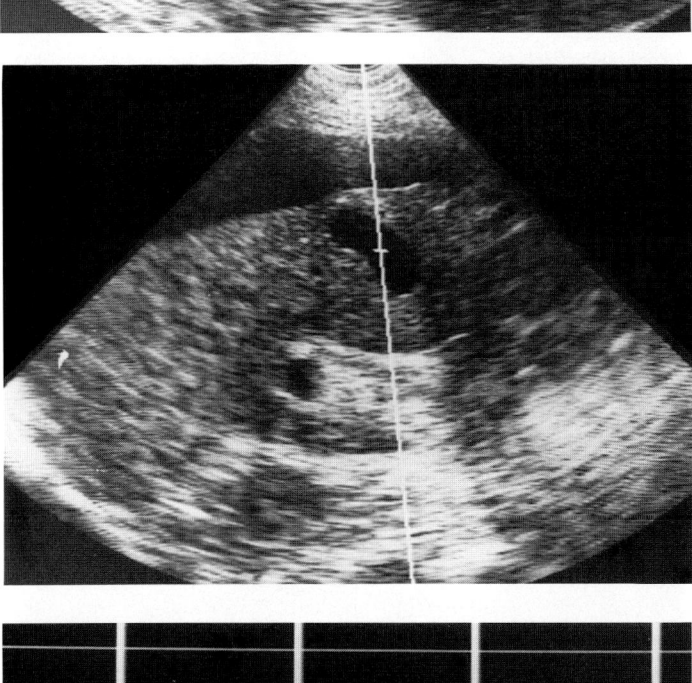

Fig. 4.26C,D. Sagittal sonograms demonstrate a tubular serpiginous structure within the liver and extending outside the hepatic margins. **E.** Doppler analysis demonstrates portal venous flow within these collateral vessels.

Fig. 4.27A–D. Budd-Chiari syndrome. **A.** Transverse ultrasound image in the region of the hepatic venous confluence with the IVC. Duplex sonography failed to show evidence of hepatic venous patency. **B.** Contrast-enhanced CT examination shows no evidence of patent hepatic veins. **C.** Similar findings are demonstrated on this MR image. *(Continued.)*

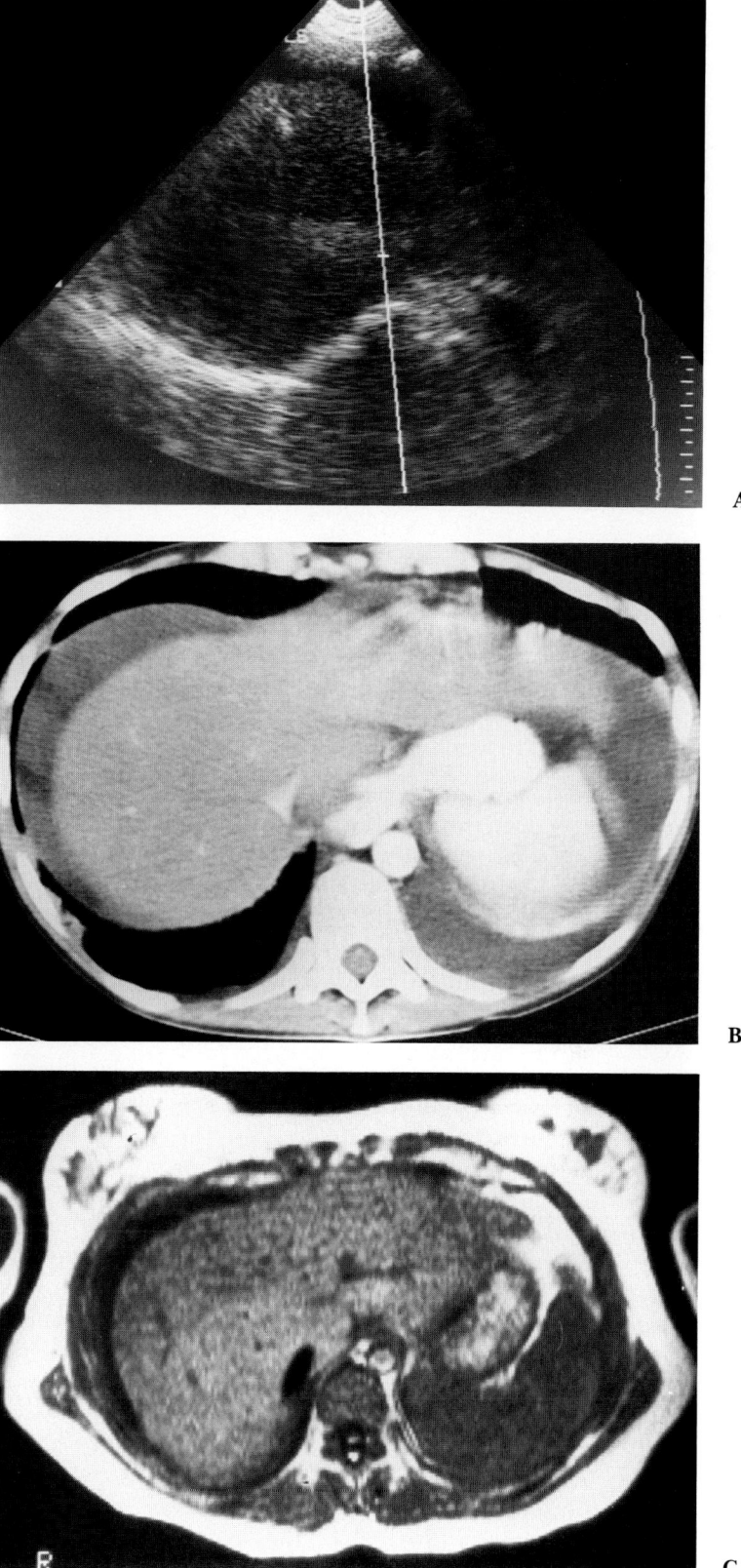

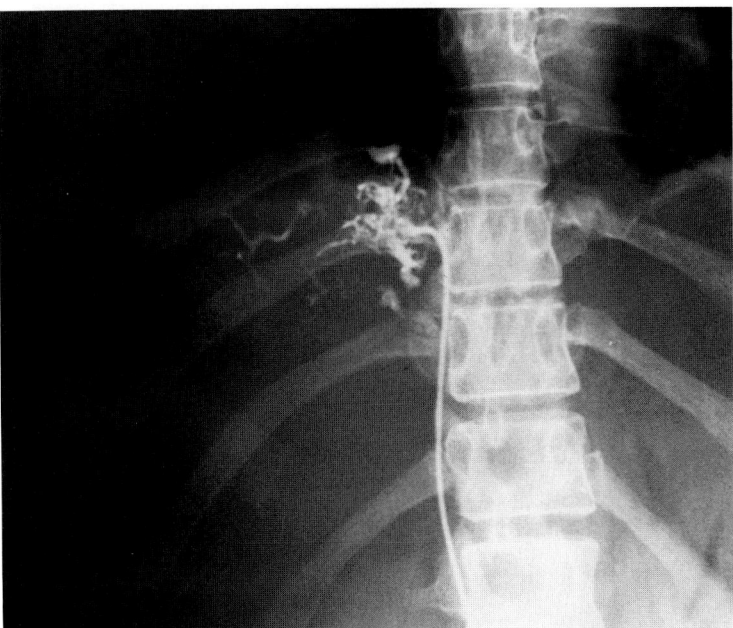

Fig. 4.27D. Confirmation of Budd-Chiari syndrome was established by hepatic venography.

Hepatic Veins

Duplex examination of the hepatic venous system is most often undertaken to assess for hepatic venous thrombosis or the Budd-Chiari syndrome. Real-time imaging may suffice to confirm patency of these vessels, particularly when dilated (35,36). However, one or more hepatic veins may be inadequately visualized on real-time imaging, even when patent. In this situation, duplex evaluation of the hepatic veins may be undertaken by imaging transversely in the superior portion of the liver (Fig. 4.27). The sample volume may then be placed in the expected locations of the right, middle, and left hepatic veins and Doppler analysis performed. This helps to establish the presence or absence of hepatic venous flow. If definitive diagnosis cannot be accomplished by ultrasound, dynamic computed tomography (CT) or even hepatic venography may be necessary.

Splenic Circulation

Significantly fewer indications have been established for Doppler evaluation of the spleen. However, certain clinical scenarios are associated with increased risk of splenic vascular injury. On the arterial side, aneurysms and pseudoaneurysms may develop. Approximately 80 to 87% of true aneurysms involving the splenic artery occur in women (18). Causative factors include atherosclerosis, infections, and both blunt and penetrating trauma. In addition, there is a frequent association of splenic artery aneurysms forming in pregnant or multiparous women. The reported incidence of rupture of true splenic aneurysms varies considerably, from 0.1 to 3% in one series (18) to 8 to 46% in another (37). When rupture occurs, it tends to be a single catastrophic event with massive intraperitoneal hemorrhage. Splenic artery pseudoaneurysms, on the other hand, develop much more frequently in men and are often associated with severe pancreatitis (18). Hemorrhage from false aneurysms is more common than from true aneurysms. It tends to be intermittent and recurrent, often with evidence of gastrointestinal bleeding. By real-time imaging, these vascular abnormalities of the splenic artery may be confused with other lesions such as cystic renal, adrenal, or pancreatic masses. Documentation of a turbulent arterial waveform within the structure may be easily and noninvasively performed using duplex ultra-

Fig. 4.28A,B. Splenic artery aneurysm. **A.** Hypoechoic soft tissue mass in the left upper quadrant, in continuity with a normal-appearing proximal splenic artery. **B.** Doppler analysis demonstrates markedly turbulent blood flow within this splenic artery aneurysm.

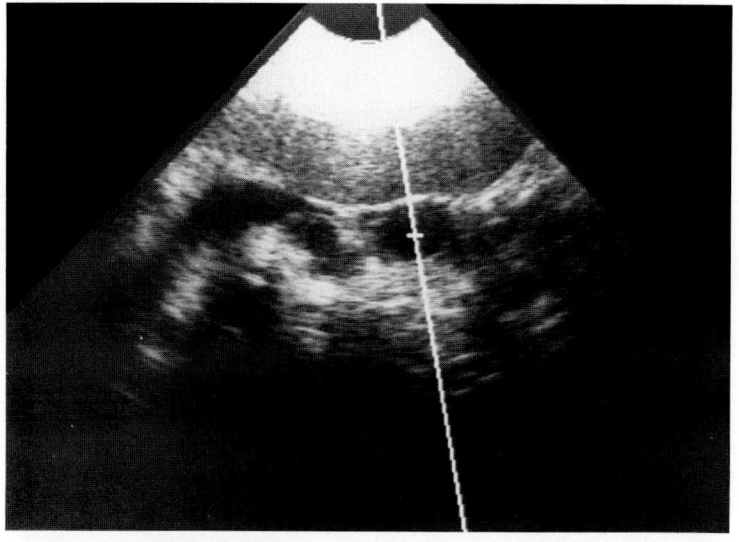

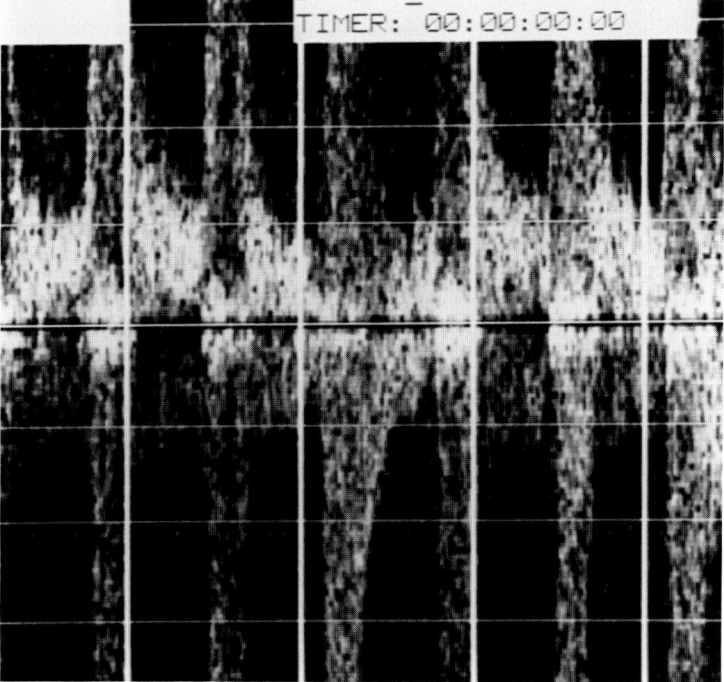

sound (37) (Fig. 4.28). As with true and false aneurysms that arise from other vessels, however, it may not always be possible to distinguish between these with duplex scanning.

A rare abnormality to involve the splenic circulation is an arteriovenous fistula. These are usually associated with aneurysms of the splenic artery (38). Patients often show manifestations of portal hypertension, due to the large volume of blood being shunted directly from the systemic into the splenoportal circulation. Sonographic findings may include those of a splenic artery aneurysm as well as dilated and tortuous splenic and portal veins.

Finally, when studying the splenic artery, it should be remembered that this vessel normally has a tortuous course, which results in turbulent flow as manifest by spectral broadening. This is

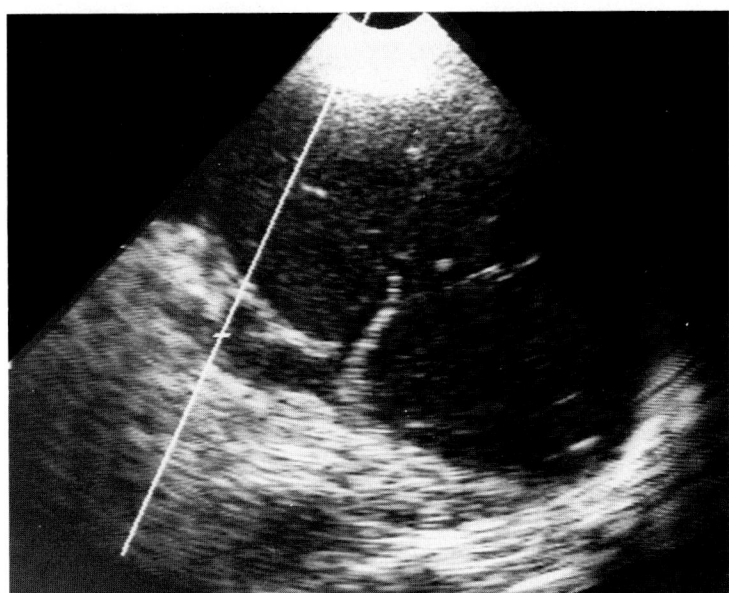
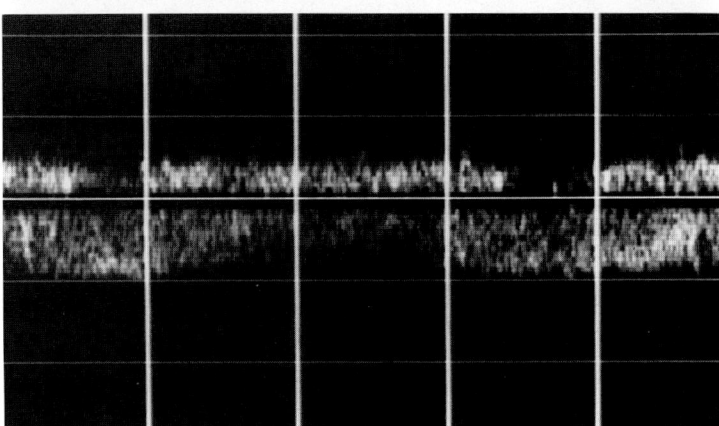

Fig. 4.29A,B. Splenic vein in portal hypertension. **A.** Transverse sonogram of an enlarged spleen in a patient with portal hypertension. Low-level internal echoes are present within the splenic vein. **B.** Doppler scanning confirms vascular patency.

a frequent finding and should not necessarily be interpreted as a manifestation of proximal splenic artery stenosis. The latter usually requires a significant increase in blood flow velocity (or Doppler shift frequency) for diagnosis from the spectral display.

The splenic vein may also be evaluated by Doppler analysis (Fig. 4.29). This vessel may be studied in the splenic hilar region or as it courses posterior to the pancreatic body and tail. One of the most common abnormalities to affect the splenic vein is partial or complete vascular occlusion. This may involve only the splenic vein, without extension into other portions of the portal venous system, as occurs with severe pancreatitis. In other circumstances, the splenic vein may contain thrombus, which is propagated from the main portal vein. On realtime ultrasound, the diagnosis may be established by increased echogenicity in the splenic vein lumen (39). Doppler sampling may be used to confirm the presence or absence of blood flow in ambiguous cases. In addition, duplex scanning of the splenic vein may be used to determine flow directionality. This is particularly applicable to patients with severe portal hypertension, who may have abnormal hepatofugal flow.

Portosystemic Shunts

Portosystemic shunts provide a means to divert blood from hypertensive splenoportal venous

Fig. 4.30A–C. Portocaval shunt. **A.** Sonogram of the right upper quadrant demonstrates a surgically created portocaval shunt. The sample volume is located within the portal vein (*arrowheads*) near the anastomosis with the IVC (*arrows*). **B.** Doppler examination of the portal vein confirms patency and demonstrates hepatopetal blood flow, with the waveform deflected above baseline. **C.** Contrast-enhanced CT scan shows changes within the liver from regenerating hepatic tissue. The portocaval shunt is again shown to be patent.

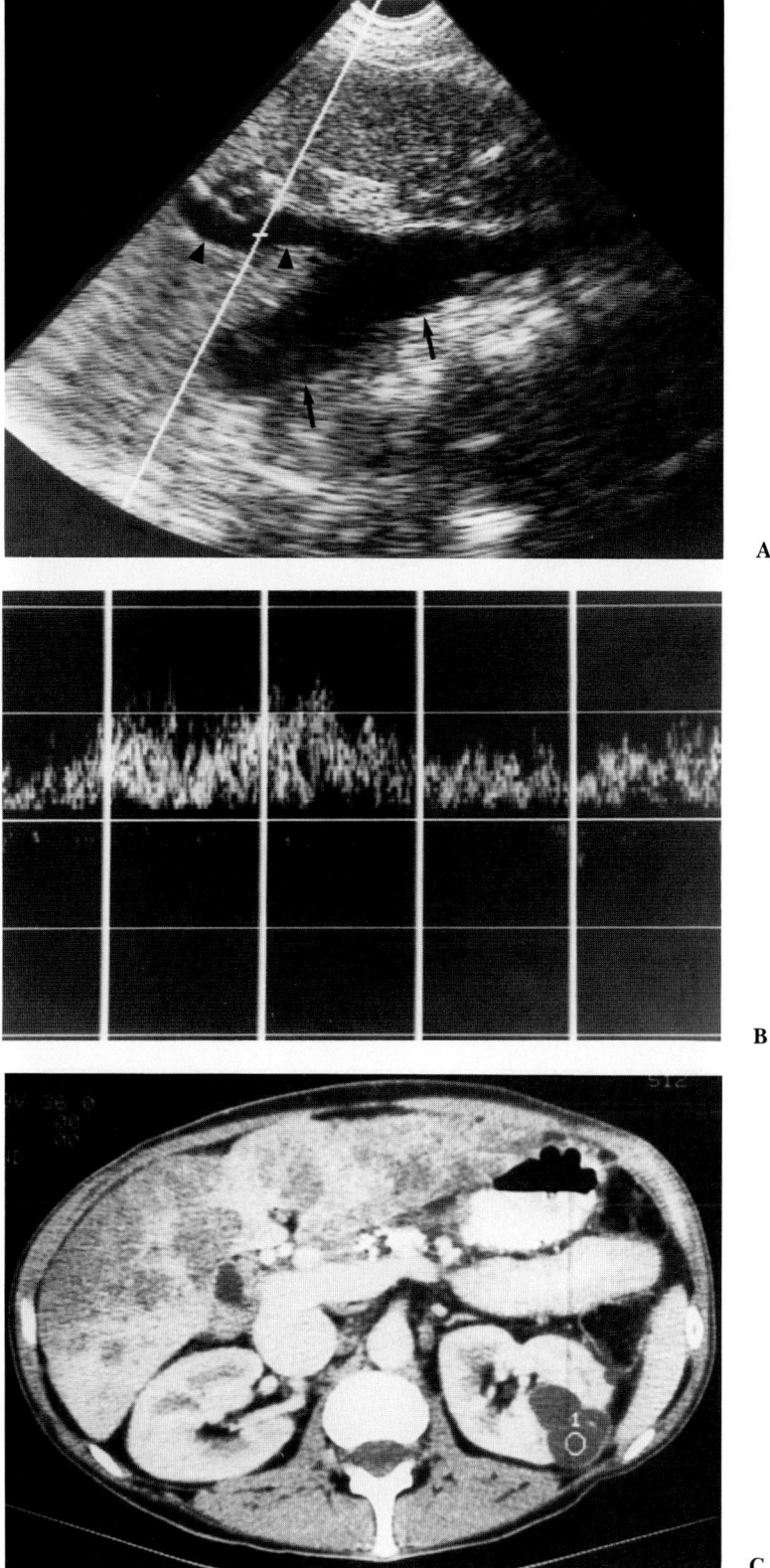

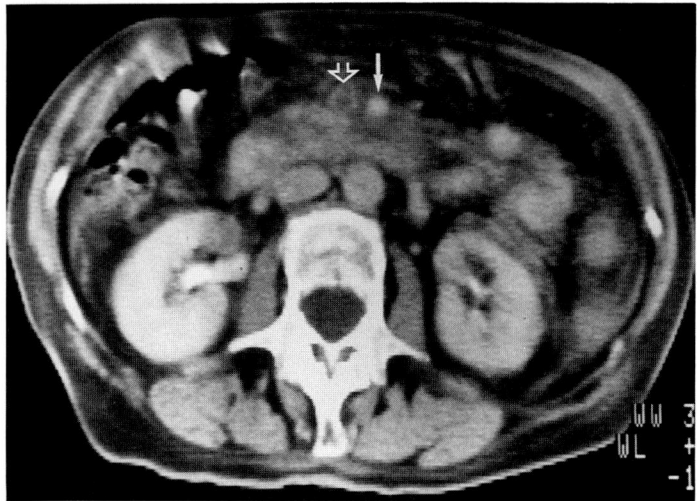

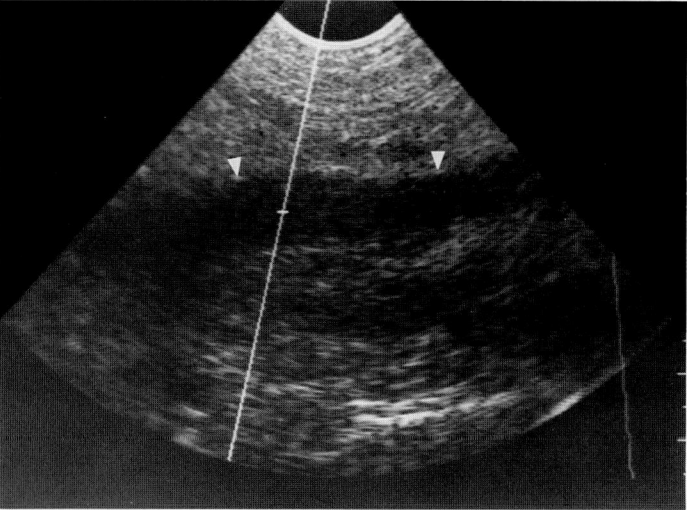

Fig. 4.31A–E. Superior mesenteric venous (SMV) thrombosis. **A.** Contrast-enhanced CT image of the mid-abdomen demonstrates a normally enhancing superior mesenteric artery (SMA) (*solid arrow*). A filling defect occupies the SMV lumen (*open arrow*). **B.** Sagittal sonogram demonstrates low-level echoes within the SMV (*arrowheads*). The Doppler cursor is positioned centrally within this vessel. **C.** Doppler analysis at **B** fails to demonstrate detectable blood flow within the central portion of the vessel. **D.** The sample volume is repositioned within the periphery of the SMV (*arrowheads*) on this sagittal image. **E.** Venous blood flow is detected along the periphery of the thrombus. This presumably represents a recanalized channel or residual lumen.

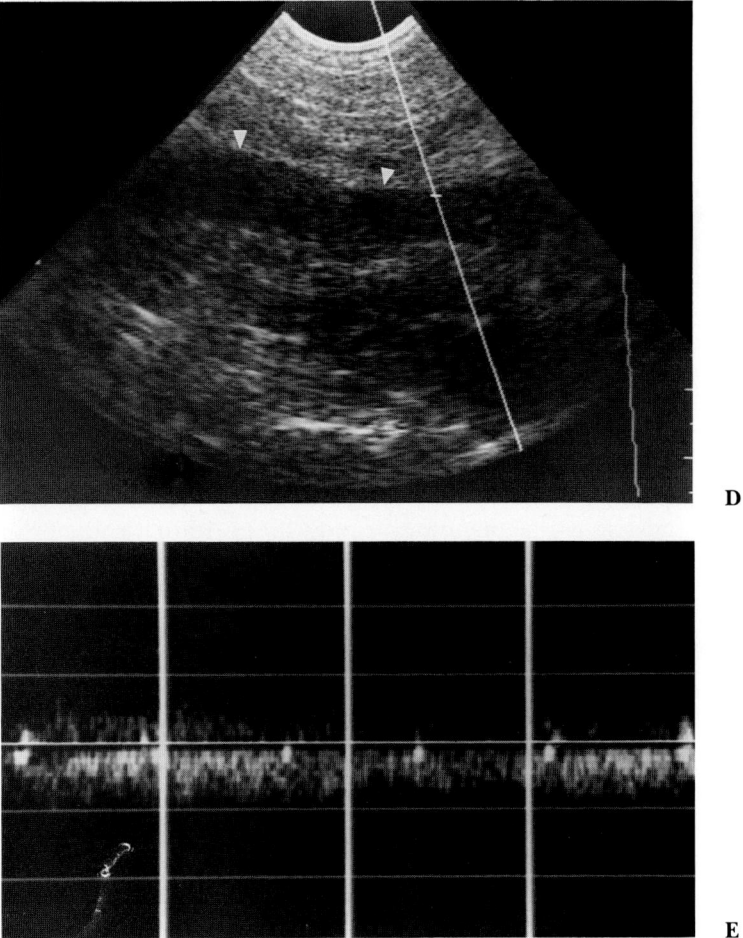

Fig. 4.31.

systems into the systemic circulation. These may develop as congenital malformations or may be spontaneously or surgically created. Duplex sonography provides an easy, noninvasive means to assess blood flow direction and patency of these shunts. Documentation of patency is particularly critical in those patients with known shunts who present with gastrointestinal bleeding, accumulating ascites, or generalized medical deterioration.

Certain extrahepatic portosystemic shunts are easier to examine than others. Portocaval shunts are usually well demonstrated sonographically, as the liver provides an excellent acoustic window (Fig. 4.30). Several other shunts are more difficult to visualize with ultrasound, due to overlying bowel gas, obesity, surgical scars, or abundant ascites. These include conventional splenorenal shunts, end-to-side distal splenorenal shunts (Warren shunts), mesocaval shunts, and omphalocaval shunts (40–42). When shunts are not well visualized on otherwise adequate examinations, performing the Valsalva maneuver may help to distend the venous structures and allow for study (40,43). In patients with long-standing portocaval shunts, dilatation of the inferior vena cava is occasionally found near the surgical anastomosis (32,43). This is attributed to the locally increased volume of blood flowing into the inferior vena cava and has been described in portocaval and mesocaval shunts.

Most intrahepatic shunts that are detected radiographically communicate between the hepatic artery and portal vein. Various etiologies for arterioportal fistulas include surgical shunt formation, abdominal trauma, penetrating wounds, liver biopsy, ruptured hepatic artery aneurysms, neoplasms (eg, hepatomas), and congenital malformations (44–46). Spontaneous formation of sinusoidal portohepatic vein shunts generally occurs in cirrhotic livers. Due to the small size of these shunts, often less than 2 mm, these are not usually visualized sonographically. Intrahepatic portohepatic venous aneurysms are rare vascular abnormalities that are usually congenital in origin. These are more commonly located in the right hepatic lobe (47). Sonographically, these appear as hypoechoic or anechoic masses, with large feeding and draining vessels (47,48). One case report underscores the importance of Doppler analysis in documenting venous flow within such a cystic appearing liver mass (46). This aneurysmal, intrahepatic portosystemic venous fistula was subsequently confirmed angiographically.

Mesenteric Circulation

The role of duplex sonography in evaluating the superior mesenteric artery and vein has not been fully defined to date. This results, in part, from frequent difficulty in adequately visualizing these vessels. Overlying bowel gas and obesity are the primary factors limiting ultrasound imaging, and under optimal circumstances, only the upper portions of the main vascular trunks are demonstrated. Therefore, other modalities, particularly invasive techniques, often preempt use of ultrasound in the evaluation of the major superior mesenteric vessels.

One application of duplex ultrasound within the mesenteric circulation is to assess for vascular occlusion when bowel ischemia is suspected. Doppler capability is particularly useful when real-time imaging demonstrates low-level echoes within these vessels. Intravascular sampling will define either a patent or occluded lumen (Fig. 4.31). Occasionally, superior mesenteric arterial or venous thrombosis sonographically presents as nonvisualized vessels, in the absence of overlying bowel gas. In this circumstance, Doppler sampling may be attempted in the expected location of these vessels.

Mesenteric venous thrombosis accounts for approximately 15% of all vascular complications involving the small bowel, and in about 50% of cases, no bowel infarction occurs (49). When the bowel remains viable, superior mesenteric venous thrombosis may be diagnosed incidentally during the course of an examination performed for other indications. The clinical presentation is often one of subacute development of abdominal pain, low-grade fever, and leukocytosis (49). The nonspecificity of these findings often poses diagnostic difficulty. In contrast, superior mesenteric arterial occlusion typically has a more immediate and severe clinical onset, often warranting angiographic evaluation with the potential for direct catheter instillation of thrombolytic agents.

Superior mesenteric arterial stenoses, when severe, may be detected by duplex sonography (50). Findings include extremely elevated peak systolic velocities and marked spectral broadening in the area of stenosis (50). Another observation that has been suggested to indicate significant stenosis is loss of the reverse flow component during diastole. This may be accompanied by an increased peak systolic velocity, exceeding that which is found in the postprandial state (51). To date, however, diagnosis of chronic mesenteric ischemia, or mesenteric angina, requires clinical findings as well as angiographic documentation of significant stenoses or occlusions involving at least two of the three major arteries supplying the gastrointestinal tract (celiac, superior mesenteric, or inferior mesenteric arteries) (50).

The inferior mesenteric circulation is extremely difficult to sonographically demonstrate, and, therefore, duplex scanning has not proven useful in the evaluation of these vessels.

Renal Circulation

Approximately 10% of the United States population is hypertensive, as defined by a diastolic blood pressure equal to or exceeding 90 mm Hg (52). Among this group, about 10% will have an identifiable and potentially correctable cause for the hypertension (52). Renal artery stenosis is the most common definable etiology. Several modalities have been used as noninvasive

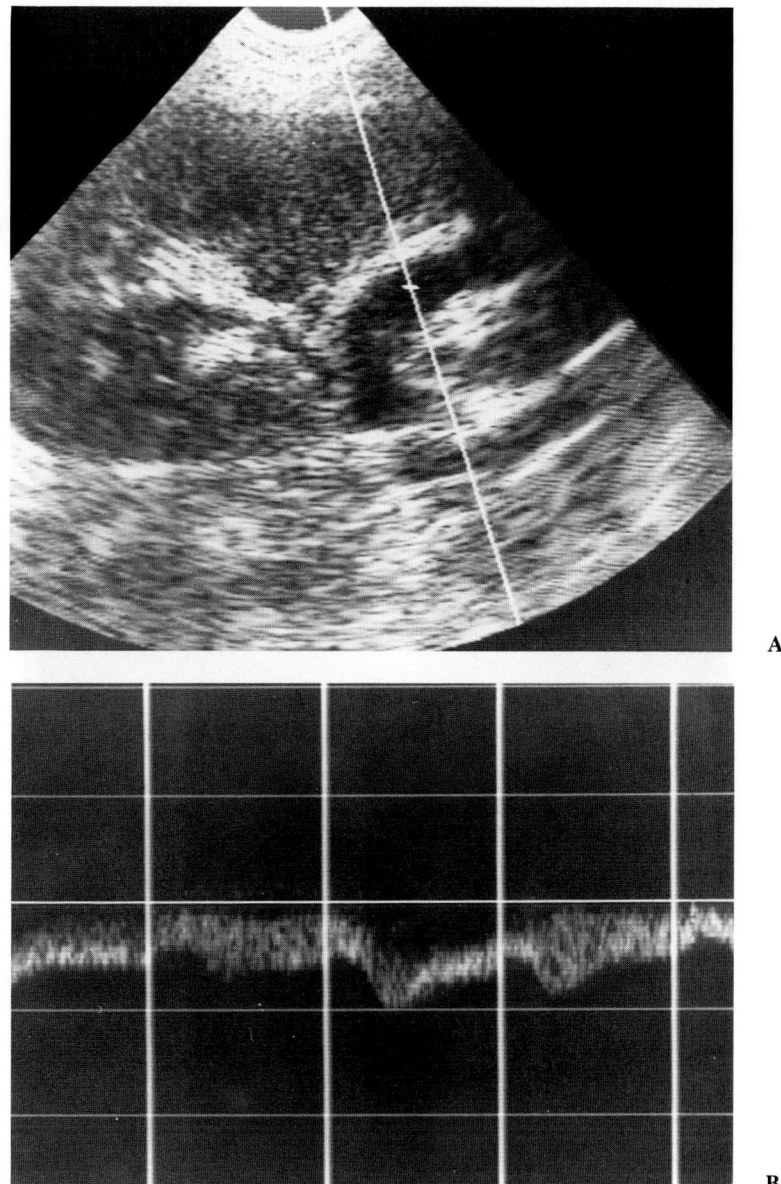

Fig. 4.32A,B. Prominent renal hilar vessels simulating hydronephrosis. **A.** Sagittal ultrasound image of the kidney demonstrates splaying of the perirenal sinus fat by an anechoic area. **B.** Doppler sampling in this area confirms a vascular waveform throughout the anechoic region, due to prominent central renal vessels.

examinations, including duplex sonography. Recent reports describe promising results in the evaluation for renal artery stenosis by Doppler (52–54). However, due to the deep retroperitoneal location of the kidneys, which are often obscured by overlying bowel gas, the main renal arteries may be difficult to visualize with ultrasound. This inconsistency in adequately imaging these vessels may limit the use of duplex sonography in mass screening of hypertensive patients for main renal artery stenosis. Larger correlative studies are needed to define the exact role that this modality will have in evaluation of renovascular hypertension.

Qualitatively, several applications have been described to evaluate renal artery hemodynamics (56). These depend on alterations in the spectral display. For example, decrease or loss of the diastolic component in the parenchymal arterial waveform helps to identify increased vascular resistance within the kidney. Turbulent, low-velocity arterial flow within a sonolucent mass are findings that suggest a true or false aneurysm or an arteriovenous fistula

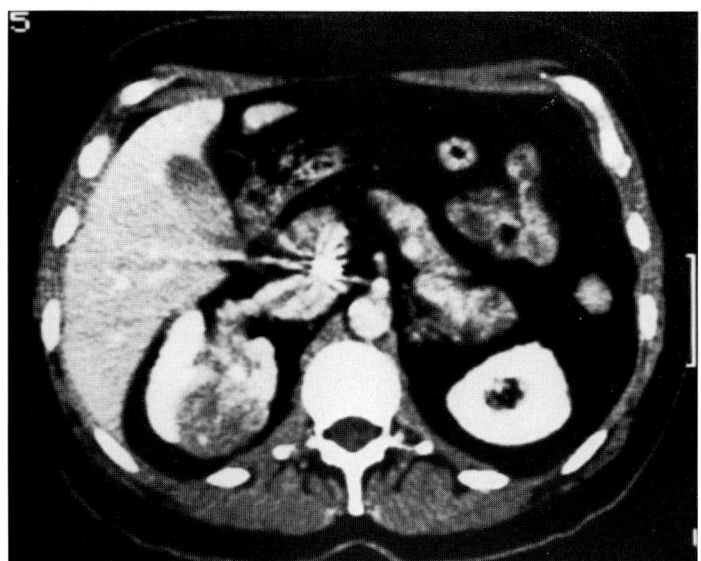

Fig. 4.33A–C. Hypernephroma. **A.** Contrast-enhanced CT scan reveals a right renal mass representing a hypernephroma. Artifact degrades images of the IVC and limits assessment of possible neoplastic infiltration of the right renal vein. **B.** Doppler sampling of the right renal vein on this transverse ultrasound (*arrowheads*). **C.** Normal waveform display in this patent renal vein.

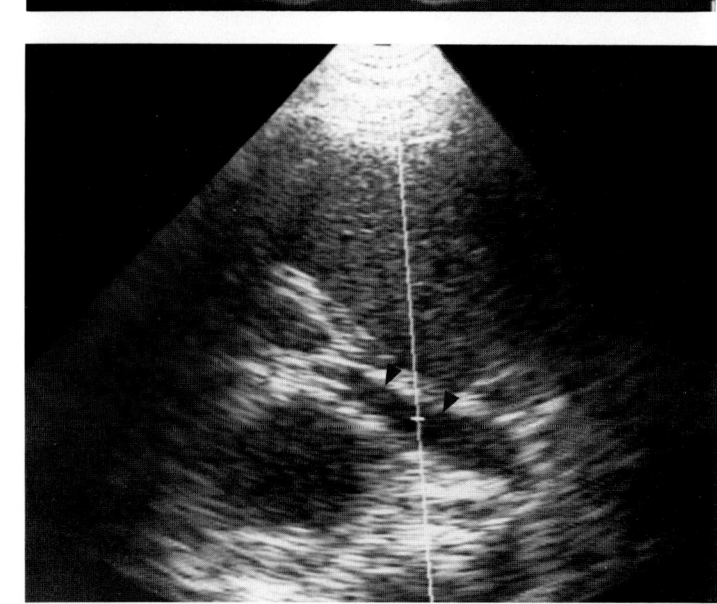

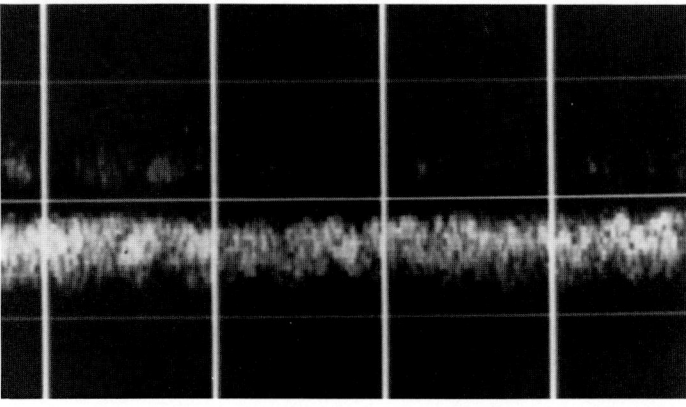

Fig. 4.34A–C. Retroaortic left renal vein. **A**. CT scan through the midabdomen demonstrates a retroaortic left renal vein. **B**. Transverse sonogram shows the left renal vein (*arrowheads*) to course posterior to the aorta (Ao) and drain into the IVC. **C**. Doppler confirms the venous tracing within this vessel.

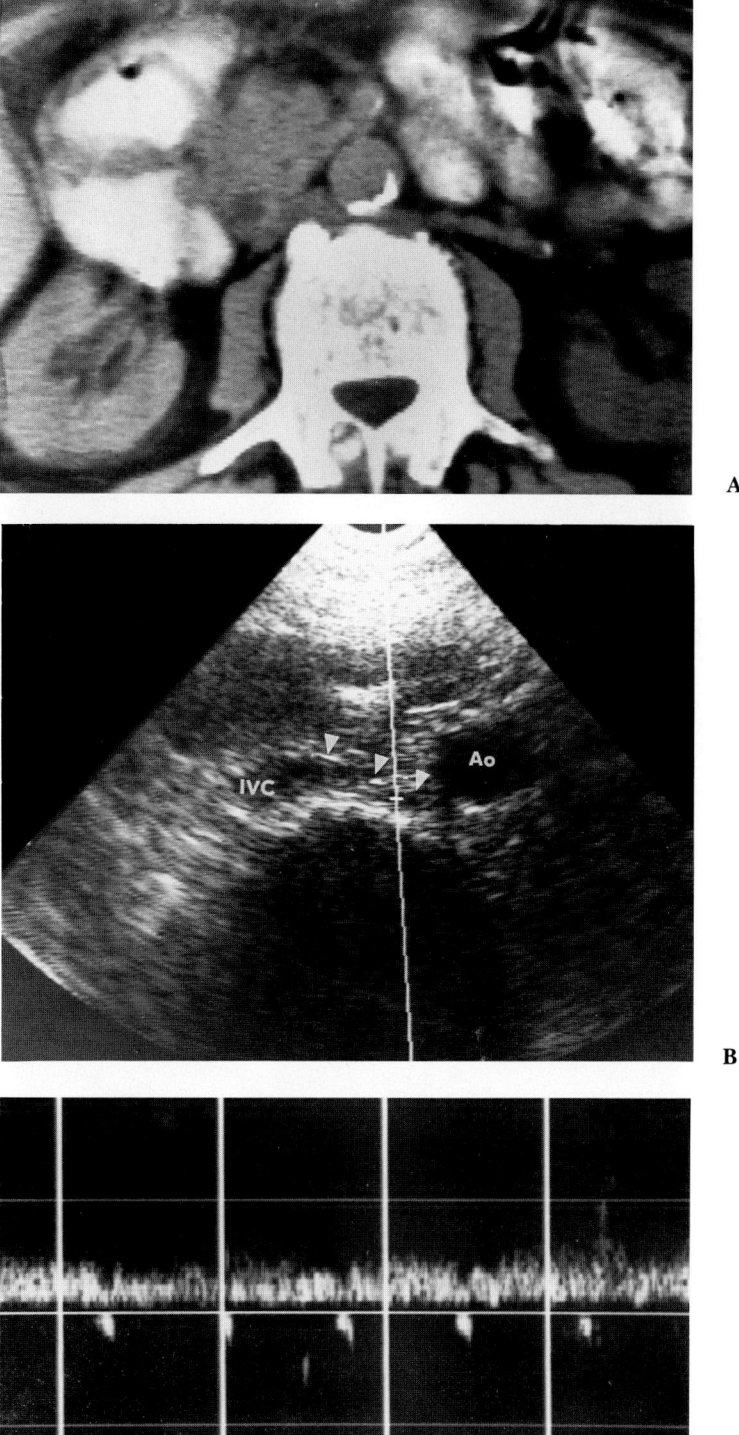

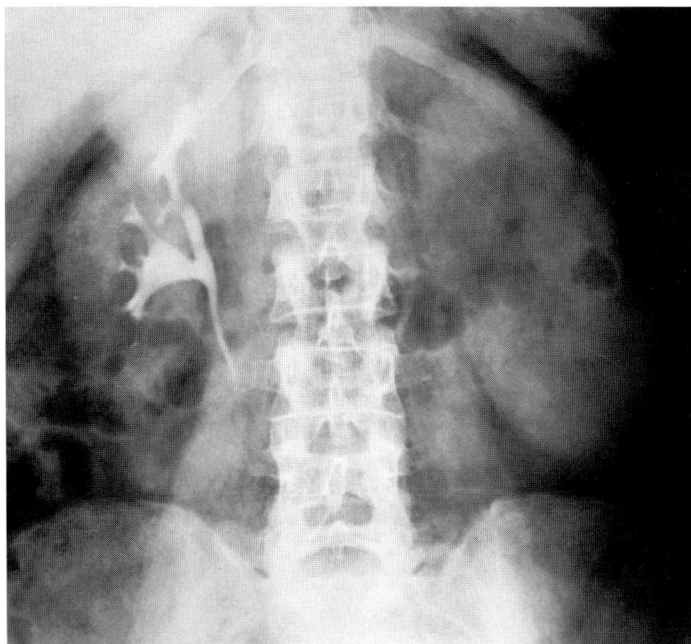

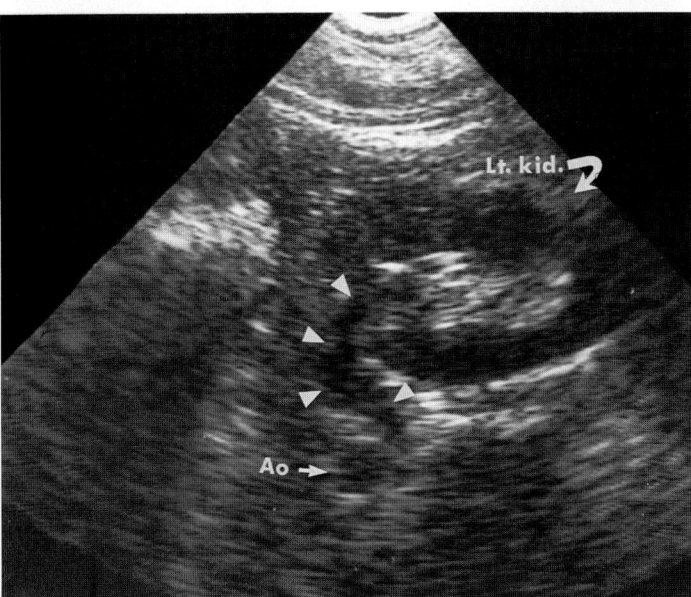

Fig. 4.35A–F. Idiopathic thrombosis within a retroaortic left renal vein. **A.** A film from an intravenous urogram demonstrates an enlarged left kidney, without contrast excretion into the left collecting system. **B.** Transverse sonogram of the left kidney (Lt. kid.) obtained through a left flank approach. The left renal vein contains low-level internal echoes as it courses posterior to the aorta (Ao). **C.** Transverse ultrasound image of the left kidney, with the sample volume positioned in the left renal vein. **D.** Doppler analysis of **C** shows venous flow around an area of thrombus. *(Continued.)*

(57,58). In addition, Doppler evaluation has been used to assist with intraoperative resection of these fistulas (58). Within the central portion of the kidneys, vascular calcifications may be confused occasionally with urolithiasis. When the Doppler sample volume is placed over the echogenic shadowing focus and a renal arterial waveform is obtained, this suggests the presence of vascular calcification. Not infrequently, prominent branching vessels within the renal hilum simulate mild hydronephrosis. Correct diagnosis is established by means of Doppler sampling in this central anechoic region. When arterial or venous waveforms are obtained from several areas, the presence of hydronephrosis may be excluded (Fig. 4.32).

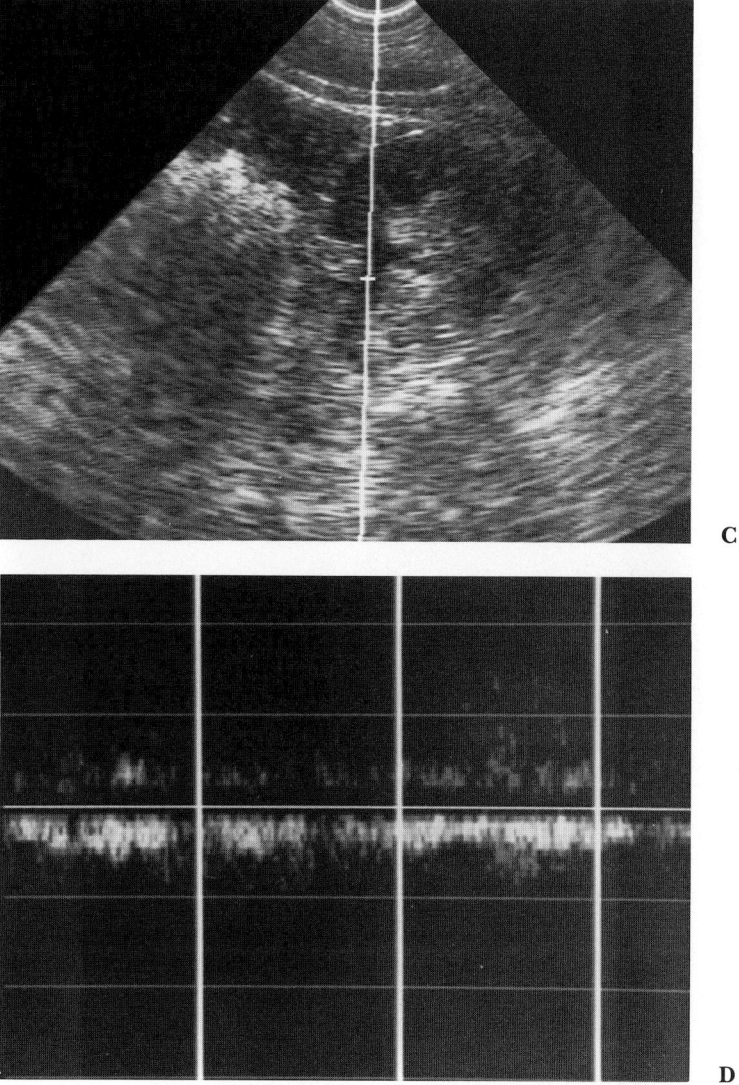

Fig. 4.35.

Pulsed-Doppler examination is also used to evaluate the main renal veins when there is suspicion of thrombus (59) (Fig. 4.33). Thrombus does not always have an echogenic appearance on real-time imaging. Lack of venous flow by Doppler examination helps to confirm the presence of thrombus. In addition, duplex sonography provides a useful adjunct to conventional real-time imaging in the diagnosis of congenital anomalies involving the renal veins. One which occurs in approximately 1.8 to 2.4% of the population is the retroaortic left renal vein (60). Duplex scanning may not only define this vessel as a venous structure, but may also be used to follow its course and confirm vascular patency (Figs. 4.34 and 4.35). Correct identification becomes important, for example, in those patients being considered for a distal splenorenal shunt (Warren shunt). A retroaortic left renal vein would contraindicate this surgery.

Finally, occasional pitfalls in real-time imaging in the renal vasculature include a prominent left renal vein, which in thin patients may mimic a left renal artery aneurysm (61). Pulsed-Doppler sampling and use of the Valsalva

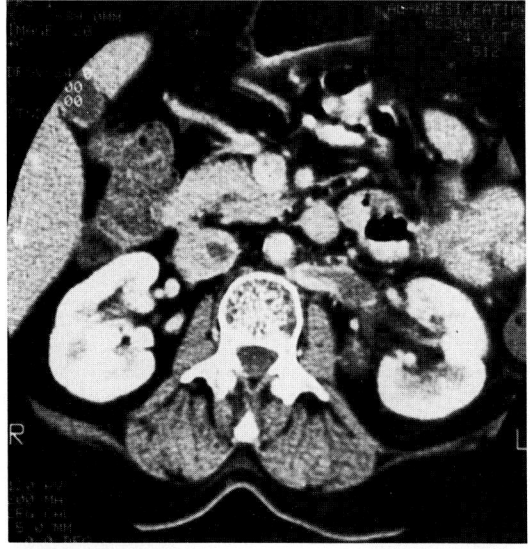

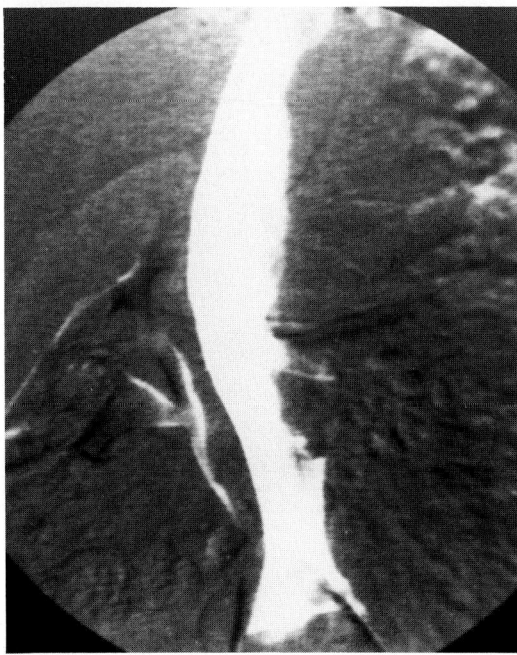

Fig. 4.35E. CT examination performed several days later demonstrates thrombus within the retroaortic left renal vein and IVC. At this time, a left pyclogram is present. **F.** Inferior venacavogram reconfirms thrombus extension along the left lateral wall of the IVC.

maneuver allow for proper interpretation on such scans.

Renal Allografts

Several complications may develop either acutely or chronically in renal allografts. Among the most common are peritransplant fluid collections (eg, urinomas, seromas, lymphoceles), anastomotic vascular strictures, obstruction of the collecting system, and development of allograft rejection. Various radiologic modalities may be used to evaluate transplants for these potential sequela. Some techniques rely solely on anatomic findings, such as dynamic CT, magnetic resonance imaging, and real-time ultrasound. Observations that are used sonographically to predict transplant rejection include: renal size; renal sinus fat; corticomedullary ratio; corticomedullary sharpness; corticomedullary conspicuity; focal parenchymal abnormalities; and pelvic wall thickening (62). Other modalities, such as radionuclide scintigraphy, offer physiologic information regarding blood flow, filtration, and excretion. Duplex sonography has the advantage of providing anatomic information through real-time imaging and blood flow data from Doppler analysis. This modality has been shown to be a valuable means for identifying acute rejection in renal allografts (63–65). Arterial Doppler waveforms in normal renal transplants demonstrate a sharp systolic peak, followed by a downward slope to a lower but continuous, antegrade diastolic blood flow component (Fig. 4.36). The presence of diastolic flow results from the low vascular impedance in the normal renal transplant. It has been shown in acute rejection that the arterial waveform is altered by the increased vascular impedance within the parenchyma. The result is a decrease in diastolic flow, often accompanied by an increased pulsatility in the arterial Doppler waveform (Fig. 4.37). Because the process of allograft rejection usually involves the entire allograft, these spectral waveform findings may be demonstrated by sampling at different sites, such as the main renal artery, in the segmental-interlobar arteries,

Fig. 4.36A,B. Normal renal transplant. **A.** Sagittal ultrasound scan of the pelvic renal transplant. **B.** Doppler waveform from the central renal sinus area shows a normal renal transplant arterial waveform, with a systolic peak and continuous diastolic blood flow.

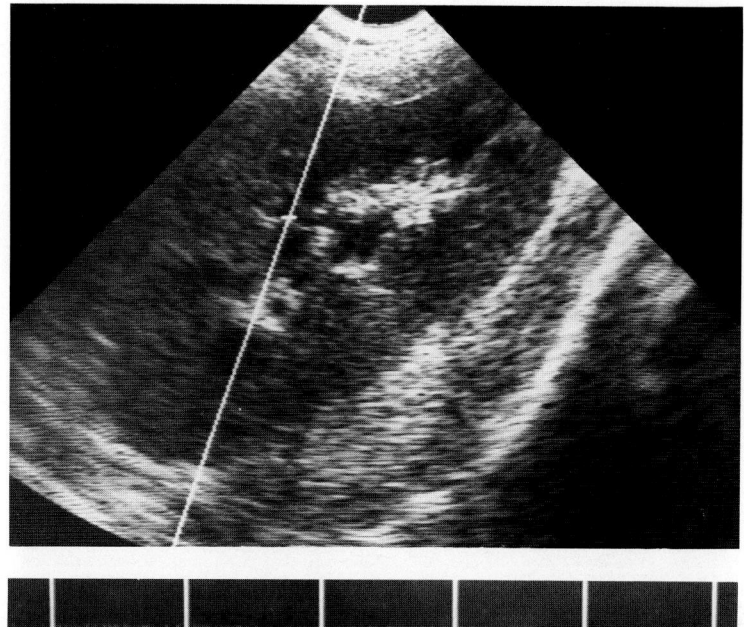

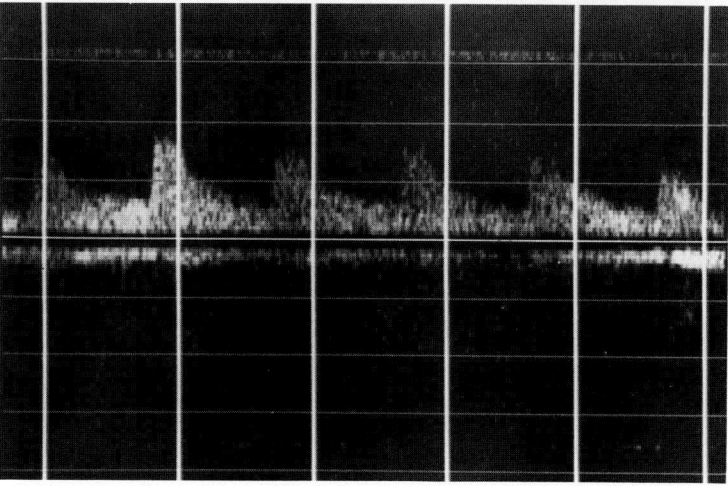

and in the arcuate arteries of the kidney. This may be quantified using the pulsatility index (PI). Acute rejection has been shown to produce a significantly higher PI than in normal transplants or in patients with either chronic rejection or acute tubular necrosis (ATN). One correlative study comparing Doppler ultrasound and magnetic resonance imaging showed duplex scanning to be significantly more sensitive, specific, and accurate in determining acute renal transplant rejection than the other modalities (66). Because of these results and its relatively low cost, duplex sonography has been recommended as a primary test for evaluating patients with possible acute renal transplant rejection. With recovery from rejection, the waveform displays return to a normal pattern. Persistently abnormal diastolic flow accompanied by changes in systolic flow, indicate a poor prognosis. In contrast to acute rejection, chronic renal transplant rejection demonstrates no significant alterations in systolic or diastolic blood flow, aside from some dampening and broadening of the systolic waveform due to deterioration in blood flow.

Another application of duplex sonography is in evaluation for stenosis involving the main renal transplant artery (Fig. 4.38). The incidence of this complication varies between 1 and 10% (67). This may become clinically manifest by either development of hypertension or a bruit auscultated over the transplant. In a study

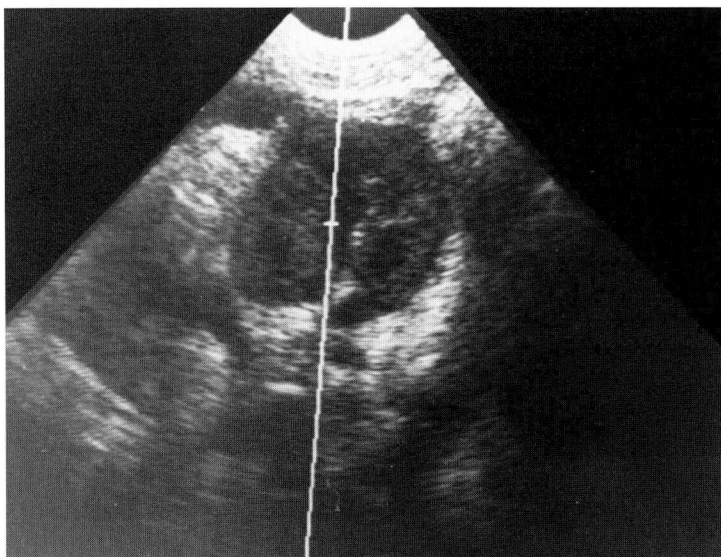

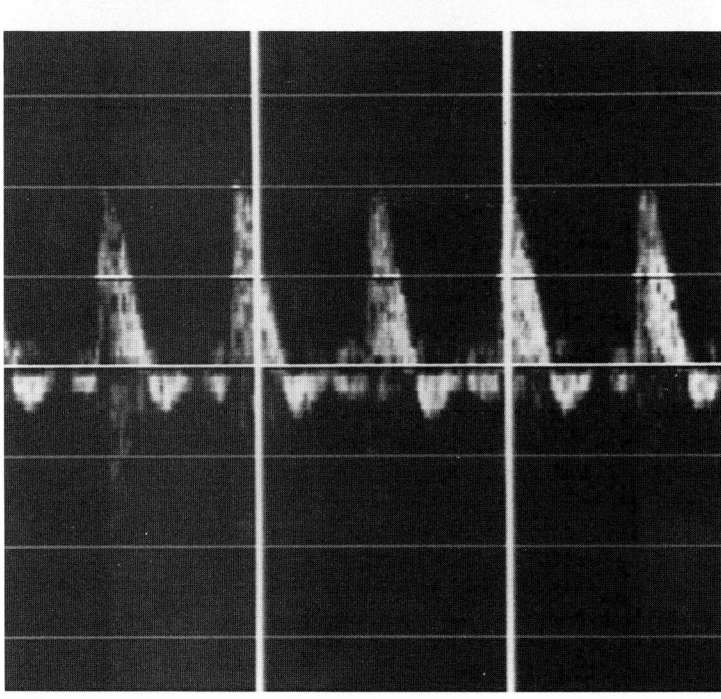

Fig. 4.37A,B. Renal transplant rejection. **A.** Transverse sonogram of the renal transplant, with Doppler sampling centrally within the kidney. **B.** The waveform demonstrates a sharp systolic peak and a reverse flow component in diastole. Subsequent biopsy confirmed renal allograft rejection.

Fig. 4.38A–E. Renal allograft artery stenosis. **A.** Transverse ultrasound image of the renal transplant, with Doppler sampling of the main renal artery. **B.** A markedly elevated frequency shift is accompanied by waveform distortion. These are findings typically seen with hemodynamically significant arterial stenosis. *(Continued.)*

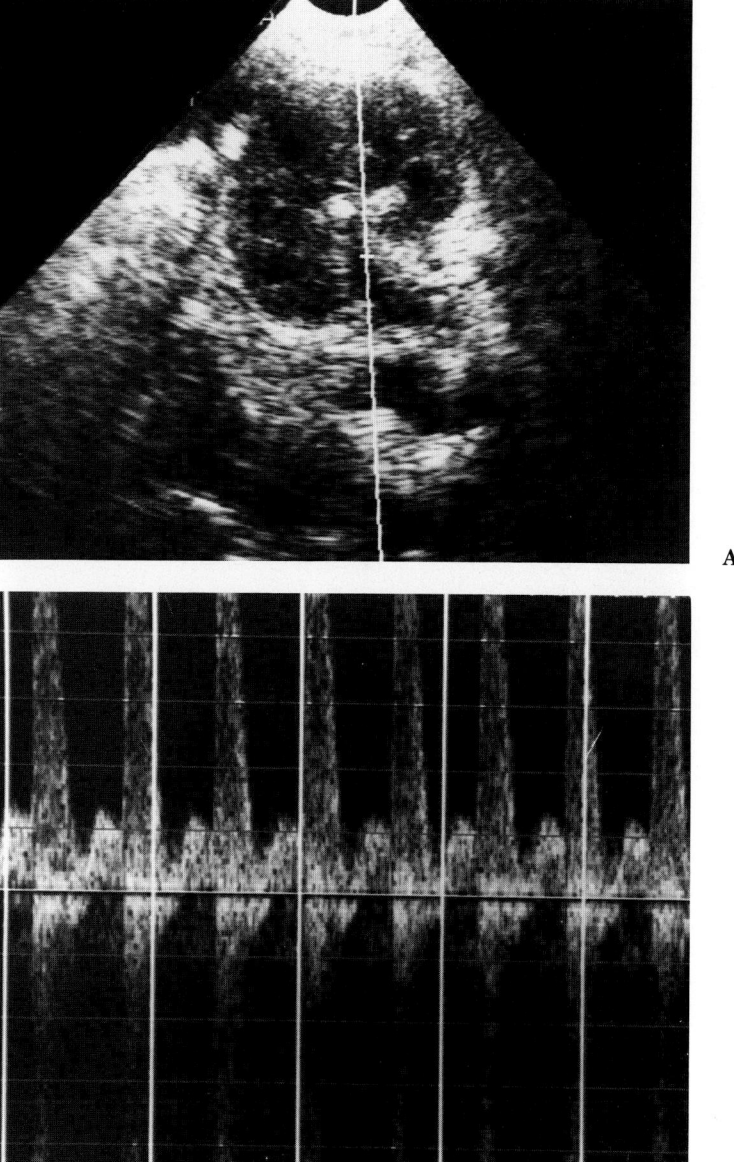

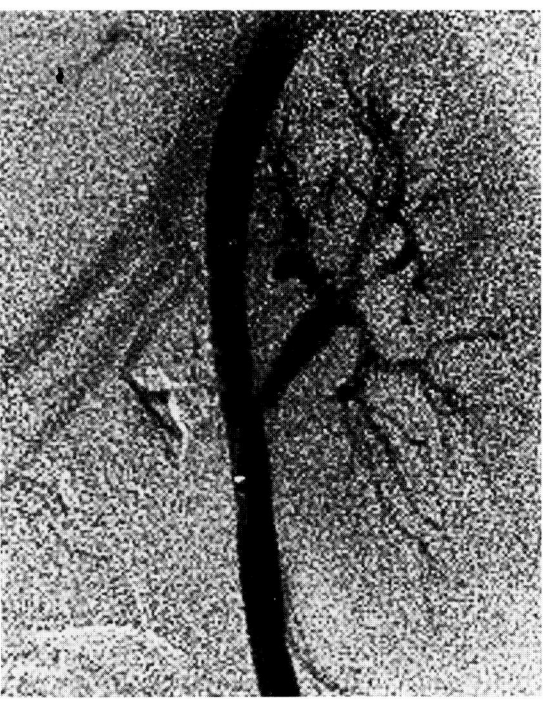

Fig. 4.38C. Arteriography confirms stenosis in the proximal segment of the main renal transplant artery. **D.** After percutaneous balloon angioplasty of this lesion, a repeat arteriogram shows successful dilatation of the stenosis.

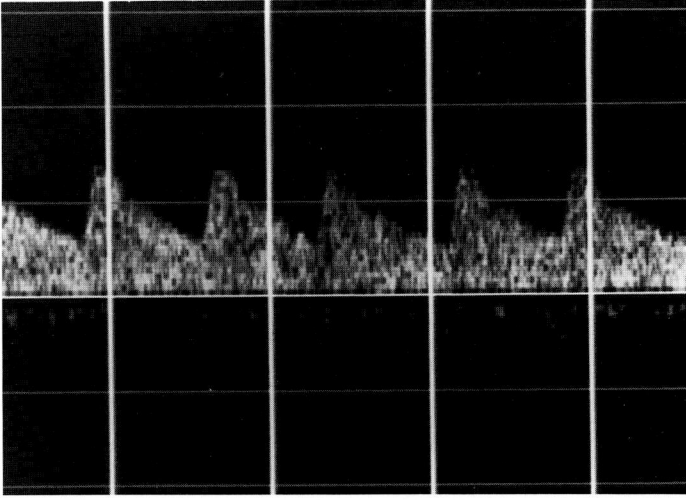

Fig. 4.38E. Repeat duplex study postangioplasty demonstrated normalization of the waveform in the main renal transplant artery.

Fig. 4.39A,B. Color-flow imaging in the abdomen. **A,B.** Clinical work is in progress to evaluate the potential role of color-flow imaging in evaluating the abdominal vasculature. Images of the portal venous system (**A**) and right renal vessels (**B**) are courtesy of Quantum Medical Systems, Inc., Issaquah, Washington. (For a color reproduction of this figure see frontmatter.)

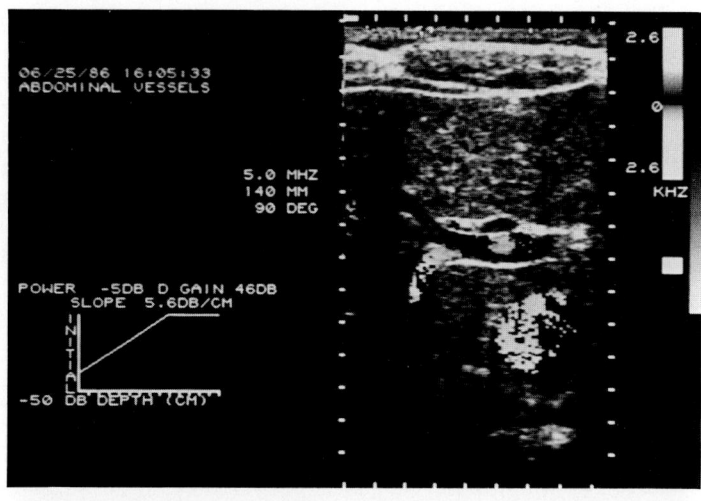

A

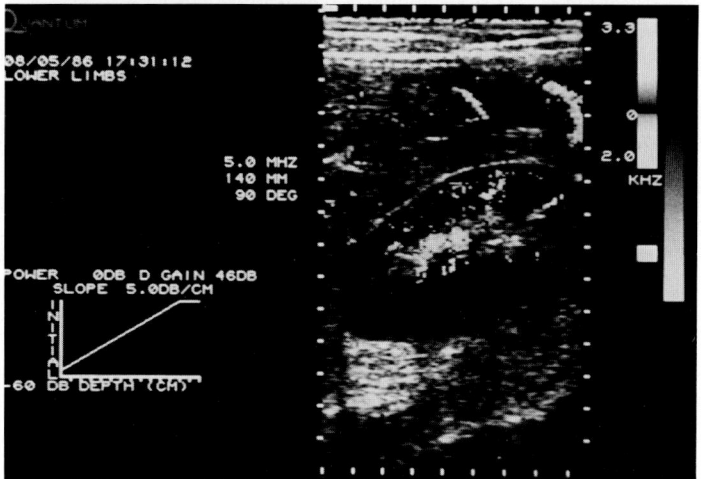

B

of seven patients with angiographically documented artery stenosis, five were diagnosed by use of Doppler ultrasound (67). Findings included a high-velocity jet at the site of stenosis (exceeding 7.5 KHz) and spectral broadening from turbulent flow (67,68). Obstruction of venous outflow from the allograft may result from either torsion of the main renal veins draining the extraperitoneal transplant or from retrograde extension of thrombus within the external iliac vein. Duplex sonography provides an easy, noninvasive means to assess for patency of the main renal transplant vein and adjacent iliac vessels (69).

Conclusion

In this chapter, normal Doppler waveforms in the abdomen have been reviewed and findings in several disease states described. This material reflects the summation of extensive clinical and technologic effort at numerous centers. At present, several potential applications of abdominal duplex sonography remain to be investigated, both qualitatively and quantitatively. In addition, color-flow imaging is emerging as a new modality (Fig. 4.39). It awaits future contributions in clinical and biotechnologic research to define further the role that duplex abdominal ultrasound will serve in the practice of medicine.

References

1. Gill RW: Measurement of blood flow by ultrasound: Accuracy and sources of error. Ultrasound Med Biol 11:625, 1985.
2. Qamar MI, Read AE, Skidmore R, et al: Pulsatility index of superior mesenteric artery blood velocity waveforms. Ultrasound Med Biol 12:773, 1986.
3. Taylor KJW, Burns PN: Duplex Doppler scanning in the pelvis and abdomen. Ultrasound Med Biol 11:643, 1985.
4. Taylor KJW, Burns PN, Woodcock JP, et al: Blood flow in deep abdominal and pelvic vessels: Ultrasonic pulsed-Doppler analysis. Radiology 154:487, 1985.
5. Wolverson MK, Nouri S, Joist JH, et al: The direct visualization of blood flow by real-time ultrasound: Clinical observations and underlying mechanisms. Radiology 140:443, 1981.
6. Cosgrove DO, Arger PH: Intravenous echoes due to laminar flow: Experimental observations. AJR 139:953, 1982.
7. Paivansalo MJ, Siniluoto TMJ: Direct visualization of laminar blood flow in abdominal aorta using real-time ultrasound. J Clin Ultrasound 14:135, 1986.
8. King DL, Van Natta FC, Thorsen K, et al: Spontaneously echogenic arterial blood flow in abdominal aortic aneurysms. AJR 138:350, 1982.
9. Wells PNT, Skidmore R: Doppler developments in the last quinquennium. Ultrasound Med Biol 11:613, 1985.
10. Baker AR, Evans DH, Prytherch DR, et al: Some failings of pulsatility index and damping factor. Ultrasound Med Biol 12:875, 1986.
11. Ralls PW, Quinn MR, Rogers W, et al: Sonographic anatomy of the hepatic artery. AJR 136:1059, 1981.
12. Qamar MI, Read AE, Skidmore R, et al: Transcutaneous Doppler ultrasound measurement of superior mesenteric artery blood flow in man. Gut 27:100, 1986.
13. Qamar MI, Read AE, Skidmore R, et al: Noninvasive assessment of the superior mesenteric artery blood flow in man (abstract). Gut 25:A546, 1984.
14. Subramanyam BR, Balthazar EJ, Raghavendra BN, et al: Sonographic evaluation of patients with portal hypertension. Am J Gastroenterol 78:369, 1983.
15. Pasto ME, Kuirtz AB, Jarrell BE, et al: The Kimray-Greenfield filter: Evaluation by Doppler real-time/ pulsed-Doppler ultrasound. Radiology 148:223, 1983.
16. Ritter SB, Bierman FZ: Noninvasive diagnosis of interrupted inferior vena cava: Gated pulsed Doppler application. Am J Cardiol 51:1796, 1983.
17. Garris JB, Kangarloo H, Sample WF: Ultrasonic diagnosis of infrahepatic interruption of the inferior vena cava with azygos (hemiazygos) continuation. Radiology 134:179, 1980.
18. Cahow CE, Gusberg RJ, Gottlieb LJ: Gastrointestinal hemorrhage from pseudoaneurysms in pancreatic pseudocysts. Am J Surg 145:534, 1983.
19. Guida PM, Moore SW: Aneurysm of the hepatic artery. Report of five cases with a brief review of the previously reported cases. Surgery 60:299, 1966.
20. Sukerkar AN, Dulay CC, Anandappa E, et al: Mycotic aneurysm of the hepatic artery. Radiology 124:44, 1977.
21. Athey PA, Sax SL, Lamki N, et al: Sonography in the diagnosis of hepatic artery aneurysms. AJR 147:725, 1986.
22. Falkoff GE, Taylor KJW, Morse S: Hepatic artery pseudoaneurysm: Diagnosis with real-time and pulsed-Doppler US. Radiology 158:55, 1986.
23. White AF, Baum S, Buranasiri S: Aneurysms secondary to pancreatitis. AJR 127:393, 1976.
24. Berland LL, Lawson TL, Foley WD: Porta hepatis: Sonographic discrimination of bile ducts from arteries with pulsed Doppler with new anatomic criteria. AJR 138:833, 1982.
25. Wing VW, Laing FC, Jeffrey RB, et al: Sonographic differentiation of enlarged hepatic arteries from dilated intrahepatic bile ducts. AJR 145:57, 1985.
26. Taylor KJW, Morse SS, Weltin GG, et al: Liver transplant recipients: Portable duplex US with correlative angiography. Radiology 159:357, 1986.
27. Freling NJM, Schuur KH, Haagsma EB, et al: Ultrasound as first imaging modality in superior mesenteric and portal vein thrombosis. J Clin Ultrasound 14:554, 1986.
28. Miller VE, Berland LL: Pulsed Doppler duplex sonography and CT of portal vein thrombosis. AJR 145:73, 1985.
29. Alpern MB, Rubin JM, Williams DM, et al: Porta hepatis: Duplex Doppler US with angiographic correlation. Radiology 162:53, 1987.
30. Weltin G, Taylor KJW, Cater AR, et al: Duplex Doppler: Identification of cavernous transformation of the portal vein. AJR 144:999, 1985.
31. Subramanyam BR, Balthazar EJ, Madamba MR, et al: Sonography of portosystemic venous collaterals in portal hypertension. Radiology 146:161, 1983.

32. Bolondi L, Mazziotti A, Arienti V, et al: Ultrasonographic study of portal venous system in portal hypertension and after portosystemic shunt operations. Surgery 95:261, 1984.
33. Huey H, Cooperberg PL, Bogoch A: Diagnosis of giant varix of the coronary vein by pulsed-Doppler sonography. AJR 143:77, 1984.
34. Moriyasu F, Nishida O, Ban N, et al: "Congestion index" of the portal vein. AJR 146:735, 1986.
35. Menu Y, Alison D, Lorphelin JM, et al: Budd-Chiari Syndrome: US evaluation. Radiology 157:761, 1985.
36. Yang PJ, Glazer GM, Bowerman RA: Budd-Chiari Syndrome: Computed tomographic and ultrasonographic findings. J Comput Assist Tomogr 7:148, 1983.
37. Derchi LE, Biggi E, Cicio GR, et al: Aneurysms of the splenic artery: Noninvasive diagnosis by pulsed Doppler sonography. J Ultrasound Med 3:41, 1984.
38. Williams DB, Payne WS, Foulk WT, et al: Splenic arteriovenous fistula. Mayo Clin Proc 55:383, 1980.
39. Weinberger G, Mitra SK, Yoeli G: Ultrasound diagnosis of splenic vein thrombosis. J Clin Ultrasound 10:345, 1982.
40. Foley WD, Gleysteen JJ, Lawson TL, et al: Dynamic computed tomography and pulsed Doppler ultrasonography in the evaluation of splenorenal shunt patency. J Comput Assist Tomogr 7:106, 1983.
41. Ackroyd N, Gill R, Griffiths K, et al: Duplex scanning of the portal vein and portosystemic shunts. Surgery 99:591, 1986.
42. Takayasu K, Moriyama N, Shima Y, et al: Sonographic detection of large spontaneous splenorenal shunts and its clinical significance. Br J Rad 57:565, 1984.
43. Holmin T, Alwmark A, Forsberg L: The ultrasonic demonstration of portocaval and interposition mesocaval shunts. Br J Surg 69:673, 1982.
44. Moeller DA, Rogers JV, Allan NK, et al: Ultrasound appearance of a traumatic hepatic artery-portal vein fistula. J Clin Ultrasound 11:237, 1983.
45. Inamoto K, Tanaka S, Yamazaki H, et al: Arterioportal fistula in hepatocellular carcinoma. J Comput Assist Tomogr 7:151, 1983.
46. Wittich G, Jantsch H, Tscholakoff D: Congenital porto-systemic shunt diagnosed by combined real-time and Doppler sonography. J Ultrasound Med 4:315, 1985.
47. Chagnon SF, Vallee CA, Barge J, et al: Aneurysmal portohepatic venous fistula: Report of two cases. Radiology 159:693, 1986.
48. Charnsangavej C, Soo CS, Bernardino ME, et al: Porto-hepatic venous malformation: Ultrasound, computed tomographic and angiographic findings. Cardiovasc Intervent Radiol 6:109, 1983.
49. Kidambi H, Herbert R, Kidambi AV: Ultrasonic demonstration of superior mesenteric and splenoportal venous thrombosis. J Clin Ultrasound 14:199, 1986.
50. Jager KA, Fortner GS, Thiele BL, et al: Noninvasive diagnosis of intestinal angina. J Clin Ultrasound 12:588, 1984.
51. Strandness DE: Ultrasound in the study of atherosclerosis. Ultrasound Med Biol 12:453, 1986.
52. Rittgers SE, Norris CS, Barnes RW: Detection of renal artery stenosis: Experimental and clinical analysis of velocity waveforms. Ultrasound Med Biol 11:523, 1985.
53. Norris CS, Barnes RW: Renal artery flow velocity analysis: A sensitive measure of experimental and clinical renovascular resistance. J Surg Res 36:230, 1984.
54. Avasthi PS, Voyles WF, Greene ER: Noninvasive diagnosis of renal artery stenosis by echo-Doppler velocimetry. Kidney Int 25:824, 1984.
55. Handa N, Fukunaga R, Uehara A, et al: Echo-Doppler velocimeter in the diagnosis of hypertensive patients: The renal artery Doppler technique. Ultrasound Med Biol 12:945, 1986.
56. Rifkin MD, Pasto ME, Goldberg BB: Duplex Doppler examination in renal disease: Evaluation of vascular involvement. Ultrasound Med Biol 11:341, 1985.
57. Chou YH, Tiu CM, Pan HB, et al: Diagnosis of renal pseudoaneurysm by pulsed Doppler ultrasound. J Clin Ultrasound 13:662, 1985.
58. Boyce WH: Ultrasonic velocimetry in resection of renal arteriovenous fistulas and other intrarenal surgical procedures. J Urology 125:610, 1981.
59. Avasthi PS, Greene ER, Scholler C, et al: Noninvasive diagnosis of renal vein thrombosis by ultrasonic echo-Doppler flowmetry. Kidney Int 23:882, 1983.
60. Kinard RE, Orrison WW: Ultrasound demonstration of the retroaortic left renal vein. J Clin Ultrasound 14:151, 1986.
61. Kurtz AB, Dubbins PA, Zegel HG, et al: Normal left renal vein mimicking left renal artery aneurysm. J Clin Ultrasound 9:105, 1981.
62. Hoddick W, Filly RA, Backman U, et al: Renal allograft rejection: US evaluation. Radiology 161:469, 1986.
63. Arima M, Takahara S, Ihara H, et al: Predictability of renal allograft prognosis during rejection crisis by ultrasonic Doppler flow technique. Urology 19:389, 1982.

64. Rigsby CM, Taylor KJW, Weltin G, et al: Renal allografts in acute rejection: Evaluation using duplex sonography. Radiology 158:375, 1986.
65. Rigsby CM, Burns PN, Weltin GG, et al: Doppler signal quantitation in renal allografts: Comparison in normal and rejecting transplants, with pathologic correlation. Radiology 162:39, 1987.
66. Steinberg HV, Nelson RC, Murphy FB, et al: Renal allograft rejection: Evaluation by Doppler US and MR imaging. Radiology 162:337, 1987.
67. Reinitz ER, Goldman MH, Sais J, et al: Evaluation of transplant renal artery blood flow by Doppler sound-spectrum analysis. Arch Surg 118:415, 1983.
68. Taylor KJW, Morse SS, Rigsby CM, et al: Vascular complications in renal allografts: Detection with duplex Doppler US. Radiology 162:31, 1987.
69. Wood RFM, Nasmyth DG: Doppler ultrasound in the diagnosis of vascular occlusion in renal transplantation. Transplantation 33:547, 1982.

5
Duplex Evaluation of Fetoplacental and Uteroplacental Circulation

MICHAEL C. HILL, IAN M. LANDE, and JOHN H. GROSSMAN, III

Fetal growth depends on a steady supply of nutrients and oxygen from the mother, and a normal uteroplacental and fetoplacental circulation is necessary for this to occur. Until recently our knowledge of blood flow in these circulations was based on animal studies, measurements taken from human abortions by hysterotomy during early pregnancy, and by examination of the fetus and placenta immediately after delivery (1–5). The measurements obtained by invasive methods were not readily repeatable and did not represent the true state of physiologic affairs. In recent years, however, Doppler ultrasound has given us a noninvasive method of evaluating blood flow to the gravid uterus and fetus. In this chapter, we briefly describe the fetoplacental and uteroplacental circulation and the application of Doppler ultrasound to normal and complicated pregnancies.

Uteroplacental Circulation

The major source of blood supply to the uterus is via the internal iliac artery and uterine arteries. A small amount of its blood supply is also received from the inferior mesenteric, middle sacral, inferior epigastric, external pudendal, and ovarian arteries (6). Branches of the uterine arteries enter the uterine substance at an acute angle and do not branch appreciably until they reach the middle third of the myometrium. Here they give off arcuate branches that form an interlacing network of blood vessels throughout the wall of the uterus (6,7). The radial arteries come off at right angles and proceed to the myometrial–endometrial junction (Fig. 5.1A). Upon entering the endometrium, they become the spiral arteries and immediately give off the basal arteries that branch in the deepest portion of the endometrium. The spiral arteries supply the intervillous spaces of the placenta with maternal blood and are drained by dilated but less numerous endometrial veins (Fig. 5.1B).

During pregnancy there is hyperplasia and hypertrophy of the uterine wall, and the arteries elongate and become coiled. At the base of the placenta, the endometrium is progressively thinned as it is invaded by the trophoblast. The trophoblast migrates along the entire length of the spiral arteries and strips it of its muscular elastic coat by the 20th postmenstrual week. This has the effect of reducing resistance to blood flow at this level. There is also little resistance to blood flow progressing from the radial artery into the intervillous space. The pressure falls from about 70 to 80 mm Hg in the former to 10 mm Hg in the latter (7).

Growth of the uterine tissues and vessels ceases at the end of the first trimester, and further lengthening is accomplished by stretching. The uteroplacental vessels gradually dilate during pregnancy to accommodate the necessary demand for increased blood flow (6). The spiral arteries increase in diameter from 200 to 300 μ in early pregnancy to 1000 μ in the last trimester. There is little resting vascular resistance in the uteroplacental circulation. The ratio of the total uterine blood flow to umbilical blood flow is 1.5 to 1.0, respectively (8). Uterine blood flow increases from 50 ml/min at the end of the first trimester to 500 to 750 ml/min at term.

Vasculature of Uterine Wall

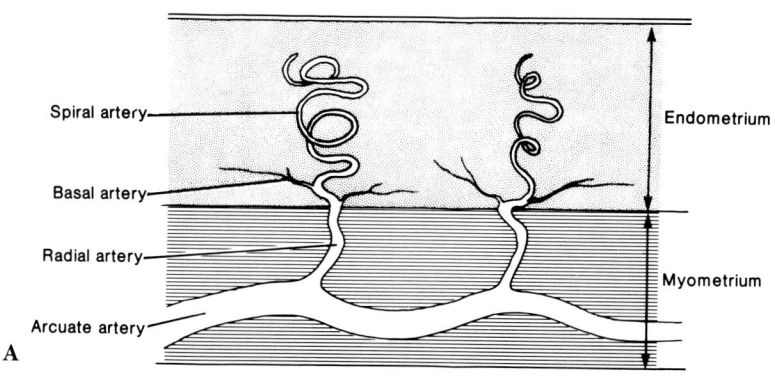

Utero-Placental Vasculature

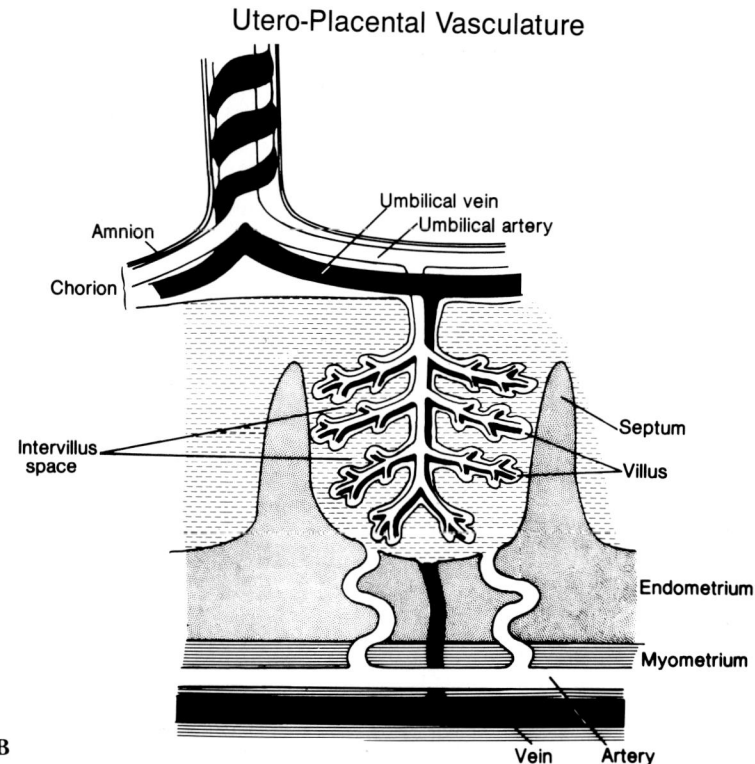

Fig. 5.1. Normal uteroplacental circulation.

Fetoplacental Circulation

Doppler ultrasound has been used for many years to monitor the fetal heart. Normal baseline fetal heart rates range from 120 to 160 beats/min and slow slightly toward term. The individual fetus tends to maintain a fairly constant heart rate within a variation of less than 10 beats/min from day to day (8).

Oxygenated blood from the placenta returns to the fetal heart via the umbilical vein (Fig. 5.2) (8). It enters the superior portion of the inferior vena cava by the ductus venosus and portal-hepatic veins. Upon entering the right atrium, approximately 70% of the blood goes via the foramen ovale into the left atrium, whereas the remainder enters the right ventricle along with most of the blood from the

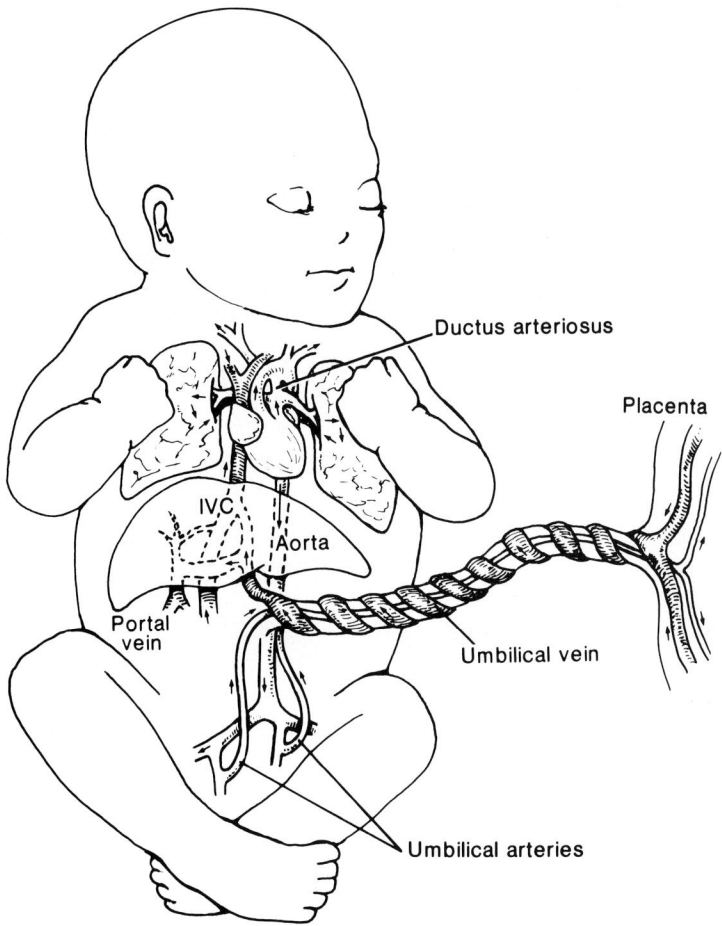

Fig. 5.2. Normal fetoplacental circulation.

superior vena cava. The right ventricular blood goes into the pulmonary artery where most passes into the descending aorta via the ductus arteriosus with only a small amount going to both lungs (Fig. 5.2).

The blood that has entered the left atrium goes into the left ventricle and ascending aorta, where it is distributed mainly to the coronary arteries and branches of the arch of the aorta to the head, neck, and upper limbs. Fifty to 60% of the blood in the descending aorta goes to the placenta via the umbilical arteries that arise from the right and left internal iliac arteries (Fig. 5.2) (3,7). The two umbilical arteries and the single umbilical vein are contained within the umbilical cord surrounded by Wharton's jelly. A single umbilical artery is present in about 1% of singleton pregnancies and in a slightly higher percentage of multiple pregnancies. This finding is associated with an increased incidence of a wide variety of congenital anomalies.

The branches of the umbilical artery and umbilical vein radiate out from the site of insertion of the cord along the fetal surface of the placenta beneath the amnion (Fig. 5.1B). Branches of the artery along with an accompanying vein penetrate the chorionic plate and enter the main stem chorionic villi. There they divide to supply individual chorionic villi. It is at this level that the exchange of nutrients and waste products takes place between the fetal and maternal circulations. The unit composed of the main stem chorionic villus and its branches is called the "fetal cotyledon." It is this capillary bed that produces the most resistance to pulsatile blood flow. As pregnancy advances, the size of the chorionic villi increases, whereas their number decreases. This is accompanied by a reduction in the thickness of the tissue layer between the fetal capillaries and the maternal intervillous spaces. These changes allow for more efficient exchange between the two circulations.

Doppler Measurement of Blood Flow

Measurement of blood flow in the fetoplacental circulation was first performed in fetal lambs. The initial measurements of blood flow in the human fetus produced disparate results and were invasive. It was not until the development of Doppler ultrasound that a noninvasive method of estimating blood flow became available (9–13).

There are many potential errors in measuring blood flow with Doppler ultrasound (Fig. 5.3) (7,14–18). They include:

1. Measurement of the vessel diameter: the accuracy in measuring the vessel diameter is particularly important because the vessel radius is squared when calculating blood flow (19). Because arteries are pulsatile, the measurement of their internal diameter can vary by as much as 20% during the cardiac cycle (14,15,17,20,21). Eik-Nes et al (14) estimated that an error of 0.4 mm in measuring a 4-mm diameter vessel may cause as much as a 25% error in estimating blood flow. To overcome this, they recommend averaging 10 measurements taken from the outer margin of the near wall to the inner margin of the far wall. Each measurement is obtained from a different freeze frame of the vessel. This method will limit the measurement error to less than 0.4 mm and compares favorably with approaches using a time-distance recorder that allows continuous measurement of the aortic diameter as it pulsates (15).
2. Proper positioning of the sample volume: the sample volume should include all the vessel lumen so that it is uniformly insonated at the same time excluding signals that arise outside the vessel (Fig. 5.3).
3. Accurate measurement of the angle between the ultrasound beam and the long axis of the vessel lumen: the angle of 45° is optimal; however, with deep lying vessels; it may be necessary to increase the angle to 65°. A trained operator can keep the angle fairly constant, to within plus to minus 5°, while sampling the vessel.
4. High pass filtering of low amplitude signals (ie, thump signals from vessel wall vibration) will cause overestimation of the mean velocity: Eik-Nes et al (15) estimated that the optimal level of high pass filtering for the measurement of fetal blood flow is around 100 Hz. Even at this level, overestimations of blood flow in the umbilical vein may approach 2.7 cm/s.
5. Distance between Doppler transducer and the vessel being examined limits the velocity that can be recorded (17). Two considerations influence the choice of a Doppler transducer: 1) as the absorption of sound is proportional to the square of the frequency, better tissue penetration is achieved using lower frequency Doppler transducers; however, 2) higher frequencies give a greater Doppler shift for a given velocity. These factors have to be balanced in choosing an appropriate Dop-

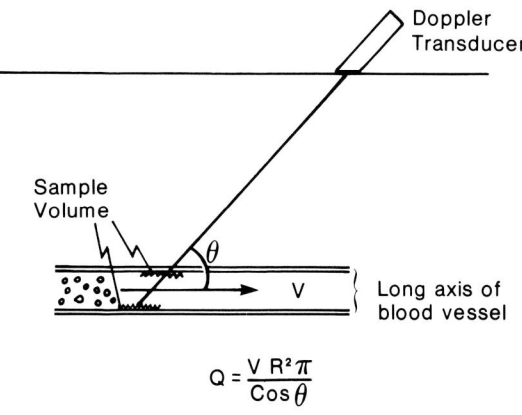

$$Q = \frac{V R^2 \pi}{\cos \theta}$$

V - Mean blood velocity
R - Radius of vessel
θ - Angle between doppler beam and vessel

Fig. 5.3. Proper technique to obtain a doppler signal from a blood vessel.

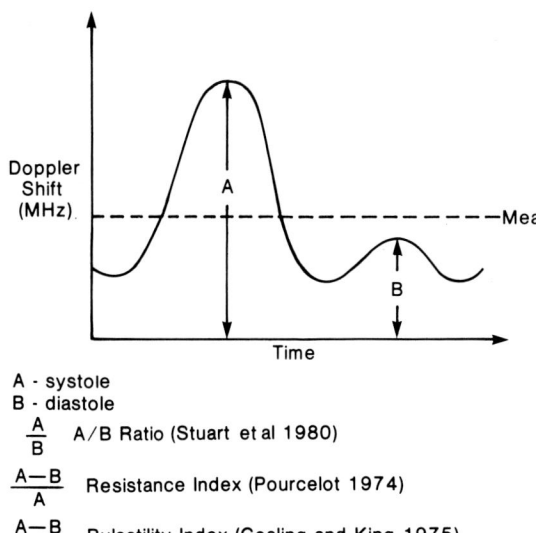

Fig. 5.4. Diagrammatic representation of a Doppler waveform and how it is used to estimate the A/B ratio, the resistance index, and the pulsatility index.

pler transducer for the evaluation of a pregnant patient.
6. Estimation of fetal weight can be notoriously inaccurate: this is a very important factor when measuring flow per kilogram per minute.

Due to the many potential errors in measuring volume blood flow using Doppler ultrasound, the technique has limitations in daily clinical practice. This has led to the development of alternatives that are easier to perform, such as flow velocity waveform analysis for the evaluation of uteroplacental and fetoplacental circulation.

Flow Velocity Doppler Waveform

Arterial blood flow is pulsatile due to contraction of the heart. The amplitude of the velocity waveform progressively decreases away from the heart and is altered by reflected waves that are produced where arteries branch. Waveforms produced at various sites differ and can be characteristic for each area (22). In arteries supplying areas of low resistance (umbilical artery, uterine artery), there is forward blood flow in diastole, whereas in arteries supplying areas of high resistance (external iliac artery), there is some reversal of blood flow in diastole (Fig. 5.9). Forward flow in diastole is a consequence of the continuing effects of cardiac contraction and the elastic recoil (complicance) of the vessel against peripheral resistance (Fig. 5.4).

Doppler waveforms in fetoplacental and uteroplacental circulation are affected by: 1) cardiac contractility, 2) viscosity of the blood, 3) elasticity of the vessel wall, 4) the peripheral resistance in the distal circulation, 5) the distance of the sampling site from the heart, and 6) the presence or absence of turbulence. There is no general consensus as to the most effective method for analyzing the waveforms produced. The ones that have been used are (Fig. 5.4): 1) the pulsatility index (PI) (23), 2) the A/B ratio (24), and 3) the resistance index (RI) (25).

In the fetoplacental circulation, these indexes appear to be independent of a normal fetal heart rate (120 to 160 beat/min) but are affected by fetal breathing movements (17,26). The waveforms do not appear to be significantly altered by uncomplicated labor (27). A single waveform should never be used for quantitative assessment, one should average a number of sequential waveforms to minimize beat-to-beat variations (17). In our practice we use the A/B ratio and obtain at least three runs containing approximately 10 waveforms each. We measure one or more ratios from each run and then average these to give the final ratio.

Normal Fetoplacental Blood Flow

The fetal circulation is characterized by a high blood flow and a low vascular resistance (3). Umbilical blood flow increases with gestational age and is dependent on the vascular resistance and pressure gradient driving the blood from the descending aorta through the placenta and back to the inferior vena cava. The increase in umbilical blood flow is not in proportion to the change in fetal body weight. For example, at 90 days' gestation umbilical blood flow in the fetal lamb is 230 ml/kg/min; this falls to 170 ml/kg/min at term, when it accounts for more than 50% of the basal cardiac output (3).

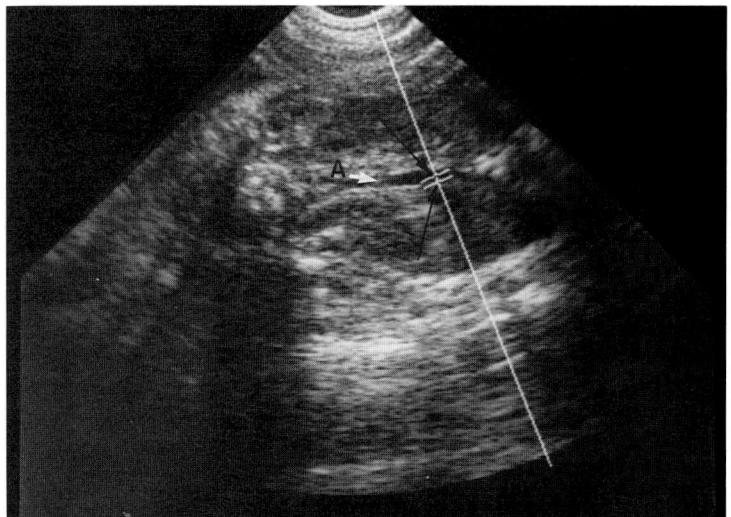

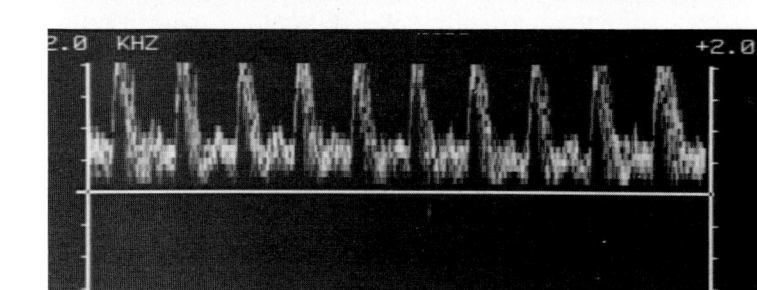

Fig. 5.5A,B. A. Doppler of the fetal aorta (A). The sample volume (*arrows*) is positioned at the level of the fetal diaphragm. **B.** Normal doppler waveform from the fetal aorta.

Fetal Aortic Blood Flow

Fetal aortic blood flow is best measured at, or just above, the level of the diaphragm (Fig. 5.5*A*). This should not be done during fetal breathing movements as they not only modulate flow velocity, especially during diastole, but decrease the diameter of the aorta in inspiration (7).

As mentioned, the diameter of the aorta should be measured from the outer margin of the near wall to the inner margin of the far wall. This diameter can change by as much as 20% during the cardiac cycle and so as many as 10 measurements should be taken and averaged (9,15,21). It has been shown that the mean aortic diameter increases in a linear fashion in the last trimester of pregnancy (16,17,20). The mean blood flow per kilogram in the upper abdominal aorta, on the other hand, remains fairly constant in the last trimester and ranges from 185 to 246 ml/kg/min (Table 5.1). The peak velocity is 97 to 118 cm/s, whereas the mean velocity is 19 to 31 cm/s. These measurements do not appear to change appreciably in uncomplicated labor nor are they altered by intravaginal prostaglandin E_2 used to induce labor (17,27,28).

Approximately 50 to 60% of blood flow in the upper abdominal aorta will eventually go to the placenta, whereas 30% is distributed to the abdominal organs. The mean blood flow in the lower fetal abdominal aorta just above the bifurcation is 184 ml/kg/min (Table 5.1) (16). Approximately 80% of the blood at this level in the aorta goes to the placenta. In contrast to blood flow in the distal aorta of the human adult, there is no retrograde flow in diastole, indicating that the placental bed is of low vascular resistance (Fig. 5.5*B*) (29).

Table 5.1. Doppler Estimation of Fetal Aortic Blood Flow

Ref.	Pt. #	Mean Velocity (cm/s)	Mean flow/kg (ml/min/kg)
9 Eik-Nes (1980)	26		191 ± 12.2
33 Wladimiroff (1981)	50	20 ± 5.0	
14 Eik-Nes (1982)	23	19 to 26	185 ± 7.6
31 Griffin (1983)	92	31.2 ± 6.4	246 ± 60
17 Marsal (1984)	64	29 ± 5.8	238.4 ± 39.9
32 Van Lierde (1984)	20	28 ± 7.0	216
29 Eldridge (1985)*	18		184 ± 20
16 Erskine (1985)	15	31.2	206 ± 8.5

*Sampling site distal fetal aorta above bifurcation.

Umbilical Vein Blood Flow

Based on the estimation of oxygen consumption, Dawes (3) calculated that the minimum blood flow in the umbilical vein of the human fetus would be 90 ml/kg/min. Estimates of blood flow in the intraabdominal portion of the umbilical vein using Doppler ultrasound vary from 107 to 125 ml/kg/min in the third trimester in uncomplicated pregnancy (Table 5.2) (9,15, 19,30–33). The blood flow velocity ranges from 13.6 to 18 cm/s (Table 5.2) (16,32,34). All of these measurements show that the rate of flow remains constant throughout the last trimester of pregnancy, with a linear increase in vessel diameter accounting for the increase in total blood flow (16). Gill et al (30), using a similar technique, showed a slight decrease in umbilical vein blood flow from 35 weeks' gestation to term.

Table 5.2. Doppler Estimation of Umbilical Vein Blood Flow

Ref.	Pt. #	Mean velocity (cm/s)	Mean flow/kg (ml/min/kg)
11 Gill (1980)	47		120 (23–35 wk)
			106 (36–40 wk)
9 Eik-Nes (1980)	26		110 ± 5.8
33 Wladimiroff (1981)	50		107
14 Eik-Nes (1982)	27		115 ± 6.9
5 Kurjak (1982)	63		107
31 Griffin (1983)	45		122 ± 4.2
32 Van Lierde (1984)	20	18.0 ± 4	117 ± 16
16 Erskine (1985)	15	12.8	125
34 Chen (1986)	163	13.6	

Maternal oxygen inhalation has little if any effect on the Doppler estimate of umbilical vein blood flow but does decrease intervillous blood flow as measured using the ^{133}Xe method (35). Similarly, umbilical vein blood flow was not altered immediately after maternal ingestion of two cups of coffee, whereas intervillous blood flow was reduced in normal pregnancies but not in hypertensive pregnancies (36).

Normal Fetoplacental Waveform Analysis

Fetal Aortic Waveform Analysis

Adequate Doppler evaluation of the fetal aorta can be obtained in more than 90% of all patients (29). The flow velocity waveform in the descending thoracic aorta shows a rapid acceleration during systole. From peak systole to end diastole, there is deceleration, at first rapid, ending in an incisura due to closure of the aortic valve. This is followed by a slower deceleration in diastole (Fig. 5.5B) (31,37). There is no reversal of flow in diastole. The upside of the velocity waveform peak depends on cardiac contractility. The downside of the velocity waveform peak and diastolic flow is determined primarily by the continuing effects of cardiac contractility along with elastic recoil (compliance) of the vessels acting against peripheral resistance (38). The A/B ratio, RI, or PI show little change throughout the third trimester except for a slight increase in end diastolic flow. This is probably due to a progressive decrease in placental vascular resistance due to an increase in placental size and in the total number of small arterial channels and tertiary stem villi (39).

Umbilical Artery Waveform Analysis

Umbilical artery waveform analysis is usually easy to perform. In the first 18 to 20 weeks of pregnancy, the umbilical artery waveform may return to the baseline during diastole (40). Beyond the 20th to the 22nd week, however, forward flow in diastole is recorded due to decreasing placental resistance (Fig. 5.6). The ratio of

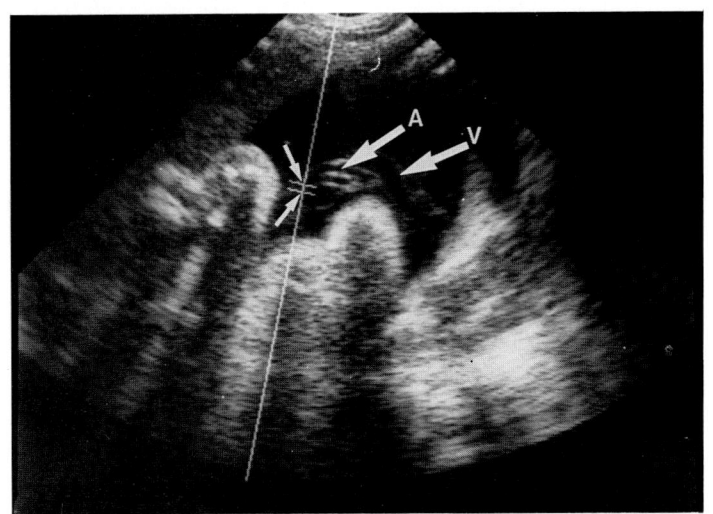
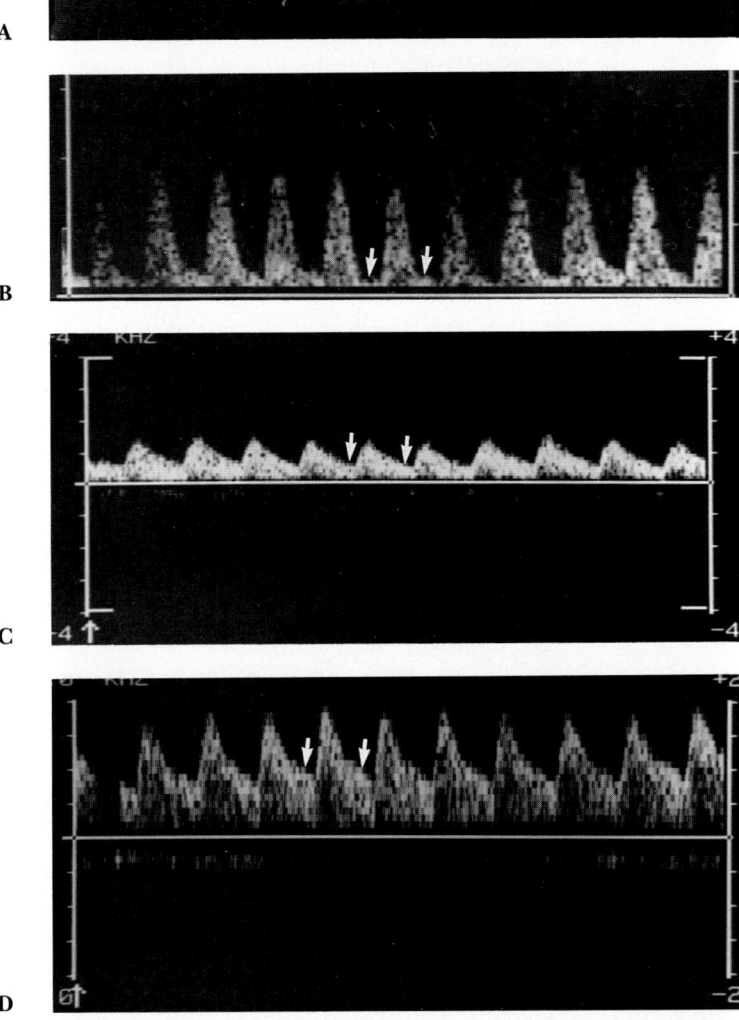

Fig. 5.6A–D. A. Doppler of the umbilical artery. Both the umbilical artery (A) and umbilical veins (V) are seen. The sample volume (*arrows*) encompasses the lumen of the umbilical artery. **B.** Normal Doppler waveform in a singleton pregnancy at 16 weeks' gestation, **(C)** 32 weeks' gestation, and at **(D)** 38 weeks' gestation. As term is approached, there is increased flow in diastole (*small arrows*).

5. Fetoplacental and Uteroplacental Circulation

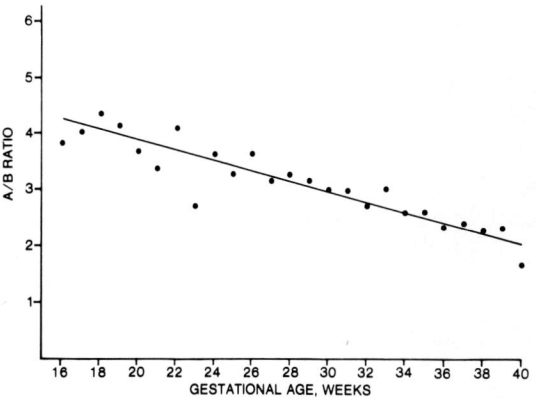

Fig. 5.7. Normal values for the A/B ratio in 107 singleton pregnancies from 16 weeks to term.

the systolic to the diastolic peak has been shown to decrease as pregnancy advances (Fig. 5.7). Before 28 weeks it is less than or equal to 5; from 28 to 34 weeks it is less than or equal to 4, and from 34 weeks to term it is less than or equal to 3.0 to 3.5 (41,42). These values will also apply to twin pregnancies where both fetuses have a birthweight appropriate for gestational age (43).

Umbilical Vein Waveform Analysis

The Doppler waveform from the umbilical vein, unlike that of the umbilical artery, is nonpulsatile and shows no variation in fetal systole or diastole (Fig. 5.8). As in the fetal aorta, however, fetal breathing movements do modulate the blood velocity signal from the intraabdominal portion of the umbilical vein. There are contradictory reports in the literature regarding the effects of fetal breathing movements on the blood flow in the umbilical vein. Marsal et al (17) state that there is a momentary decrease in umbilical blood flow velocity with inspiration and an increase with expiration, whereas Chiba et al (26) stated the exact opposite. Blood flow changes also can be found in the adjacent portion of the fetal inferior vena cava with fetal respiration.

Normal Uteroplacental Waveform Analysis

In the nonpregnant uterus during the proliferative phase of the menstrual cycle, the waveform from the parauterine arteries obtained vaginally shows a prominent early diastolic notch with little or no end diastolic flow. In the secretory phase, however, some end diastolic flow is present giving an A/B ratio of approximately 8. This is also present during the first 10 weeks of pregnancy. There is a sharp decrease in the ratio to 2.6 to 3.0 at the beginning of the second trimester (44). These measurements are taken via the abdominal wall and reflect changes in the arteries in the uterine wall. The diastolic notch disappears from the 20th to 26th week of gestation, unless one uterine artery is supplying the majority of the blood to the placenta (44). The normal ratio after 26 weeks averages 2.0 plus to minus 0.3 (Fig. 5.9).

Normal flow velocity waveforms are easily obtained from the branches of the maternal uterine artery in the uterine wall where the placenta has implanted (7,44–46). When possible, the central portion of the placental bed should be sampled; however, with posterior placentation, a more peripheral portion may have to be used. One cannot determine whether one is sampling a radial or an arcuate vessel. There is a small increase in diastolic flow velocity in relation to peak systolic velocity in the latter half of pregnancy (45,46). The uterine artery waveform analysis is more likely to be affected by maternal causes of poor fetal growth, such as, maternal hypertension (45,46). Trudinger et al (46) stated that a poor fetal outcome is better predicted with an umbilical artery waveform analysis than with a waveform analysis of the branches of the uterine artery (46).

Use of Doppler in Complicated Pregnancy

Adequate Doppler evaluation of the fetal descending aorta and intraabdominal portion of the umbilical vein can be obtained in 80 to 90% of cases. Evaluation of the umbilical cord vessels is somewhat more successful. The main difficulties arise when there is excessive fetal movement or where the fetus is spine up with a posterior placenta. Assessment is also more difficult in very obese patients, in multiple pregnancy, in late pregnancy, with oligohydram-

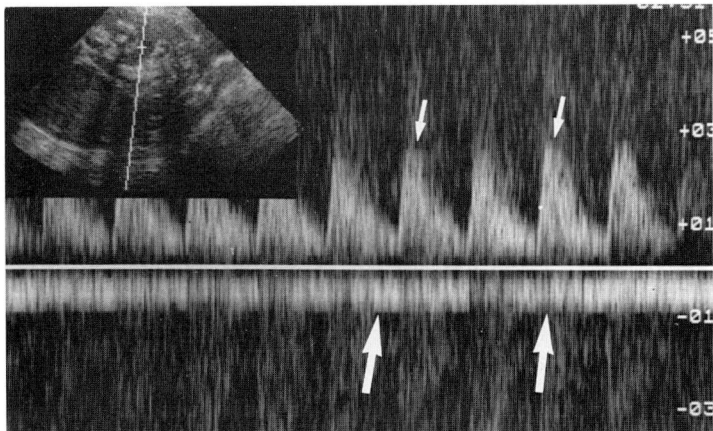

Fig. 5.8. Doppler waveform of the umbilical vein (*large arrows*) in comparison to the waveform from the umbilical artery (*small arrows*). The nonpulsatile waveform of the umbilical vein is easy to distinguish from the pulsatile waveform in the umbilical artery.

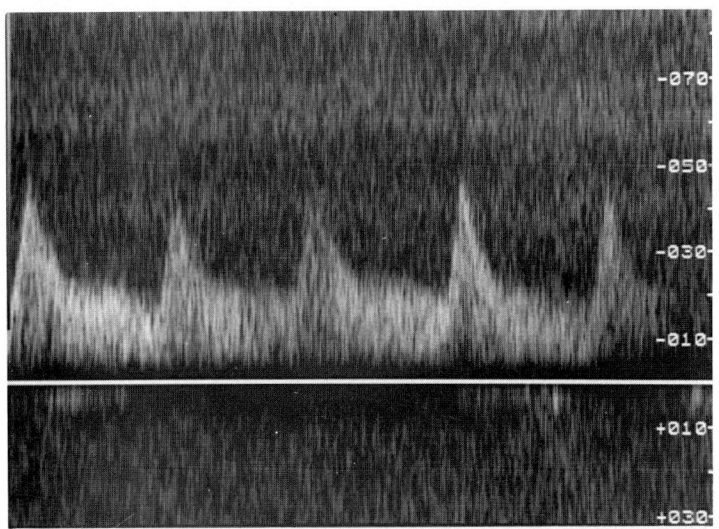

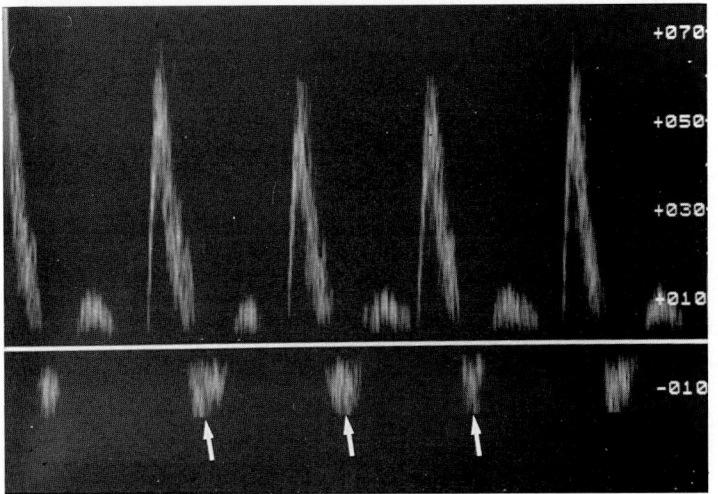

Fig. 5.9A–C. A. Doppler waveform of the uterine artery in comparison to the waveform in (**B**) the maternal external iliac artery, and the (**C**) fetal umbilical artery in the same patient. There is a short period of reversal of flow (*small arrows*) in the maternal external iliac artery, but not in the uterine artery or umbilical artery.

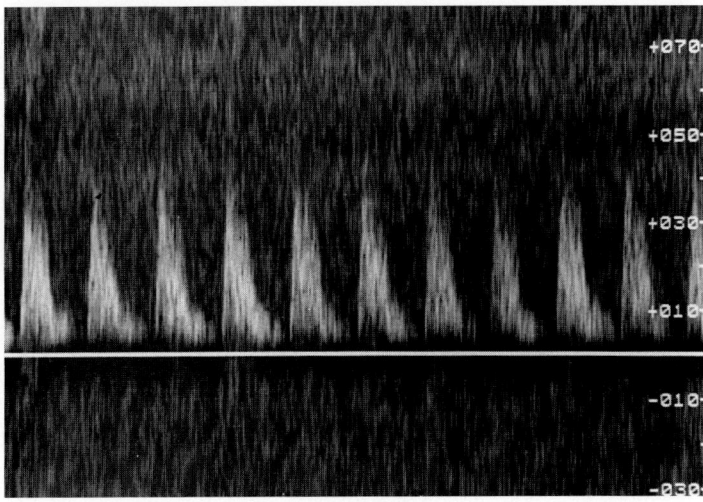

Fig. 5.9.

Intrauterine Growth Retardation

nios, and sometimes with polyhydramnios, which allows the fetus a wide area of movement.

It has been shown experimentally in sheep that acute and chronic hypoxia cause selective vasoconstriction mediated by alpha-adrenergic innervation to low priority areas such as the gut and lung. This is accompanied by increased blood flow to high priority areas including the brain, myocardial circulation, and adrenal glands (1,47,48). Wladimiroff et al (49) showed, using Doppler ultrasound, that there is increased vascular resistance in the fetal aorta and umbilical artery in intrauterine growth retardation (IUGR) accompanied by decreased resistance in the fetal carotid arteries. This explains the "head sparing" effect that occurs in the growth-retarded fetus (7).

Approximately 45 to 62% of fetal cardiac output goes to the umbilical-placental circulation, and, thus, vasoconstriction in this vascular system would be expected to have an effect on blood flow in the descending aorta (7,14). In the early stages of fetal growth failure with increased placental resistance, Thompson et al (38) postulated that the fetus can initially compensate by increasing cardiac contactility. It also has been shown in fetal lambs that oxygen consumption can be maintained when umbilical artery blood flow is reduced by half (2,4). Further reductions in blood flow lead to a progressive fall in fetal oxygen consumption. As umbilical blood flow is reduced, the degree of oxygen extraction from the blood increases.

In IUGR the most striking finding in the flow velocity waveform of the descending thoracic aorta is a reduction in the end diastolic velocity (Fig. 5.10) (37,50). There is also a reduction in the peak systolic velocity, but this is less marked. In the study of Griffin et al (37), nine of 20 fetuses with IUGR had no recordable flow during end diastole, whereas in another six, it was reduced. The mean PI in this group of fetuses was 2.78, which was significantly above the normal mean, whereas in 75% it was greater than two standard deviations above normal. The magnitude of difference did not correlate with birthweight. The flow velocity waveform provided an earlier warning of fetal compromise than did cardiotocography.

The pulsatility index and A/B ratio from the umbilical artery also can be used to diagnose IUGR (Figs. 5.10, 5.11) (38,51,52). With increasing placental resistance the diastolic flow decreases. The absence of diastolic flow and especially reversal of flow in diastole indicates that the fetus is at risk for intrauterine death (Fig. 5.12) (51). These changes are most likely due to increased placental vascular resistance from placental villous vasoconstriction and placental villous infarction. Giles et al (39)

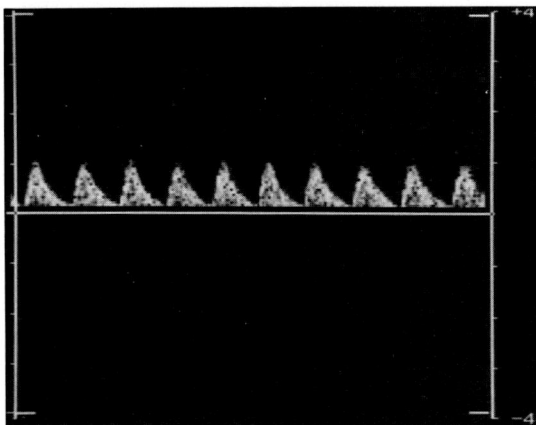

Fig. 5.10. Doppler of the umbilical artery shows an increased A/B ratio (6.7) in this 32 week' singleton pregnancy with IUGR, secondary to maternal hypertension. There was mild oligohydramnios, but the BPD, abdominal circumference, and femur length were all within the range of normal for gestational age.

found a correlation between high resistance umbilical artery waveforms and a reduction in the stem villi. Fleischer et al (53), in a study of 189 patients between 18 and 42 weeks of gestation, found that an abnormal A/B ratio (greater than or equal to 3) had a positive predictive value of 49% for IUGR, which increased to 66% if the patient was hypertensive. The negative predictive value of the test was 95%.

It is difficult to separate the small normally growing fetus from one with a low growth rate who is at risk for poor outcome. Trudinger et al (46,55) and Rochelson et al (54) have shown that the small for gestational age fetus with a normal A/B ratio of the umbilical artery is at much lower risk than a similar fetus with an abnormal ratio. The latter group has a much increased incidence of pregnancy-induced hypertension, Cesarian section for fetal distress, perinatal death, and postnatal complications requiring admissions to the neonatal intensive care unit (46,54,55).

Jouppila and Kirkinen (56) found a reduction in the size and blood flow in the intraabdominal umbilical vein in 10 of 11 growth-retarded fetuses. Similar findings with IUGR have been reported by Kurjak and Rajhvajn (5) and Gill et al (30). In the study by Gill et al (30), 15 were called "false positives" for IUGR based on the umbilical vein blood flow. Six of these had a birthweight below the 20th percentile, whereas another five were delivered early because of flattening of their growth curve, thus preventing the development of more evident IUGR. The accuracy of diagnosing IUGR was increased when the measurement of umbilical vein blood flow was obtained on more than one occasion. This approach was more accurate in diagnosing IUGR than serial biparietal diameter (BPD) measurements, and changes in umbilical vein blood flow were recorded up to 3 weeks before BPD measurements indicated a flattening of growth. The combination of low flow with low flow/kg was associated with late flattening of growth, IUGR, fetal death, and increased complications after birth (30).

Abnormal maternal uterine artery waveforms have been associated with 60% of growth retarded fetuses in a study by Trudinger et al (45,46). These waveforms are more often affected when there is a maternal cause for poor fetal growth such as maternal hypertension (7). However, overall, they are not as accurate in predicting IUGR as umbilical artery waveform analysis (45,46). In a study of 53 patients with complicated pregnancy in the last trimester, the patients with an abnormal flow velocity waveform had an increased incidence of hypertension and were delivered earlier of smaller infants than those with a normal flow velocity waveform. The former group had a higher incidence of Cesarian section and their infants were in poorer condition at birth (7). Changes in the uteroplacental flow velocity waveform can precede changes in fetal growth by as much as 9 weeks. Cohen-Overbeek et al (7) reported that the maternal arcuate artery Doppler waveform shows a higher than normal resistance in patients with high blood pressure, proteinuria, and IUGR. The small for gestational age fetus with a normal uterine artery waveform, on the other hand, is at a significantly lower risk than those with an abnormal waveform.

Intrauterine Fetal Death

The nonstress test along with the fetal biophysical profile are presently used to assess fetal well-being. Trudinger et al (57) showed that umbilical artery waveform analysis detects fetal compromise more accurately than does fetal heart rate monitoring. As mentioned, if the Doppler

Fig. 5.11A,B. A. Doppler of the umbilical artery shows an increased A/B ratio (7.0) at 30 weeks' gestation in a singleton pregnancy complicated by preeclampsia. **B.** A follow-up study at 32 weeks shows absence of flow (*arrows*) in diastole. The fetus was delivered by Cesarean section at 35 weeks due to lack of fetal growth.

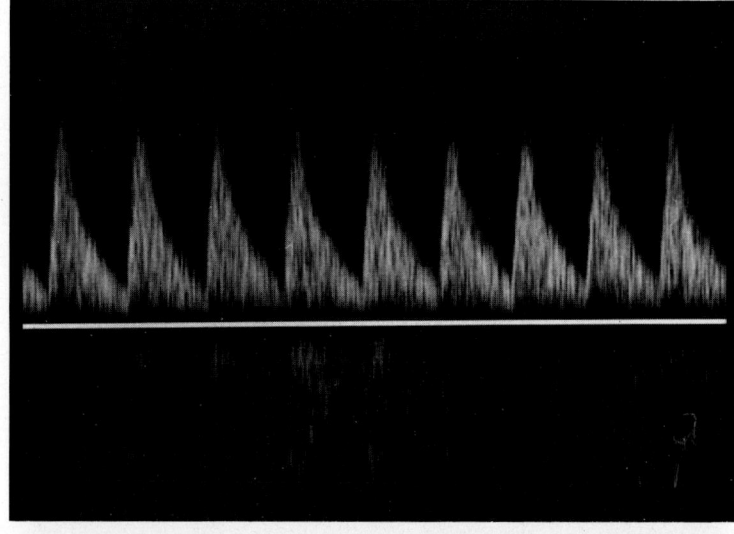

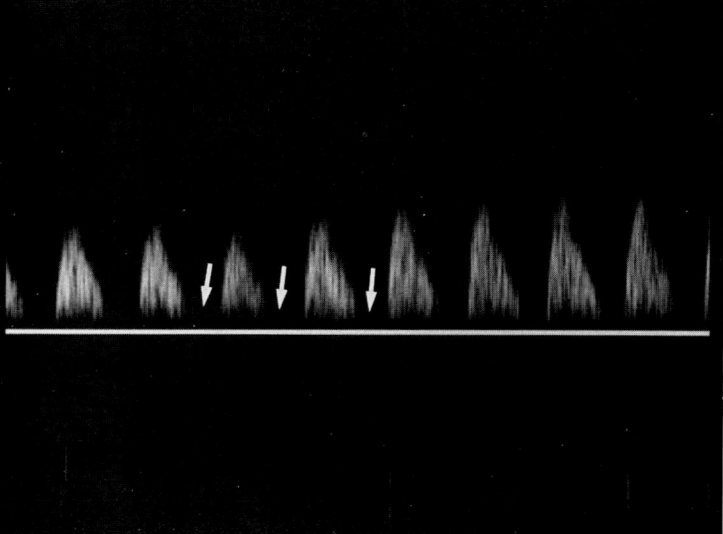

waveform from the umbilical artery shows no flow in diastole, then this has a grave prognostic significance for the fetus (Fig. 5.11) (46,55,58). This is especially so if there is retrograde flow in diastole (Fig. 5.12). In a case reported by Erskine et al (59), however, the Doppler waveform was normal the day before the intrauterine death of a normal term fetus.

Rochelson et al (58) recently reported on 10 patients with absent flow in diastole appearing between 31 to 36 weeks' gestation. Six patients had pregnancy-induced hypertension and four had lethal congenital anomalies. All delivered before 37 weeks, usually (70%) by Cesarian section, and there were four perinatal deaths. The finding of an abnormal Doppler waveform from the umbilical artery may precede the onset of maternal hypertension by up to 2 weeks and defines a high-risk state that demands constant monitoring. Such findings also have been reported by Fitzgerald et al (60), Erskine and Ritchie (51), and Trudinger et al (39,46,55).

Complicated Twin Pregnancy

Doppler waveform analysis of the umbilical artery will be normal in a twin gestation where the birthweights are appropriate for gestational age (43). On average, however, the A/B ratio is

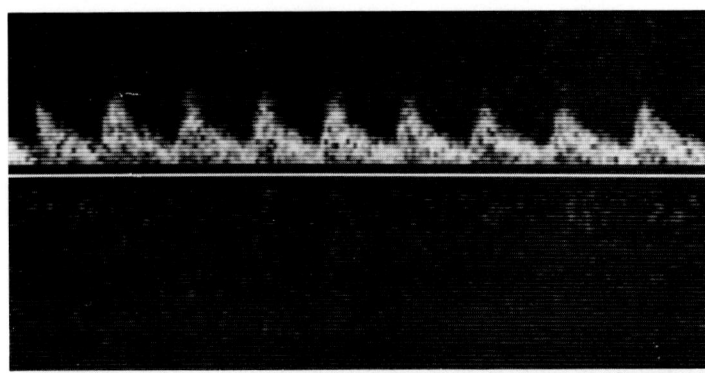

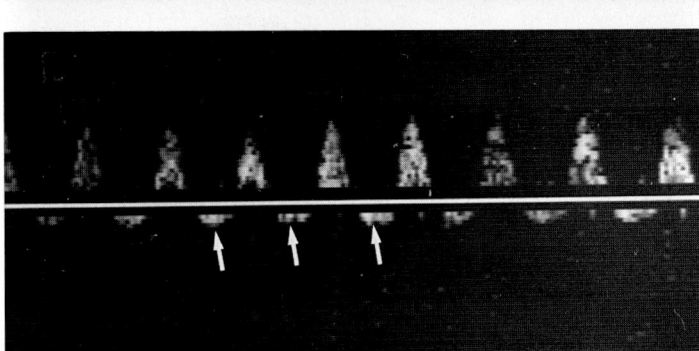

Fig. 5.12A,B. Twin gestation at 31 weeks. **A.** The twin on the left had a normal A/B ratio in the umbilical artery. **B.** The right twin had reversal of flow (*arrows*), and on a follow-up sonogram 48 hours later, this twin was dead.

slightly elevated in comparison to a normal singleton pregnancy (61). This may explain the lower growth profile of a twin gestation in the last trimester in comparison to a singleton gestation. When the average of all A/B ratios taken in the last 2 months of pregnancy are correlated with birthweight, it is found that a difference of 0.4 between the twins indicates a weight difference equal to or greater than 350 g (61). This does not apply if both twins are growth retarded.

An abnormally elevated A/B ratio is found in twins with IUGR (43). In a study of twins by Giles et al (43), when it was dichorionic (43 twins), the A/B ratio was elevated in 12 of 18 where at least one twin was small for gestational age. The incidence of IUGR was more common with monochorionic twins (18 twins), and the A/B ratio was elevated in 7 of 12 such twins.

If there is a twin-to-twin transfusion, Farmakides et al (61) have found that the recipient twin will have a low A/B ratio in comparison to the donor twin, who will have a high ratio. On the other hand, Giles et al (43), in their study of twins found no difference in the A/B ratio in the twin-to-twin transfusion syndrome. The diagnosis, however, is aided by the sonographic detection of a discrepancy in their size (43,61).

Fetal Cardiac Arrhythmia

Fetal aortic blood flow is affected by cardiac arrhythmias. With extra systolic beats, there is a lower peak velocity and mean velocity. The first post extrasystolic beat shows an increase in blood flow velocity that does not fully compensate for the extrasystolic beat. This compensation does, however, take place over the ensuing three to four beats (Fig. 5.13) (17,62). Time-averaged mean blood flow in the normal range also can be found in atrioventricular heart block. The increased stroke volume after a prolonged diastolic ventricular filling phase shows that the fetal heart operates according to the Frank-Starling law.

Congenital Fetal Anomalies

The Doppler findings in congenital fetal anomalies have been contradictory (49,52,58,63). In a study of 26 patients who gave birth to an infant

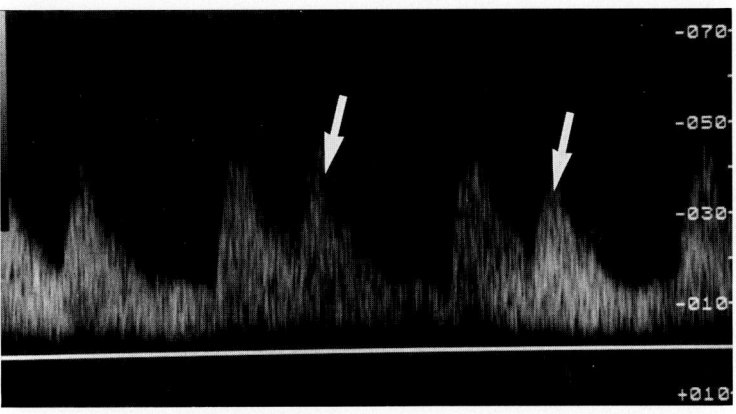

Fig. 5.13. Doppler waveform of the umbilical artery showing extrasystolic beats (*arrows*) in a 35 week normal fetus. These were documented on two subsequent sonograms, but were not present after birth.

with a major congenital anomaly, Trudinger et al (63), showed an elevated A/B ratio in the umbilical artery in 13, consistent with increased resistance in the placental circulation. They postulated that this was secondary to obliteration of the small arteries in the placenta, possibly triggered by the abnormal fetus. A uterine artery waveform analysis was performed in 16 patients in this study, and, in each case, it was normal.

A malformed fetus with a normal placenta may have a normal pulsatility index (49,52). Wladimiroff (64) determined the pulsatility index in the umbilical artery and fetal internal carotid arteries in 10 patients with IUGR and marked oligohydramnios. In six patients it was abnormal, consistent with placental insufficiency, and at birth moderate to marked placental infarcts were present in four. The remaining patients in the study had normal P/l, and all of these infants at birth had structural congenital anomalies and normal placentas. Thus, it appears that the Doppler findings with fetal anomalies depend on the placental, rather than the fetal, changes present.

Rhesus Isoimmunization

In cases of Rhesus isoimmunization, it has been shown that umbilical vein blood flow increases, and there is a direct relationship between this increase and the severity of the disease (30,65). Not only is the velocity of blood flow increased, but so is the diameter of the umbilical vein. This increase in velocity could be to compensate for insufficient tissue oxygenation and/or due to a decrease in blood viscosity from the reduction in red cell mass.

Maternal Bleeding

Jouppila and Kirkinen (66) studied umbilical vein blood flow in 19 patients with third-trimester bleeding. In each case the severity of the bleeding did not warrant an emergency Cesearian section. Ten had some degree of partial previa, five were diagnosed as having a partial placental abruption, and in the remaining four no cause for the bleeding was determined. At the time of evaluation, the fetal heart rate was within normal limits in each case, and at birth there was no evidence of fetal anemia. The umbilical vein blood flow exceeded the 90th percentile in more than 60%. They postulated that such changes not only depended on the amount of fetal blood lost but on the gestational age, as a large fetus can afford to lose more blood than a smaller one. Gill et al (30) also showed increased umbilical vein blood flow in antepartum hemorrhage that returned to normal within 2 weeks after the cessation of bleeding.

Maternal Complications

Brosens (67,68) found failure of migration of the trophoblast along the spiral arteries in all the placental bed biopsies performed on patients with pregnancy-induced hypertension and found only partial migration in 50% of normotensive patients with IUGR. Normally this process helps to reduce resistance to blood flow at this level, and so its absence or partial absence will reduce this effect. In hypertensive and preeclamptic patients, pathologic changes have been demonstrated in the myometrial arteries and decidual arterioles (69). These consist of increased connective tissue in the media and, to a lesser extent, the intima, with varying degrees of stenosis of the lumen (70). In severe cases there may be obliteration of the lumen by intravascular thrombosis; acute arteritis as well as fibrinoid necrosis also may be seen.

In severe maternal hypertension, Trudinger et al (45) have shown a decrease in the uteroplacental diastolic flow velocity waveform in 9 of 12 patients. In the three "normal" patients, the hypertensive state had not yet led to Doppler detectable changes in placental resistance. If such patients were followed at frequent intervals, the waveform could be used to tell when pathologic hypertensive changes had occurred in the placenta. It is also possible that Doppler waveform analysis could be used to monitor response to medical antihypertensive therapy. It is interesting to note that the umbilical artery waveform analysis was abnormal in only two of the 16 hypertensive patients in this study. This, again, emphasizes that the uteroplacental circulation is more affected by maternal disease, whereas the fetoplacental circulation is more affected by fetal disorders. Fleischer et al (71) showed good correlation between a normal pregnancy outcome in hypertensive patients with an A/B ratio less than or equal to 2.6 in branches of the uterine artery alongside the lower uterine segment. Normally, there is a small notch in the early diastolic component of the waveform that disappears around the 26th week of pregnancy. If the A/B ratio was above 2.6, and especially if the notch failed to disappear, the pregnancy was more likely to be complicated by maternal preeclampsia, IUGR, premature birth, and stillbirth. The positive and negative predictive values for uterine artery waveform analysis were 93 and 91%, respectively (71).

In diabetic pregnancies, the umbilical vein blood flow has been found to be increased; however, this is most likely due to the larger than normal babies in this group (30). In a study by Bracero et al (72), of 43 diabetic patients a positive correlation between the A/B ratio in the umbilical artery in the last trimester and the serum glucose level was demonstrated. When both were increased, there was an increased incidence of stillbirths and neonatal morbidity.

In maternal anemia, Doppler evaluation of umbilical vein blood flow has had contradictory results. Jouppila et al (66) reported on seven cases, six with moderate iron deficiency anemia, and one with severe anemia due to hereditary spherocytosis. In the former group, the umbilical vein blood flow was above the 90th percentile in half, whereas it was normal in the latter patient with severe anemia.

Maternal smoking has been associated with impaired fetal growth, decreased birthweight, increased perinatal mortality, and long-term impairment of mental and physical development. It has been shown to reduce intervillous blood flow, and histologic evaluation of the placenta in chronic smokers has shown findings consistent with underperfusion. Jouppila et al (73) found little change in the Doppler estimation of blood flow in the fetal descending thoracic aorta or intraabdominal portion of the umbilical vein during the last trimester immediately after the smoking of one cigarette. A more detailed study is necessary, however, before reaching a definite conclusion.

Summary

Doppler waveform analysis of uteroplacental and fetoplacental circulation provides clinically useful information in managing pregnancy. The uteroplacental circulation is affected earlier in maternal disease states such as hypertension, whereas the fetoplacental circulation is more affected by fetal disorders. In IUGR, the changes in the Doppler waveform can precede by weeks any sonographically detectable change in fetal growth. In the last trimester of pregnancy, the absence of flow in the umbilical artery in diastole signals the presence of fetal compromise. Such infants are born earlier, are small for gestational age, are frequently growth retarded, and have a higher incidence of congenital anomalies and in-utero death. This warning is even more grave when there is reversal of flow in diastole.

All of the questions regarding the role of Doppler ultrasound in the management of high-risk pregnancy have not been answered; however, some of these answers are on their way.

References

1. Block PSB, Llanos AJ, Creasy RK: Response of the growth retarded fetus to acute hypoxemia. Am J Obstet Gynecol 148:879, 1984.
2. Dawes GS, Mott JC: Changes in oxygen distribution and consumption in foetal lambs with variations in umbilical blood flow. J Physiology 170:524, 1964.
3. Dawes GS: The umbilical circulation. *In* Fetal and Neonatal Physiology. Chicago, Year Book Medical Publishers, 1968, pp 66–78.
4. Itskovitz J, LaGamma EF, Rudolph AM: The effect of reducing umbilical blood flow on fetal oxygenation. Am J Obstet Gynecol 145:813, 1983.
5. Kurjak A, Rajhvajn B: Ultrasonic measurements of umbilical blood flow in normal and complicated pregnancies. J Perinat Med 10:3, 1982.
6. Ramsey EM, Donner MW: Placental Vasculature and Circulation. Philadelphia, Saunders, 1980.
7. Cohen-Overbeek T, Pearce JM, Campbell S: The antenatal assessment of utero-placental and fetoplacental blood flow using Doppler ultrasound. Ultrasound Med Biol 2:329, 1985.
8. Walsh SZ, Meyer WW, Lind J: The Human Fetal and Neonatal Circulation. Springfield, IL, Charles C Thomas, 1974.
9. Eik-Nes SH, Brubakk AO, Ulstein MK: Measurement of human fetal blood flow. Br Med J 280:283, 1980.
10. Fitzgerald DE, Drumm JE: Noninvasive measurement of human fetal circulation using ultrasound: A new method. Br Med J 2:1450, 1977.
11. Gill RW: Fetal blood flow. *In* White DN (ed): Recent Advances in Perinatal Pathology and Physiology. Chichester, England, Research Studies Press, 1980, pp 161–174.
12. McCallum WD, Williams CS, Napel S, et al: Fetal blood velocity waveforms. Am J Obstet Gynecol 132:425, 1978.
13. McCallum WD: Fetal cardiac anatomy and vascular dynamics. Clin Obstet Gynaecol 24:837, 1981.
14. Eik-Nes SH, Marsal K, Brubakk AO, et al: Ultrasonic measurement of human fetal blood flow. J Biomed Eng 4:28, 1982.
15. Eik-Nes SH, Marsal K, Kristofferson K: Methodology and basic problems related to blood flow studies in the human fetus. Ultrasound Med Biol 10:329, 1984.
16. Erskine RLA, Ritchie JWK: Quantitative measurement of fetal blood flow using Doppler ultrasound. Br J Obstet Gynaecol 92:600, 1985.
17. Marsal K, Lindblad A, Lingman G, et al: Blood flow in the fetal descending aorta; intrinsic factors affecting fetal blood flow, i.e. fetal breathing movements and cardiac arrhythmia. Ultrasound Med Biol 10:339, 1984.
18. Trudinger BJ, Thompson RS, Giles WB: Doppler ultrasound and blood flow in obstetrics. *In* Saunders RC, Hill MC (ed): Ultrasound Annual 1986. New York, Raven Press, 1986, pp 39–65.
19. Griffin DR, Teague MJ, Tallet P, et al: A combined ultrasonic linear array scanner and pulsed Doppler velocimeter for the estimation of blood flow in the foetus and adult abdomen. II. Clinical evaluation. Ultrasound Med Biol 11:37, 1985.
20. Eriksen PS, Gennser G, Linstrom K: Physiological characteristics of diameter pulses in the fetal descending aorta. Acta Obstet Gynecol Scand 63:355, 1984.
21. Tonge HM, Struijk PC, Wladimiroff JW: Blood flow measurements in the fetal descending aorta: Technique and clinics. Clin Cardiol 7:323, 1984.
22. Taylor KJW, Burns PN, Woodcock JP, et al: Blood flow in deep abdominal and pelvic vessels: Ultrasonic pulsed-Doppler analysis. Radiology 154:487, 1985.
23. Gosling RG, King DH: Ultrasound angiology. *In* Marcus AW, Adamson L (eds): Arteries and Veins. Edinburgh, Churchill Livingston, 1975, pp 61–98.
24. Stuart B, Drumm J, Fitzgerald DE, et al: Fetal blood velocity-waveforms in normal pregnancy. Br J Obstet Gynaecol 87:780, 1980.
25. Pourcelot L: Application Clinques des l'examin Doppler transcutanie. *In* Peronneau P (ed): Veliometric Ultrasonor Doppler 34:625, 1974.
26. Chiba Y, Utsu M, Kanzaki T, et al: Changes in venous flow and intratracheal flow in fetal breathing movements. Ultrasound Med Biol 11:43, 1985.
27. Stuart B, Drumm J, Fitzgerald DE, et al: Fetal blood velocity waveforms in uncomplicated labour. Br J Obstet Gynaecol 88:865, 1981.
28. Lindblad A, Ekman G, Marsal K, et al: Fetal circulation 60 to 80 minutes after vaginal prostaglandin E_2 in pregnant women at term. Arch Gynecol 237:31, 1985.
29. Eldridge MW, Berman W Jr, Greene E: Serial echo Doppler measurements of human fetal abdominal aortic blood flow. J Ultrasound Med 4:453, 1985.
30. Gill RW, Kossoff G, Warren PS, et al: Umbilical venous flow in normal and complicated pregnancy. Ultrasound Med Biol 10:349, 1984.
31. Griffin D, Cohen-Overbeek T, Campbell S: Fetal and uteroplacental blood flow. *In* Campbell S (ed): Clin Obstet Gynaecol. London, Saunders 10:565, 1983.

32. Van Lierde M, Oberweis D, Thomas K: Ultrasonic measurement of aortic and umbilical blood flow in the human fetus. Obstet Gynecol 63:801, 1984.
33. Wladimiroff JW, McGhie J: Ultrasonic assessment of cardiovascular geometry and function in the human fetus. Br J Obstet Gynaecol 88:870, 1981.
34. Chen HY, Chin-Cheng L, Cheng YT, et al: Antenatal measurement of fetal umbilical venous flow by pulsed Doppler and B-mode ultrasonography. J Ultrasound Med 5:319, 1986.
35. Jouppila P, Kirkinen P, Koivula A, et al: The influence of maternal oxygen inhalation on human placental and umbilical venous blood flow. Eur J Obstet Gynecol Reprod Biol 16:151, 1983.
36. Kirkinen P, Jouppila P, Koivula A, et al: The effect of caffeine on placental and fetal blood flow in human pregnancy. Am J Obstet Gynecol 147:939, 1983.
37. Griffin D, Bilardo K, Masini L, et al: Doppler blood flow waveforms in the descending thoracic aorta of the human fetus. Br J Obstet Gynaecol 91:997, 1984.
38. Thompson RS, Trudinger BJ, Cook CM: Doppler ultrasound waveforms in the fetal umbilical artery: Quantitative analysis technique. Ultrasound Med Biol 5:707, 1985.
39. Giles WB, Trudinger BJ, Baird RJ: Fetal umbilical artery flow velocity waveforms and placental resistance: Pathological correlation. Br J Obstet Gynaecol 92:31, 1985.
40. Reuwer PJ, Nuyen WC, Beijer HJ, et al: Characteristics of flow velocities in the umbilical arteries, assessed by Doppler ultrasound. Eur J Obstet Gynaecol Reprod Biol 17:397, 1984.
41. Friedman DM, Rutkowski M, Snyder JR, et al: Doppler blood velocity waveforms in the umbilical artery as an indicator of fetal well-being. J Clin Ultrasound 13:161, 1985.
42. Schulman H, Fleischer A, Sterm W, et al: Umbilical velocity wave ratios in human pregnancy. Am J Obstet Gynecol 148:986, 1984.
43. Giles WB, Trudinger BJ, Cook CM: Fetal umbilical artery velocity time waveforms in twin pregnancies. Br J Obstet Gynaecol 92:490, 1985.
44. Schulman H, Fleischer A, Farmakides G, et al: Development of uterine artery compliance in pregnancy as detected by Doppler ultrasound. Am J Obstet Gynecol 155:1031, 1986.
45. Trudinger BJ, Giles WB, Cook CM: Uteroplacental blood flow velocity-time waveforms in normal and complicated pregnancy. Br J Obstet Gynaecol 92:39, 1985.
46. Trudinger BJ, Giles WB, Cook CM: Flow velocity waveforms in the maternal uteroplacental and fetal umbilical placental circulation. Am J Obstet Gynecol 152:155, 1985.
47. Cohn HE, Sacks EJ, Heyman MA, et al: Cardiovascular responses to hypoxemia and acidemia in fetal lambs. Am J Obstet Gynecol 120:817, 1974.
48. Peeters LLH, Sheldon RE, Jones M, et al: Blood flow to fetal organs as a function of arterial flow content. Am J Obstet Gynecol 135:638, 1980.
49. Wladimiroff JW, Tonge HM, Steward PA: Doppler ultrasound assessment of cerebral blood flow in the human fetus. Br J Obstet Gynaecol 93:471, 1986.
50. Jouppila P, Kirkinen P: Increased vascular resistance in the descending aorta of the human fetus in hypoxia. Br J Obstet Gynaecol 91:853, 1984.
51. Erskine RLA, Ritchie JWK: Umbilical artery blood flow characteristics in normal growth retarded fetuses. Br J Obstet Gynaecol 92:605, 1985.
52. Reuwer PJ, Bruinse HW, Stoutenbeek P, et al: Doppler assessment of the feto-placental circulation in normal and growth retarded fetuses. Eur J Obstet Gynaecol Reprod Biol 18:199, 1984.
53. Fleischer A, Schulman H, Farmakides G, et al: Umbilical artery velocity waveforms and intrauterine growth retardation. Am J Obstet Gynecol 151:502, 1985.
54. Rochelson BL, Schulman H, Fleischer A, et al: The clinical significance of Doppler umbilical artery velocimetry in the small for gestational age fetus. Am J Obstet Gynecol 156:1223, 1987.
55. Trudinger BJ, Giles WB, Cook CM, et al: Fetal umbilical artery flow velocity waveforms and placental resistance: Clinical significance. Br J Obstet Gynaecol 92:23, 1985.
56. Jouppila P, Kirkinen P: Umbilical vein blood flow as an indicator of fetal hypoxia. Br J Obstet Gynaecol 91:107, 1984.
57. Trudinger BJ, Cook CM, Jones L, et al: A comparison of fetal heart rate monitoring and umbilical artery waveforms in the recognition of fetal compromise. Br J Obstet Gynaecol 93:171, 1986.
58. Rochelson B, Schulman H, Farmakides G, et al: The significance of absent diastolic velocity in umbilical artery velocity waveforms (in press).
59. Erskine RLA, Ritchie JWK, Zaltz A, et al: Failure of nonstress test and Doppler-assessed umbilical arterial blood flow to detect imminent intrauterine death. Am J Obstet Gynecol 154:1109, 1986.
60. Fitzgerald DE, Stuart B, Drumm E, et al: The assessment of the feto-placental circulation with continuous wave Doppler ultrasound. Ultrasound Med Biol 10:371, 1984.
61. Farmakides G, Schulman H, Saldana LR, et al: Surveillance of twin pregnancy with umbilical arterial velocimetry. Am J Obstet Gynecol 153:789, 1985.

62. Lingman G, Dahlstrom JA, Eik-Nes SH, et al: Haemodynamic evaluation of fetal heart arrhythmias. Br J Obstet Gynaecol 91:647, 1984.
63. Trudinger BJ, Cook CM: Umbilical and uterine artery waveforms in pregnancy associated with major fetal abnormality. Br J Obstet Gynaecol 92:666, 1985.
64. Wladimiroff JW, Tonge HM, Stewart PA, et al: Severe intrauterine growth retardation; assessment of its origin from fetal arterial flow velocity waveforms. Eur J Obstet Gynecol Reprod Biol 22:23, 1986.
65. Kirkinen P, Jouppila P, Eik-Nes SH: Umbilical vein blood flow in Rhesus isoimmunization. Br J Obstet Gynaecol 90:640, 1983.
66. Jouppila P, Kirkinen P: Umbilical vein blood flow in the human fetus in cases of maternal and fetal anemia and uterine bleeding. Ultrasound Med Biol 10:365, 1984.
67. Brosens I: Morphological changes in the uteroplacental bed in pregnancy hypertension. *In* Symonds EM (ed): Hypertensive States in Pregnancy, Clin Obstet Gynecol, Vol. 4. London, Saunders, 1977, pp 573–594.
68. Brosens I, Dixon HG, Robertson WG: Fetal growth retardation and the arteries of the placental bed. Br J Obstet Gynaecol 84:656, 1977.
69. Fox H: Placental pathology. *In* Studd JWW (ed): Prog Obstet Gynaecol 3:47, 1984.
70. Dixon HG, Robertson WB: A study of the vessels of the placental bed in normotensive and hypertensive women. J Obstet Gynaecol Br Emp 65:803, 1958.
71. Fleischer A, Schulman H, Farmakides G, et al: Uterine artery Doppler velocimetry in pregnant women with hypertension. Am J Obstet Gynecol 154:806, 1986.
72. Bracero L, Schulman H, Fleischer A, et al: Umbilical artery velocimetry in diabetes and pregnancy. Obstet Gynecol 68:654, 1986.
73. Jouppila P, Kirkinen P, Eik-Nes S: Acute effect of maternal smoking on the human fetal blood flow. Br J Obstet Gynaecol 90:7, 1983.

6
Duplex Sonography of Peripheral Arteries

EDWARD G. GRANT

The evaluation of the carotid bifurcation with duplex sonography is a commonly used and well-established procedure. The use of duplex elsewhere in the peripheral arterial system, however, has been limited. The reasons for the relative lack of enthusiasm for duplex sonography outside of the carotids are many and depend on the specific site in question. Considering the potential of duplex sonography as a noninvasive adjunct in peripheral vascular diagnosis, duplex will undoubtedly prove to be a more popular examination in the future.

In an attempt to limit this chapter to more practical applications we shall describe the use of duplex in the peripheral arteries from three specific standpoints. First, the role of duplex sonography in the evaluation of atherosclerotic disease of the aortoilial and femoropopliteal systems is discussed. Although not frequently used in most centers, duplex sonography can add a great deal to the noninvasive diagnosis of atherosclerotic disease of the legs.

A second, and very promising, use for duplex is in the evaluation of postsurgical/traumatic vascular lesions. This somewhat poorly defined classification involves a wide array of pathology, the common feature of which is usually an iatrogenic origin. The duplex evaluation of arterial bypass grafts, arteriovenous fistulae for hemodialysis, and pseudoaneurysms is discussed in this section. A brief note on the duplex evaluation of congenital peripheral arteriovenous malformations (AVMs) forms the final portion of this chapter. Although congenital AVMs are uncommon, their duplex features should be pathogonomonic.

Duplex Evaluation of Atherosclerosis in the Legs

Atherosclerosis is a disease that typically involves the entire arterial system. The classic manifestations of the disease depend, however, almost entirely on which vessel is involved and the specific site of involvement in any given artery. In the peripheral arterial tree, focal atherosclerotic lesions tend to develop in areas that are most prone to constant endothelial injury such as arterial bifurcations or areas of posterior fixation (1). In the legs, focal atherosclerosis commonly affects the aortic bifurcation, the common iliac bifurcation, and the common femoral bifurcation. The classic site for peripheral vascular disease associated with posterior fixation is the mid/distal superficial femoral artery in the region of Hunter's canal.

Considering the most frequent locations for atherosclerosis and the presently available options or surgical intervention, we limit our discussion to the duplex evaluation of the major arteries between the aortic bifurcation and the calf. Before beginning any duplex examination in the legs, careful attention should be given to the clinical history and physical findings in an effort to tailor the examination. A complete evaluation of the arterial tree between the aortic bifurcation and calf can be extremely time consuming and a more directed evaluation is advisable. For the purpose of discussion, however, we describe an evaluation of one side of the body from the aortic bifurcation to the calf.

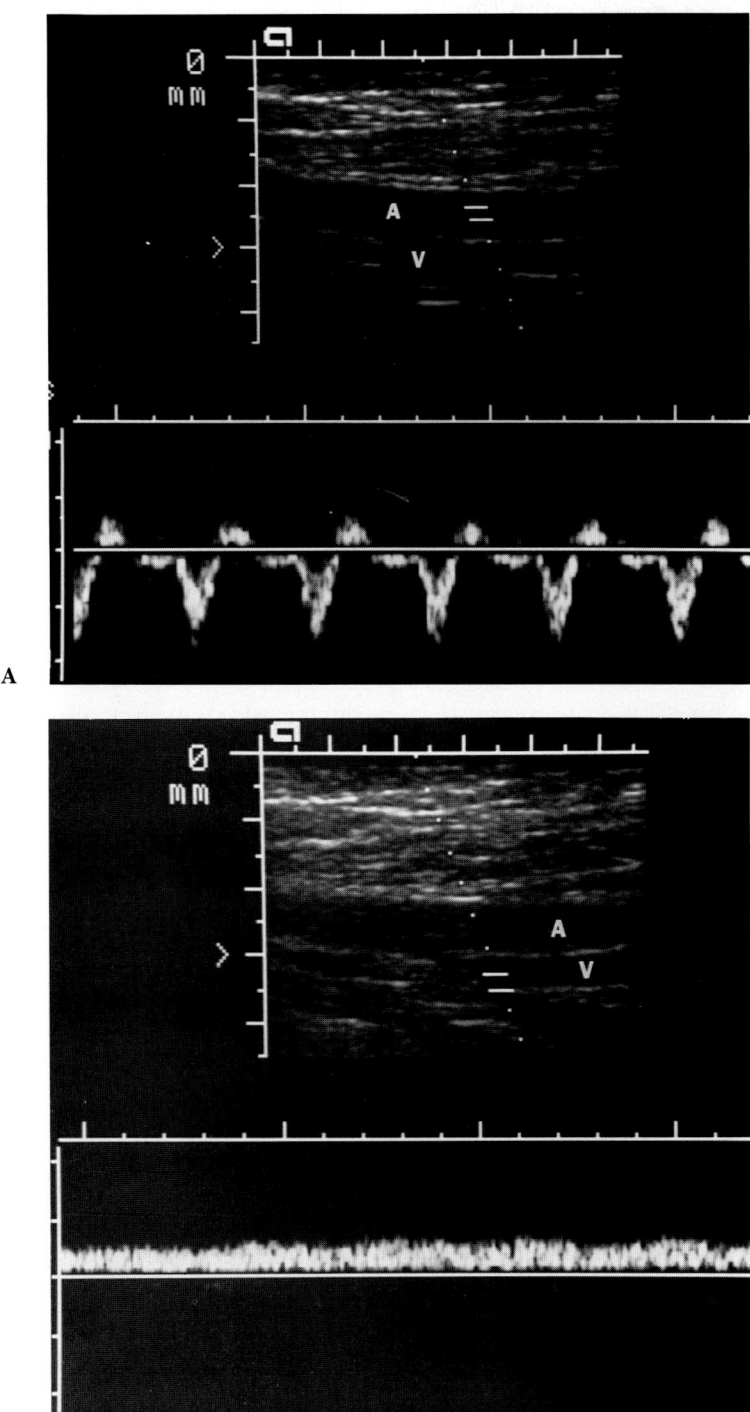

Fig. 6.1A,B. Longitudinal sections in the groin show the relationship of the common femoral artery (A) and vein (V). Doppler signals are characteristic. Femoral artery (**A**) exhibits triphasic waveform; vein exhibits monotonous forward flow. Note mild respiratory variation in venous trace (**B**).

Fig. 6.2A–C. Proximal iliac artery stenosis. Section through mildly ectatic distal aorta (A) and proximal common iliac artery (I) depicts irregular atherosclerotic plaque (*arrows*) (**A**). Doppler evaluation reveals markedly abnormal waveform. Note extreme elevation of the peak kilohertz shift and considerable spectral broadening (**B**). Arteriogram (**C**) confirms high-grade stenosis.

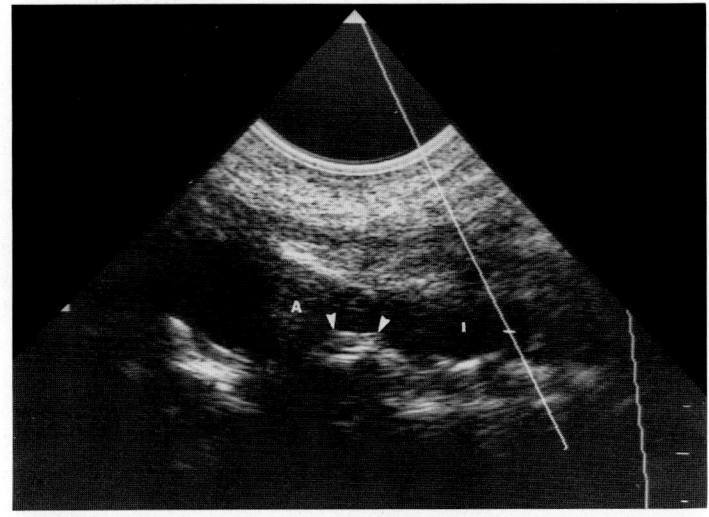

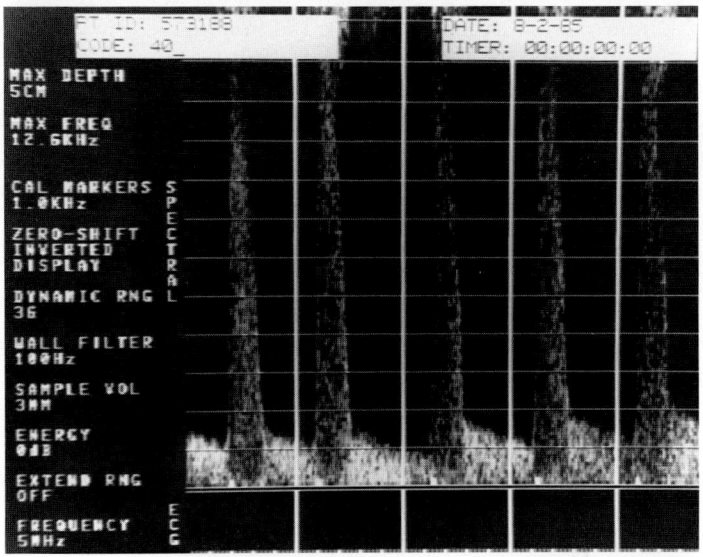

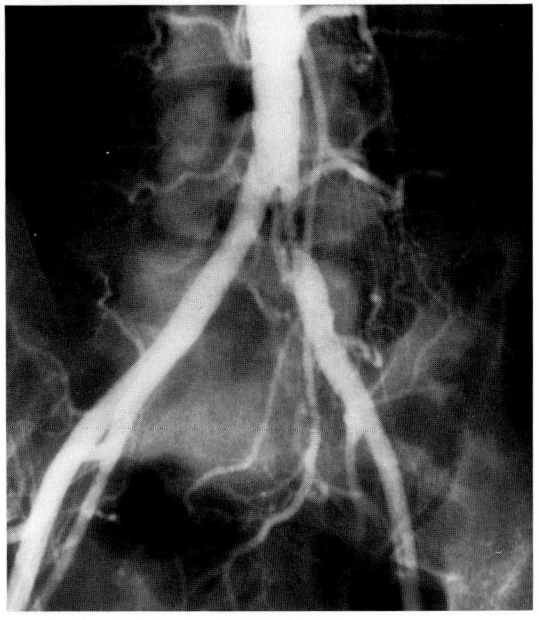

We begin most arterial evaluations in the region of the groin, where the common femoral artery lies in a superficial location as it emerges from beneath the inguinal ligament. The femoral pulse, if present, should be easily palpated, facilitating the correct placement of the transducer. In the groin, the common femoral artery should be visualized in almost every patient, even the most obese. The examination is best begun by scanning in a transverse orientation. In this location, the artery usually lies medial and superficial to the vein. To visualize the vein, one must scan very lightly, lest it be compressed and invisible. Doppler samples from the two vessels will obviously confirm their venous or arterial nature (Fig. 6.1*A,B*). Turning longitudinally on the artery, one may then proceed either proximally into the region of the pelvis, or distally toward the common femoral bifurcation.

Proceeding proximally, the iliac artery immediately dives deep into the pelvis. The iliac gradually assumes a more superficial location as it travels along the sacrum. The more proximal portions of the iliac vessel are, therefore, usually more accessible to the sonographer. In patients in whom the entire course of the iliac artery cannot be followed proximally, the origins may almost always be located by following the abdominal aorta into each of its two branches (Fig. 6.2A–C). Unfortunately, lesions of the mid/distal iliac arteries are frequently obscured by bowel gas. Because the origins of the internal iliac arteries are found in this inaccessible area, they are often impossible to visualize. Lesions of this vessel are of great importance because they may be associated with impotence (2). Graded compression, similar to what has been described in the evaluation of appendicitis (3), may be effective in aiding evaluation of the deeper portions of the right iliac artery. The left iliac artery, however, tends to be covered by colon and, therefore, often totally inaccessible to the sonographer. The use of abdominal (deep Doppler) transducers is essential in attempting to evaluate the iliac arteries. Despite meticulous technique, and the use of various transducers and sonographic maneuvers, we have been unable to adequately evaluate the entirety of the iliac artery in an unacceptably high number of patients. In the occasional patient suspected of having iliac artery aneurysms, full bladder technique may improve accuracy somewhat. We have not found a full bladder to be of any assistance in the evaluation of stenoses.

Scanning distal to the inguinal ligament, one quickly encounters the bifurcation of the common femoral artery into the superficial femoral artery (SFA) and profunda femoris (Fig. 6.3A,B). This bifurcation is an important site for focal atherosclerotic lesions. As is often the case, where arteries divide the two vessels thus formed exhibit somewhat different arterial traces. The superficial femoral artery is the successor to the common femoral artery and transmits the expected sharply triphasic waveform. The profunda, on the other hand, supplies a large muscular bed and, acting more like an end-organ vessel, tends to exhibit a somewhat dampened waveform. Evaluation of the origin of the profunda is extremely important. Although symptoms referable to occlusion of the profunda are unusual, this artery does serve as the major collateral pathway (via the geniculate arteries of the knee), when the superficial femoral artery is diseased.

Moving distally, one can frequently advance rapidly along the proximal/mid SFA as it courses along the medial portion of the thigh. As the SFA proceeds through the adductor canal, however, it may become difficult to locate. Unfortunately, atherosclerotic lesions in this area are not unusual. The final portions of the examination may be rapidly completed by scanning behind the knee, as the popliteal artery is usually relatively superficial. Unlike in the region of the groin, the popliteal artery lies superficial to the corresponding vein. Again, compression and Doppler evaluation will allow easy differentiation of the two. If further evaluation of the trifurcation vessels (posterior tibial, peroneal, and anterior tibial arteries) is warranted, they may be located with duplex in the appropriate anatomic area (Fig. 6.4A,B). In general, however, evaluation of the arteries of the calf and foot is more easily accomplished using nonduplex Doppler.

When a diagnostic quality scan is possible, atherosclerotic lesions between the aortic bifurcation and the knee should be identified with relative ease. To date, however, only Jager et al (4) have attempted to set forth criteria by which one may diagnose such stenoses. As is true elsewhere in the body, one should identify a focal increase in peak systolic flow velocity. Specific kilohertz shifts or velocities, as used in the carotid arteries, are difficult to apply in the legs. According to Jager (4), the most reliable sign seems to be a 1.5- to 2-fold focal increase in flow velocity. High-grade stenoses of the arteries of the legs tend to generate markedly increased systolic velocities (Fig. 6.5A–E). Ancillary findings in stenoses of the legs include a dampened waveform distal to the lesion and distortion of the typical triphasic waveform. Distortion of the waveform is usually first manifested by loss of the negative component and eventually by flow throughout diastole. The former is common in early atherosclerosis and may be found throughout the peripheral vasculature. Loss of the negative component probably reflects the

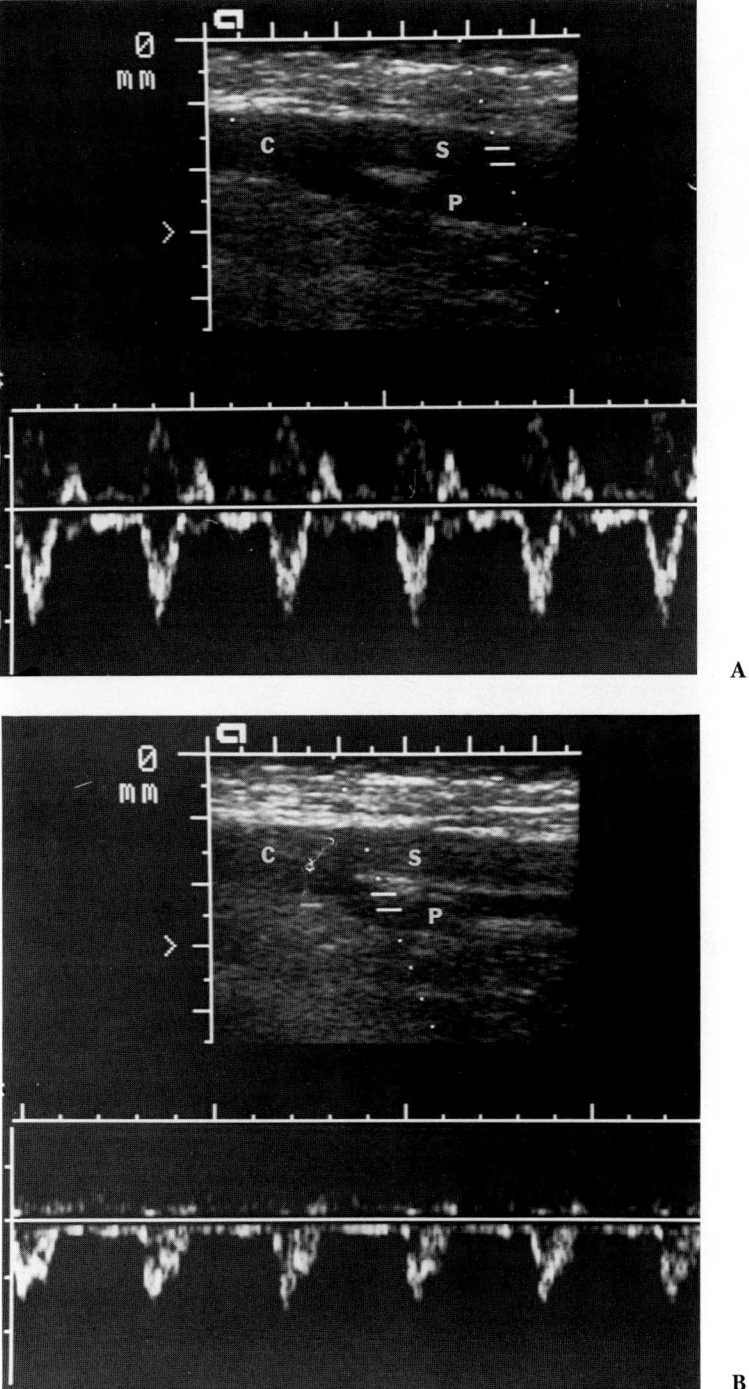

Fig. 6.3A,B. Normal superficial femoral/profunda bifurcation. The common femoral artery (C) bifurcates just distal to the region of the inguinal ligament and hip joint. The superficial femoral artery (S) continues through the anterio/medial portion of the thigh, eventually becoming the popliteal artery. The profunda (P) dives deep into the leg to supply the musculature of the posterior thigh. Note that the Doppler waveform of the profunda (**B**) appears considerably more dampened and less triphasic than the superficial artery (**A**). This difference may be the result of the profunda immediately supplying a large vascular bed, whereas the superficial femoral artery continues distally with relatively few branches before the knee. The origin of the profunda femoris should always be evaluated carefully, as this vessel represents an important collateral pathway in patients with disease of the superficial femoral artery.

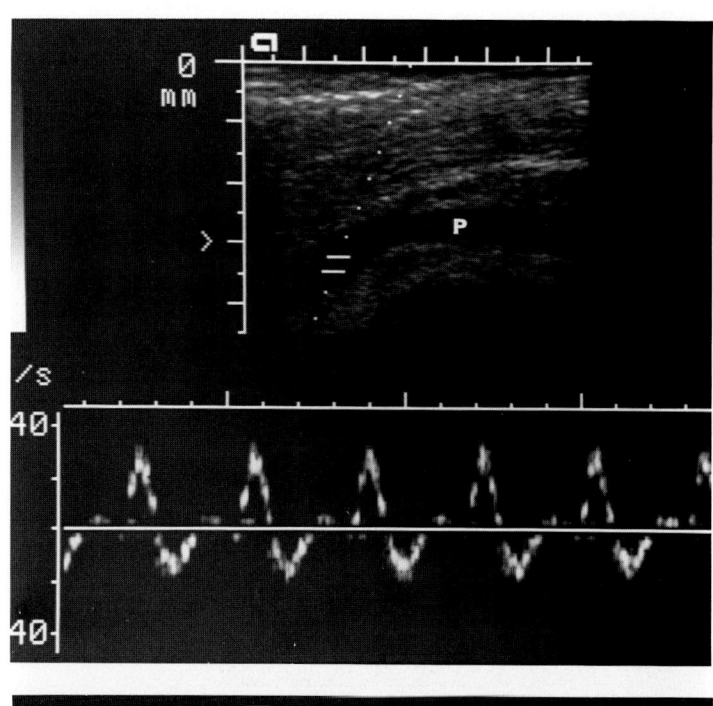

Fig. 6.4A,B. Popliteal artery. The popliteal artery (P) should be easily located behind the knee. A strong triphasic Doppler signal should be present (**A**). Meticulous scan technique will enable one to follow the artery into its distal branches (*arrows*) (**B**).

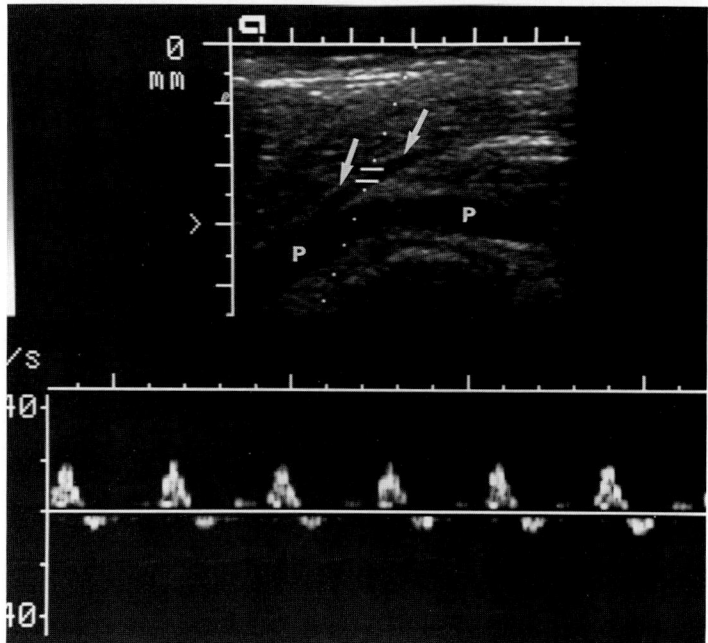

Fig. 6.5A–E. Common femoral artery stenosis. As the common femoral artery (C) curves over the hip joint (**A**) a markedly abnormal Doppler waveform is encountered (**B**). Note extremely high peak systolic velocity and marked spectral broadening; diastolic flow velocity (*arrows*) is also elevated. Distal to the lesion, a dampened waveform is present. *(Continued.)*

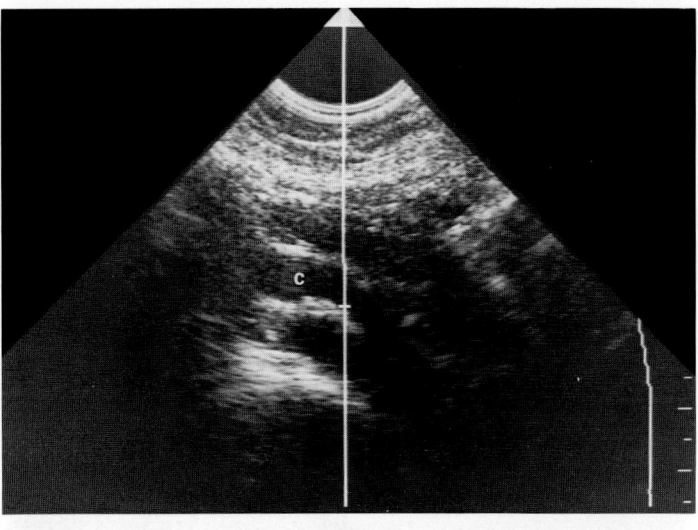

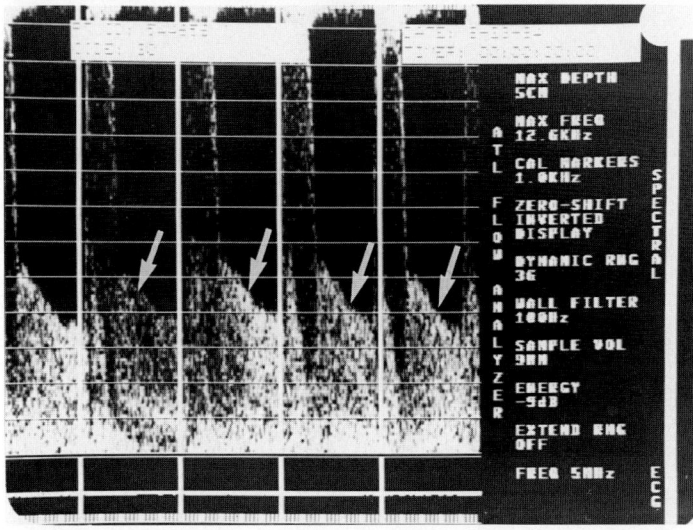

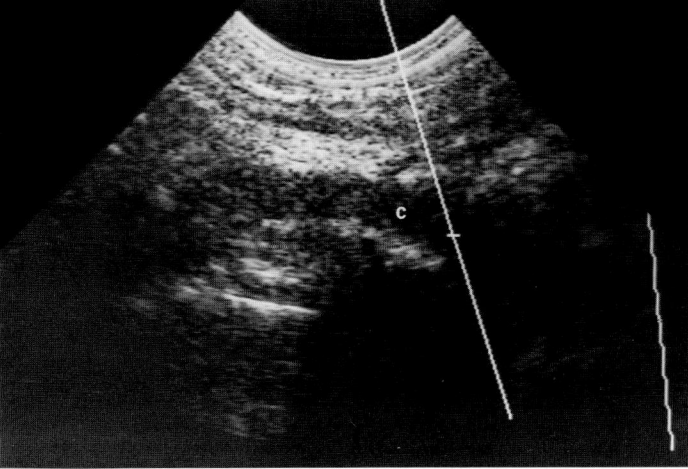

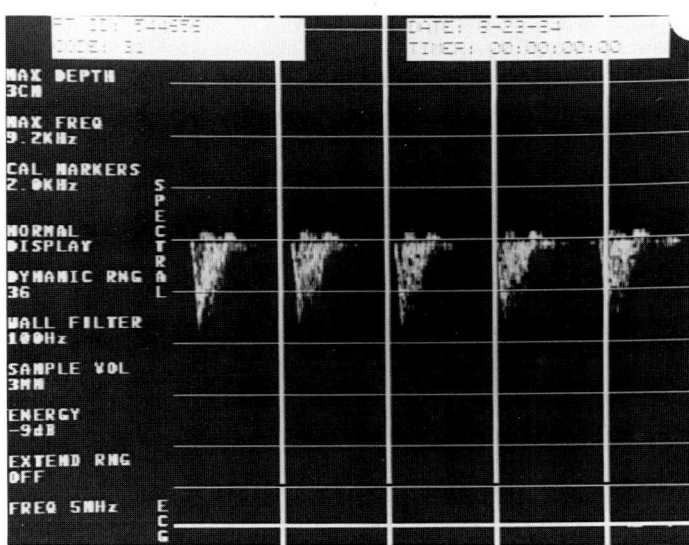

Fig. 6.5D. Negative component and diastolic flow are absent. Arteriogram confirms duplex findings (**E**).

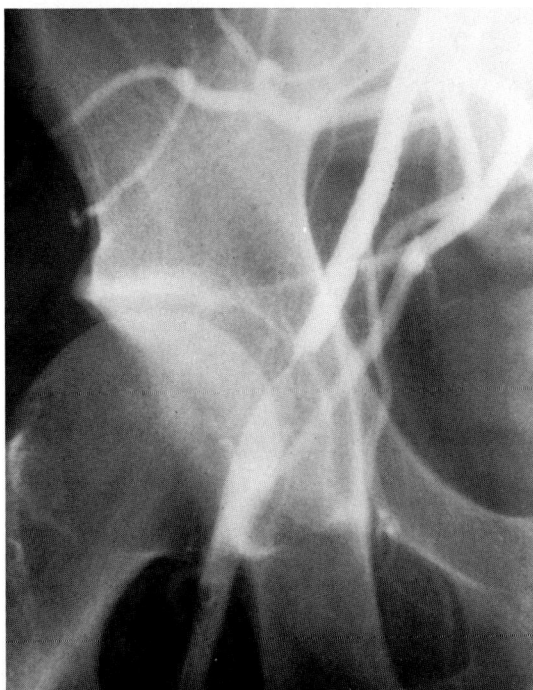

decrease in the vessel elasticity that accompanies generalized atherosclerosis. Rising diastolic flow velocity, on the other hand, most likely indicates peripheral vasodilitation in response to a focal stenotic lesion.

An overall duplex evaluation of the arteries of the legs can be time consuming and fraught with inaccuracies. In our hands, in fact, it has been an inadequate method for such an evaluation. Evaluation of selected regions of interest, however, may yield sufficient information to make such an evaluation worthwhile. Aside from the search for focally suspected disease, it may also be of value, for example, in extremely debilitated patients in whom arteriography would pose a considerable risk or in the simple evaluation of complete occlusion (Fig. 6.6A–F). We have found that duplex sonography also may be used to evaluate response to percutaneous transluminal angioplasty (Fig. 6.7A–F), and it may represent a simple, noninvasive technique to follow the long-term success of these procedures (5). With further experience, the use of duplex in the peripheral arteries may increase. Although duplex may yield valuable information in selected patients, at present its use is certainly not routine.

Aneurysms

Although typically associated with atherosclerosis, the actual mechanisms through which peripheral arterial aneurysms develop are poorly understood. Aneurysms most commonly affect the abdominal aorta and popliteal arteries. Although uncommon, aneurysms also may be identified in the iliac and femoral vessels (6). Among aneurysms of the pelvis and legs, those that occur in the iliac arteries are usually the most difficult to diagnose because of their deep location. Conversely, aortic, femoral, and

Fig. 6.6A–F. Complete occlusion of superficial femoral artery (**A**). Debilitated, elderly nursing home patient presents with cold leg. Evaluation of common femoral artery (**C**) shows a mildly abnormal waveform (**B**). Profunda femoris (P) (**C**) shows appropriately directed trace. *(Continued).*

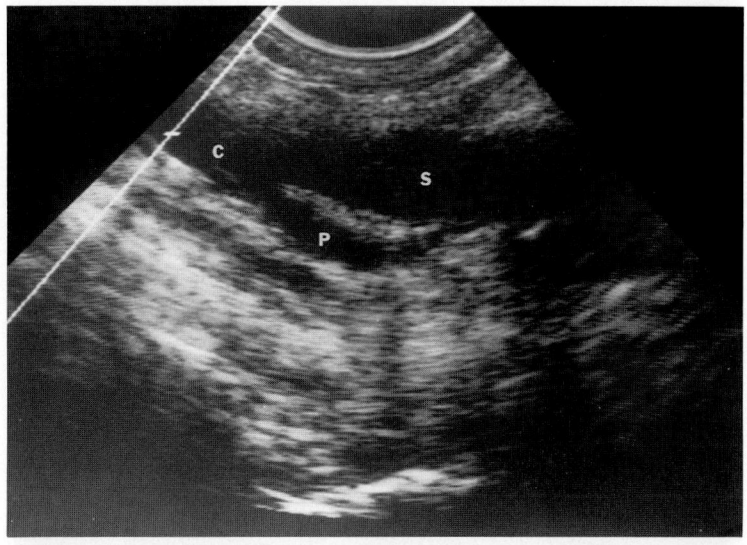

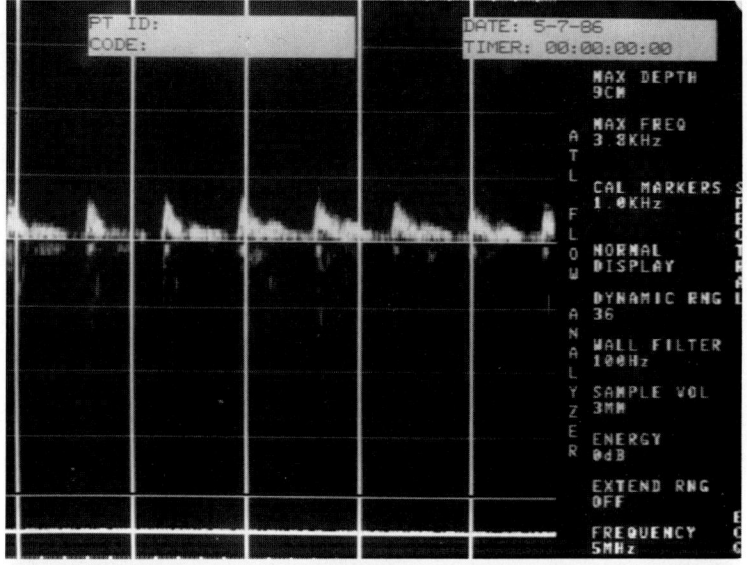

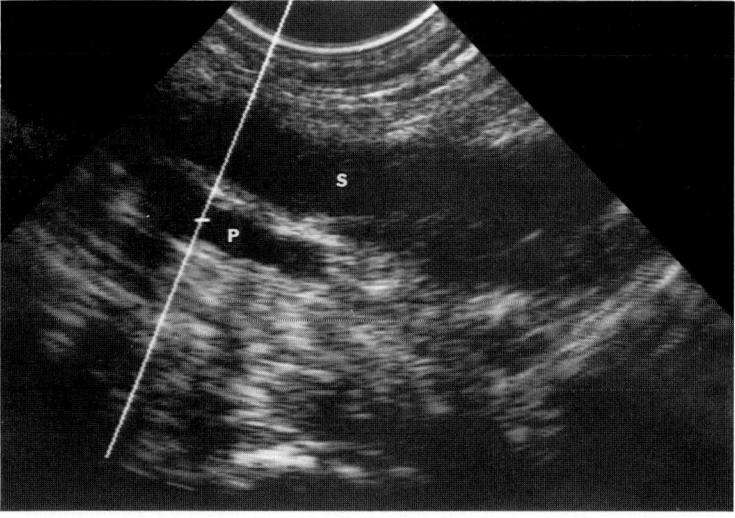

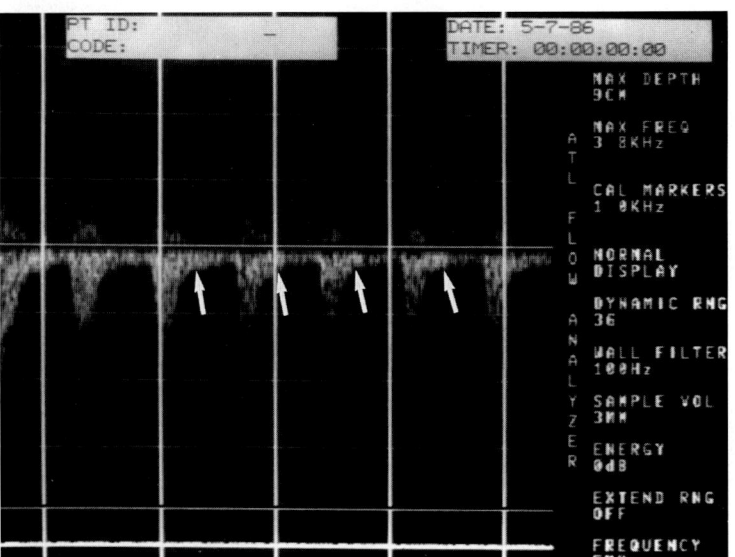
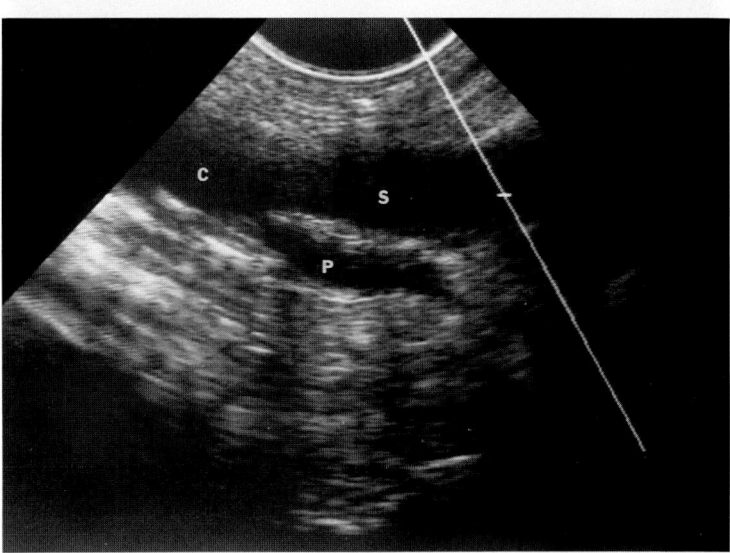

Fig. 6.6D–F. Note flow throughout diastole (*arrows*). Superficial femoral artery (S) (**E**) shows complete absence of Doppler trace (**F**).

Fig. 6.7A–F. Common femoral stenosis pre- and postangioplasty. Initial evaluation in 44-year-old runner with recent onset of claudication reveals a focal area of extremely abnormal flow in mid/distal SFA (**A,B**). Arteriogram confirms a segmental lesion (*arrows*) (**C**). *(Continued.)*

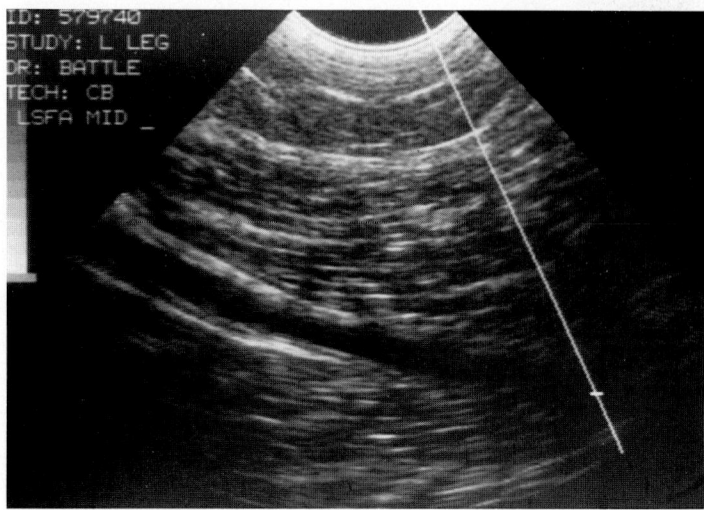

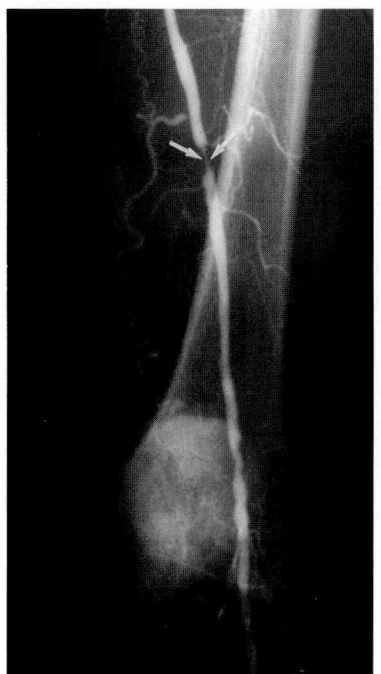

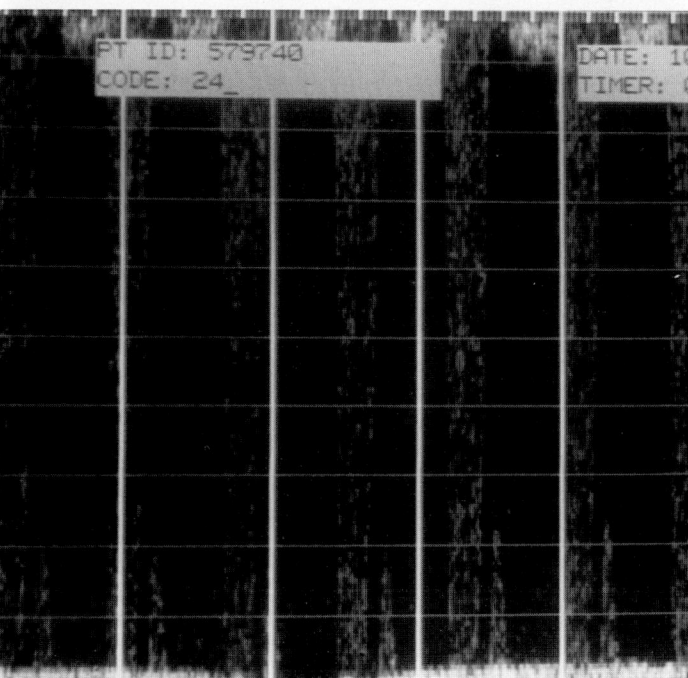

popliteal artery aneurysms are easily recognized by sonography (7), and ultrasound has been the recommended modality even before the advent of duplex sonography.

Simple real-time imaging will adequately identify all peripheral aneurysms that can be diagnosed using ultrasound without the addition of Doppler. Duplex, however, has the ability to clearly define the arterial nature of a cystic mass suspected of representing an aneurysm if the arterial connections cannot be clearly visualized (Fig. 6.8A–C). This is of particular value in the pelvis, whereas popliteal and femoral artery aneurysms are usually easily diagnosed using real-time alone (Fig. 6.9A,B). When attempting to diagnose an aneurysm, it should be kept in mind that internal flow patterns may be very unusual. Flow velocity may vary considerably from one portion of the aneurysm to the next. Turbulence and reversed flow are

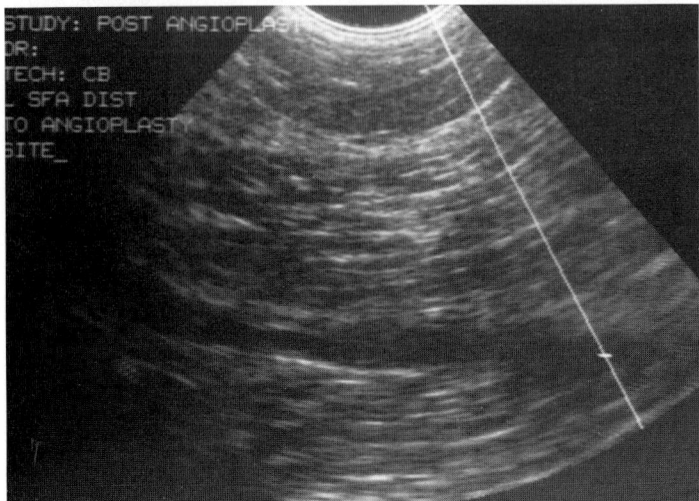

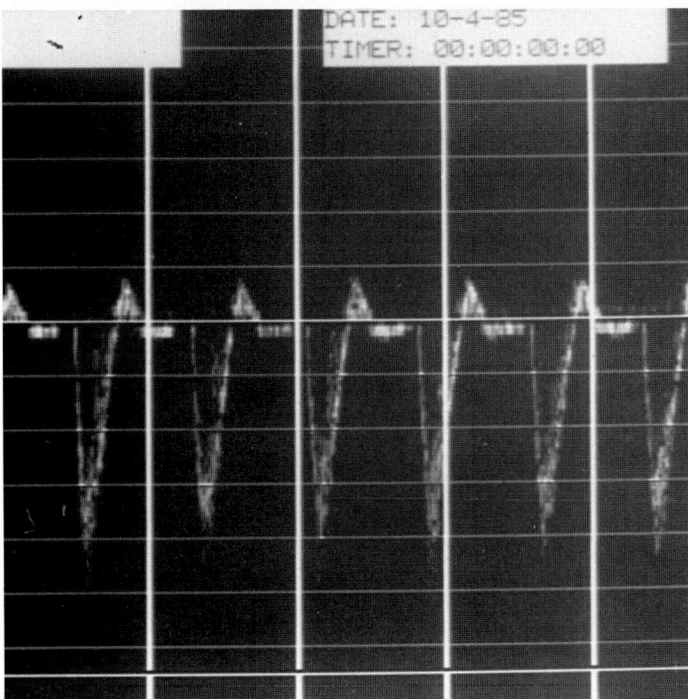
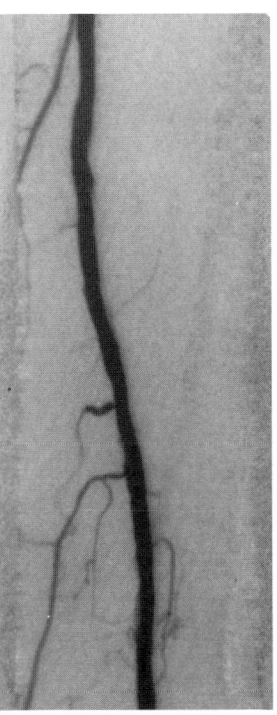

Fig. 6.7D–F. Postangioplasty Doppler patterns are normal (**D,E**). Angiogram (**F**) shows excellent result of angioplasty.

common. We have found that the amount and location of mural thrombus and the size of the lumen have a considerable effect on flow (8).

Iatrogenic/Traumatic Vascular Lesions

Under this heading, we discuss the evaluation of arterial bypass grafts, hemodialysis shunts (A-V fistulae), and pseudoaneurysms. In each of these entities, duplex sonography may produce pivotal diagnostic information noninvasively. In many cases, duplex may actually be the only evaluation necessary before surgery. The superficial location of bypass grafts, hemodialysis shunts, and pseudoaneurysms makes all of these lesions amenable to evaluation with high-resolution duplex sonography.

Fig. 6.8A–C. Iliac artery aneurysm: Cystic mass (C) (**A**) is identified in upper pelvis of a 72-year-old man. Patient previously had abdominal aortic aneurysm resected. Doppler evaluation (**B**) shows extremely dampened waveform. CT (**C**) confirms that mass is an iliac artery aneurysm (*arrowheads*).

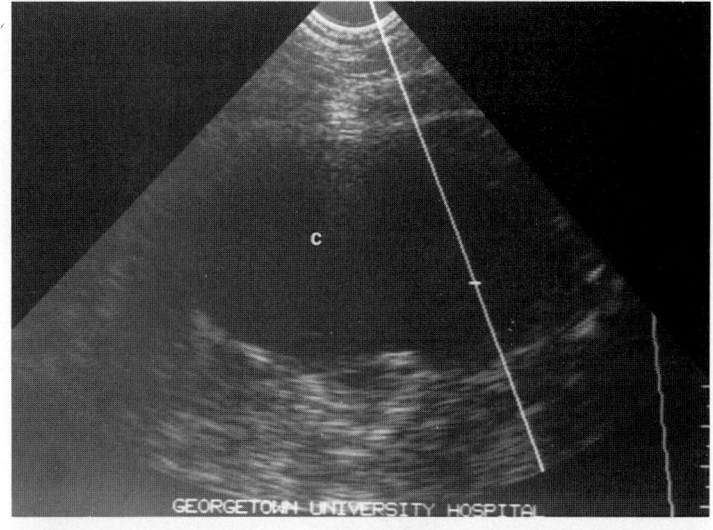

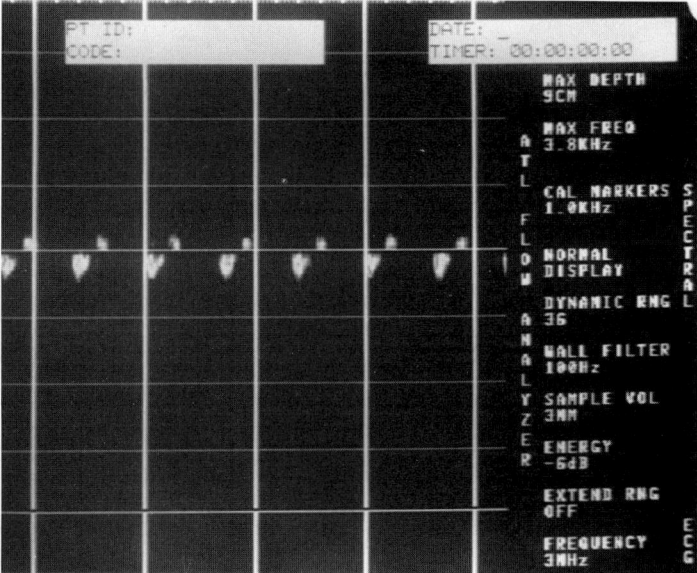

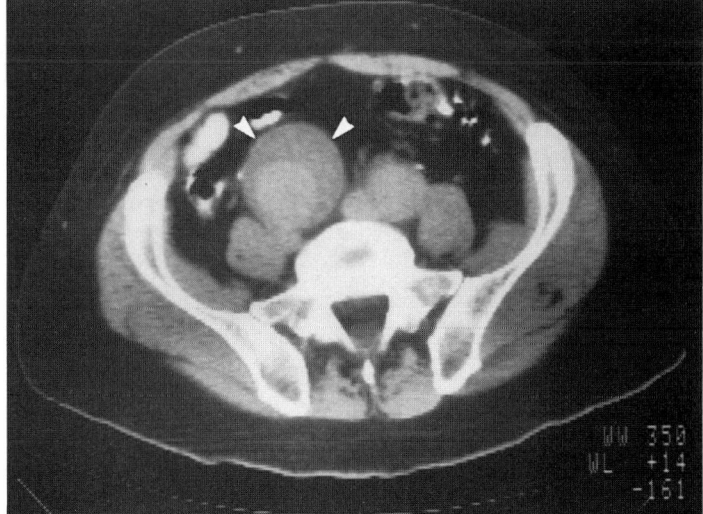

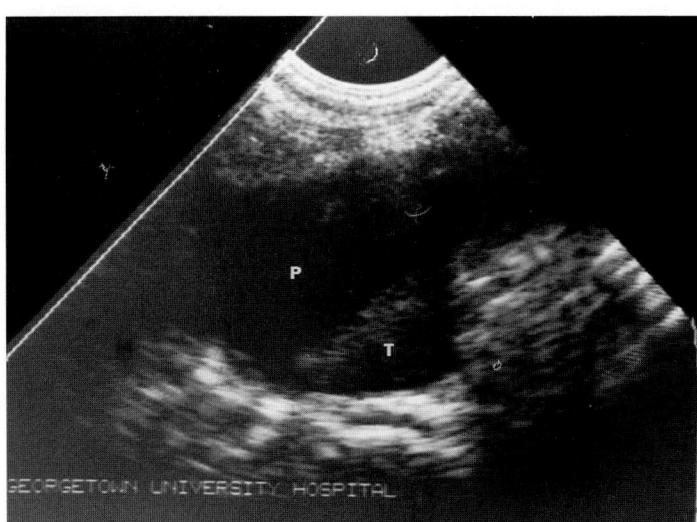

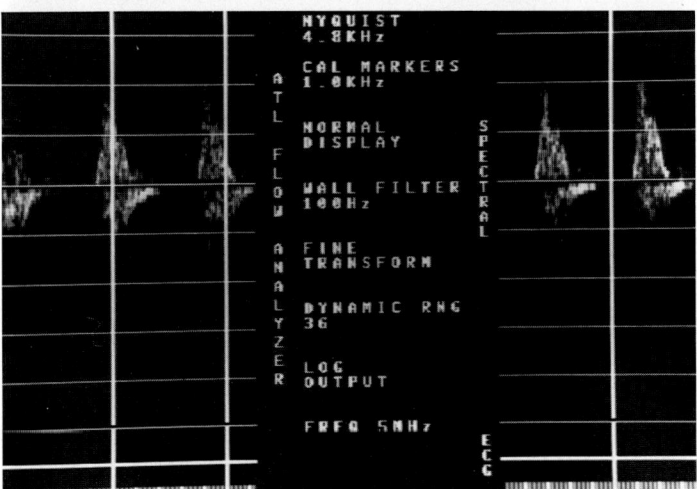

Fig. 6.9A,B. Popliteal artery aneurysm. Pulsatile mass in popliteal fossa represents an outpouching of the popliteal artery(**A**) (P). Note posterior thrombus (T). Doppler evaluation reveals relatively normal flow through the aneurysm (**B**).

Arterial bypass grafts are frequently located directly beneath the skin. Although many grafts are palpable, a conversation with the vascular surgeon should be sought before performing the duplex evaluation. Both the anatomy and the material used in the graft should be determined. Knowledge of the postoperative vascular anatomy will allow one to greatly shorten the time required for the examination and frequently eliminate considerable confusion. Although bypass grafts may be located between almost any two arteries, the most frequently evaluated grafts are femoropopliteal bypasses. These are easily located in the medial thigh directly beneath the surgical scar. Evaluation of the graft is quite simple if it is an autogenous (usually saphenous) vein, provided one does not apply too much pressure on the transducer. Evaluation becomes slightly more difficult if the graft is synthetic. The most commonly used material is polytetrafluoroethylene (Gortex). Unfortunately, this substance causes considerable attenuation of the second beam, which may degrade the diagnostic quality of the examination. With these relatively minor rules in mind, evaluation for suspected graft stenosis of complete occlusion should be fast and provide essential diagnostic information.

Flow patterns in arterial bypass grafts exhibit a clear-cut arterial waveform, although it may be somewhat dampened. Graft stenosis is generally found at one of the anastamotic sites (Fig. 6.10A–D) or may occasionally be seen in association with thrombus propagating around an

Fig. 6.10A–D. Bypass graft. Left femoropopliteal saphenous vein graft is evaluated in patient with recurrent symptoms. (**A**) The origin of the graft (*arrow*) exhibits a focal region of markedly increased flow velocity (**B**). (Each graticule corresponds to a 2 KHzΔ shift). More distally within the graft (**C**), more normal waveforms are identified (**D**). *(See next page.)*

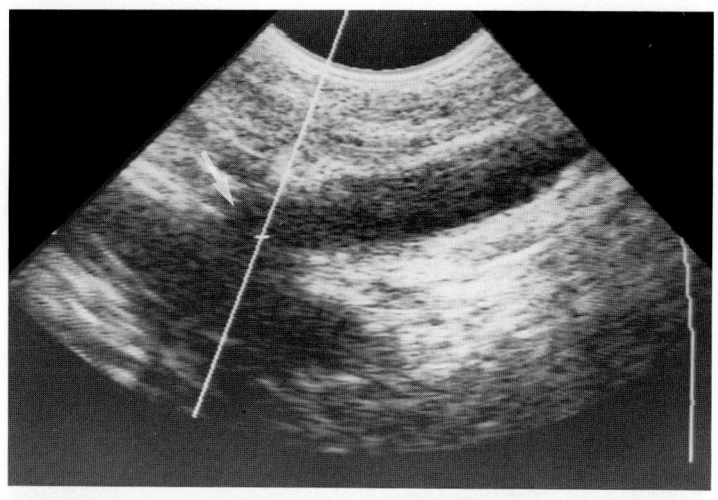

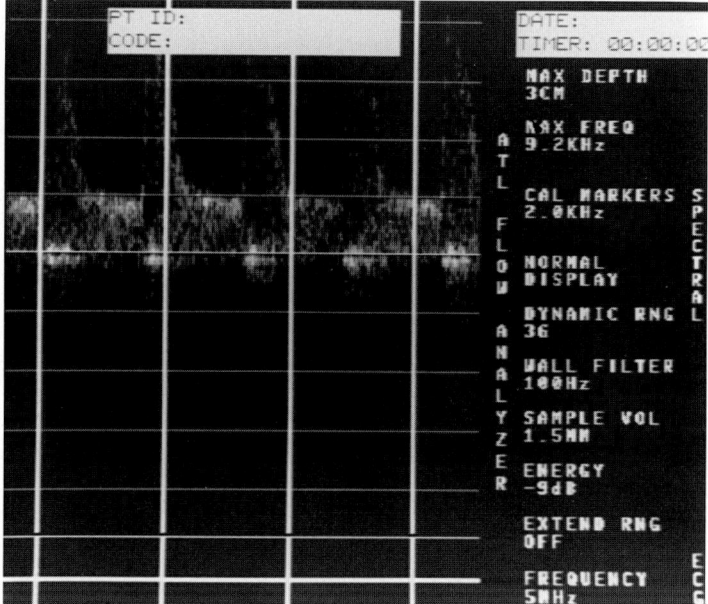

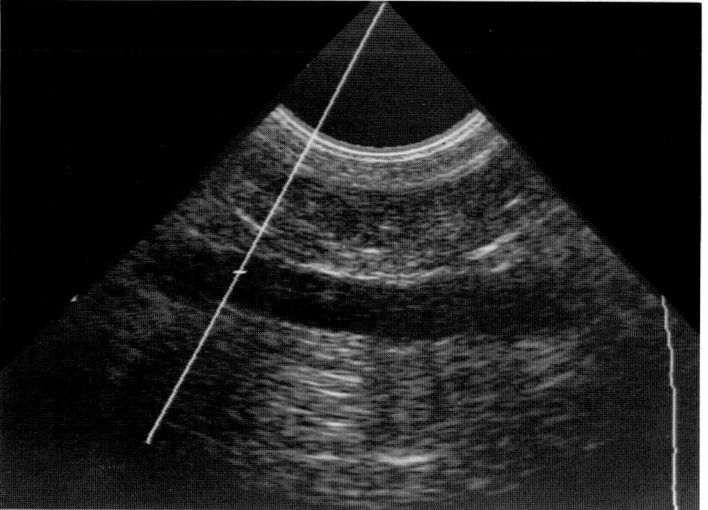

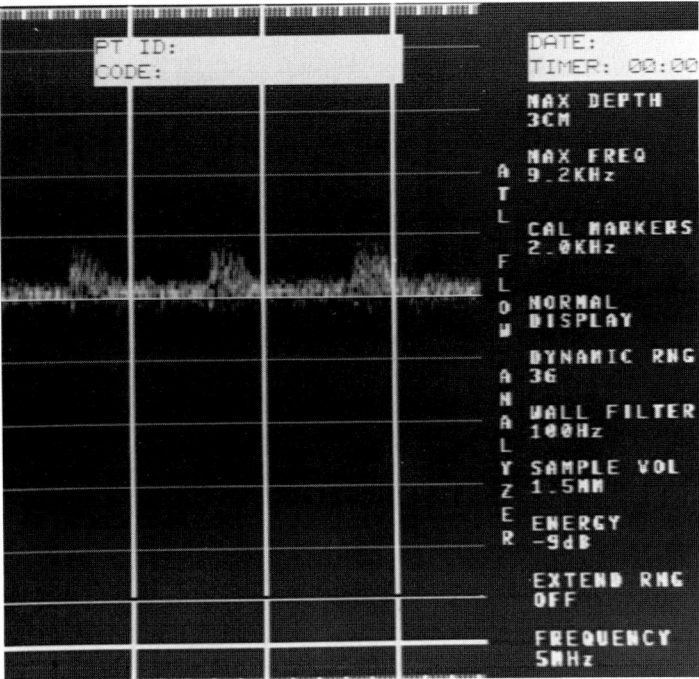

Fig. 6.10.

overlooked venous valve leaflet (9). As elsewhere in the body, stenosis is usually heralded by a marked increase in peak systolic velocity and spectral broadening. Total graft occlusion should be diagnosed easily with duplex sonography. Thrombus in a bypass graft is frequently anechoic; the diagnosis, therefore, depends almost entirely on Doppler (Fig. 6.11A–E).

Hemodialysis shunts also are evaluated easily using duplex sonography (10). Again, these man-made fistulae are superficially located and easily palpable. Similar to bypass grafts, they may be comprised of either synthetic material or, more commonly, native vessel. Complete thromboses, stenoses, ectasia, and most other graft malfunctions may be adequately and definitely evaluated using duplex sonography (Fig. 6.12A–D). We have found duplex to be particularly useful in the evaluation of palpable masses that occasionally develop around graft sites. The differentiation between infection around the shunt and intrinsic ectasia or pseudoaneurysm should be accomplished easily. In each of these cases the sonographic findings will dictate the treatment: infection warrants shunt removal, severe ectasia may lead to high output failure and necessitate shunt revision, and pseudoaneurysms may be easily clipped and resected.

Whereas pseudoaneurysms represent a possible complication of hemodialysis shunts, they may form at any vascular anastomosis or after a penetrating wound. In our practice, they are most commonly iatrogenic; elsewhere the most common etiology may be intravenous drug use. Both pseudoaneurysms and mycotic aneurysms may occur in the latter group of patients. Regardless of the etiology, patients with pseudoaneurysms most frequently present with a pulsatile mass. A careful history will usually reveal recent vascular surgery, arteriography, multiple arterial punctures (usually for blood gas levels), or intravenous drug use. Sonography should initially differentiate between a collection around the artery (hematoma or pus) and a true vascular abnormality. One must then determine whether the suspected aneurysm involves a main vessel or a branch. Finally, both venous and arterial flow in the area should be examined to eliminate the possibility of arterial

Fig. 6.11A–E. Graft occlusion. Elderly woman presents with cold legs and absence of pulses below the groin. Patient had history of bilateral aortofemoral and femoro-popliteal grafts. Duplex evaluation of right graft (R) (**A**) confirms absence of flow (**B**). Note typical striated appearance of Gortex graft (*arrowheads*). Evaluation of left graft (L) in proximal thigh (**C**) also reveals total occlusion (**D**). Arteriogram (**E**) confirms occlusion of both grafts. *(See next page)*

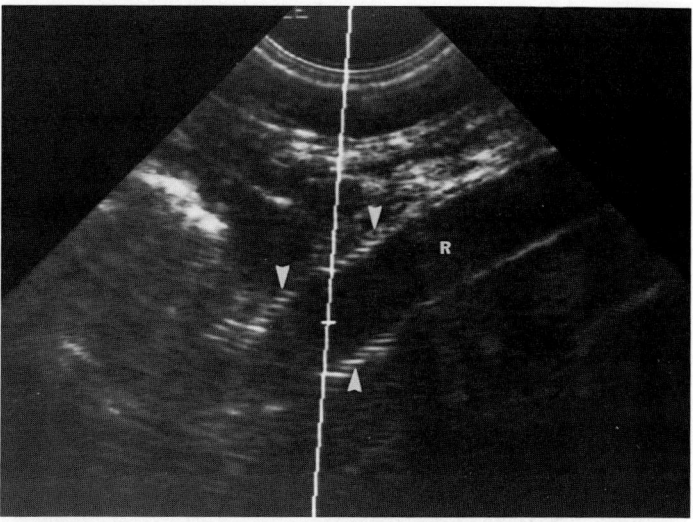

A

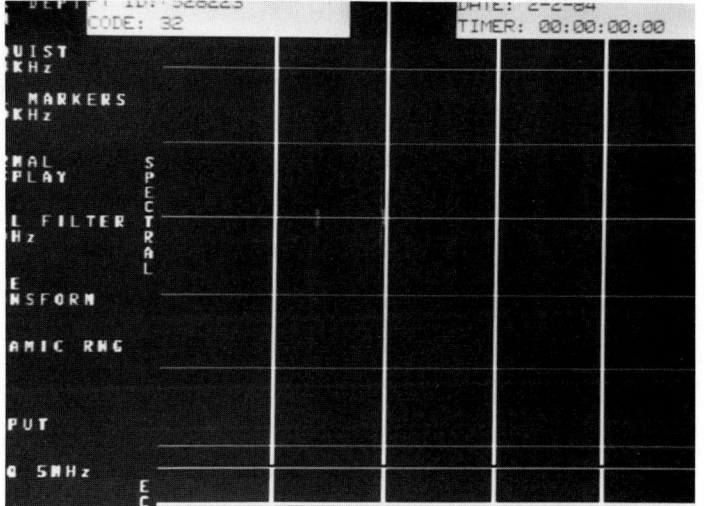

B

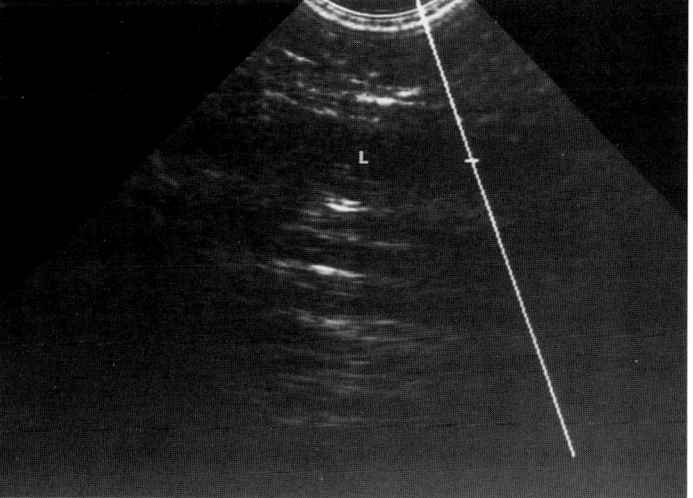

C

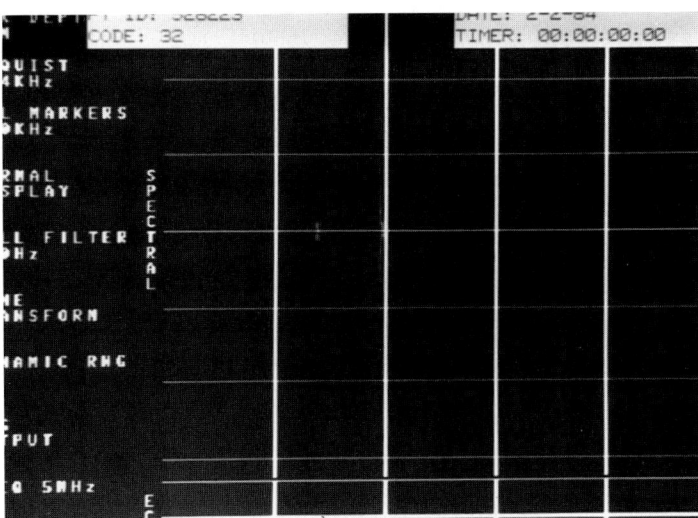

compromise or venous thrombosis. Formation of an abscess around a graft is a dreaded complication; abscess formation mandates immediate removal. Identification of aneurysmal dilatation of a major vessel, on the other hand, requires either bypass or resection; major surgery is implied (Fig. 6.13A–C). Conversely, identification of a pseudoaneurysm that does not involve the main artery implies a benign surgical procedure in which the feeder vessel may be easily clipped and the aneurysm removed. This may be done under local anesthesia (Fig. 6.14A–G). In general, the duplex evaluation of pseudoaneurysms/vascular masses has been well-accepted and provides easily accessible yet essential information.

Congenital Arteriovenous Malformations

Congenital arteriovenous malformations represent an abnormal communication between a peripheral artery and vein. Although they may be present at birth, they frequently do not manifest clinical symptoms until childhood. Most frequently, a parent will notice that one extremity is larger than the other. Specific clinical symptoms and signs may be present in some cases, but, in general, arteriography has been required for confirmation. Duplex sonography represents an excellent screening modality in

Fig. 6.11.

Fig. 6.12A–D. Hemodialysis shunt evaluation. Patient presents with enlarging mass-like area over existing hemodialysis arteriovenous fistula. Mass consists of markedly dialated vascular channels (**A,C**) (V). Doppler confirms high flow rate (**B**). Shunt eventually required revision; the high flow rate (**B,D**)was believed responsible for congestive heart failure. *(See next page.)*

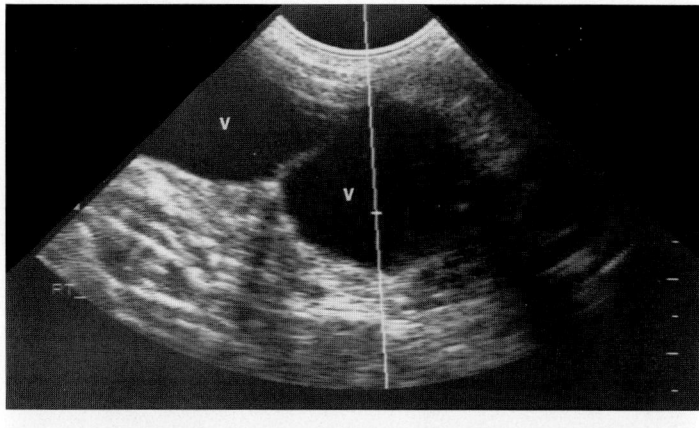

A

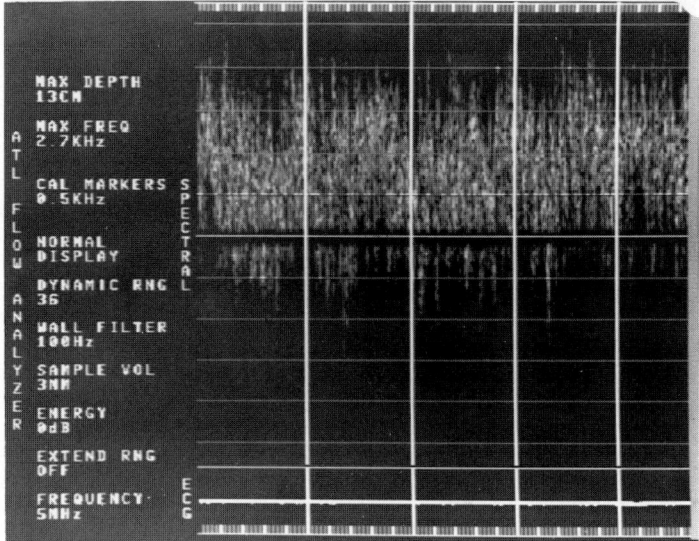

B

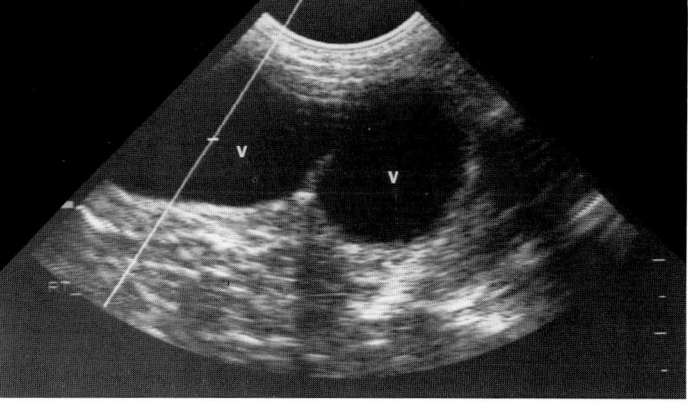

C

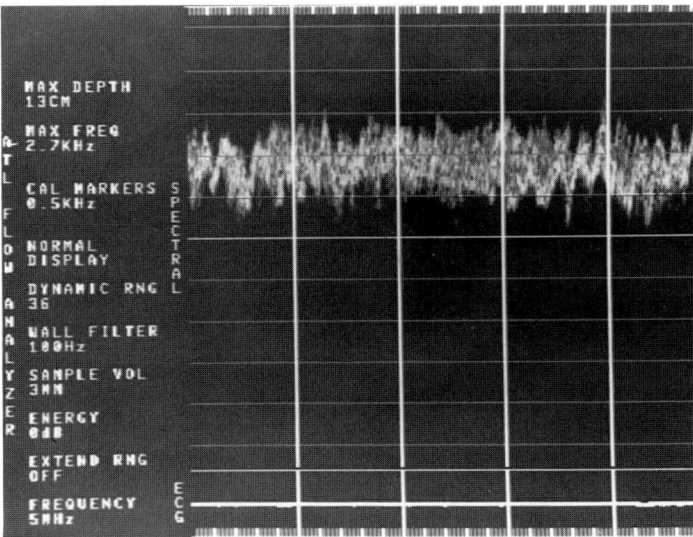

D

Fig. 6.12.

patients suspected of arteriovenous malformation. In general, we have found it quite useful in children with one leg that is larger than the other, regardless of the etiology. Pathologically, arteriovenous malformations are formed by a nest of dilated, intertwined vessels. These are usually depicted by real-time imaging as a group of serpiginious cystic spaces. The realtime findings alone, however, are not diagnostic. Other abnormalities, including resolving hematomas and even sarcomas, occasionally may present a similar picture. Duplex sonography provides the diagnosis by identifying characteristic flow in many of the abnormal vascular channels. As is suspected, increased arterial inflow and pulsatile venous outflow is frequently identified (Fig. 6.15*A–F*). Although uncommon, patients suspected of peripheral arteriovenous malformations should undergo screening with duplex sonography before arteriography.

Summary

The evaluation of the peripheral arterial system with duplex sonography has received relatively little attention. In the evaluation of atherosclerotic lesions, the difficulty and time-consuming nature of the evaluation has undoubtedly prevented duplex from becoming a major diagnostic tool. In the evaluation of bypass grafts and postsurgical/traumatic lesions, duplex sonography offers noninvasive yet often definitive information that can be essential in preoperative planning. Finally, peripheral arteriovenous malformations are rare, yet, duplex sonography offers an excellent and frequently definitive modality for their evaluation. As familiarity and expertise with peripheral arterial duplex sonography increases, we may eventually find that it offers more diagnostic information than is presently known.

Fig. 6.13A–C. Mycotic aneurysm. Erythematous, painful swelling in groin of 24-year-old drug addict is caused by focal dilatation of the common femoral artery (C) (**A**). Dampened but relatively normal flow through the area is confirmed by duplex evaluation (**B**). Arteriogram (**C**) confirms the presence of a large aneurysm of the native vessel in the area of the palpable abnormality. Lesion required surgical resection and grafting and proved to represent a mycotic aneurysm.

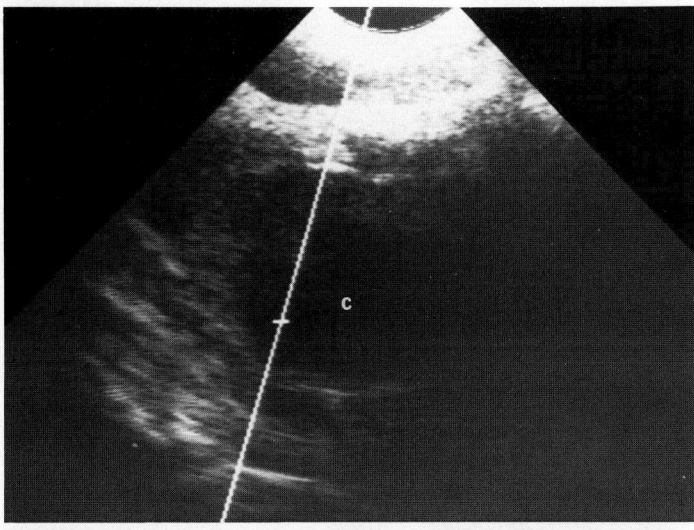

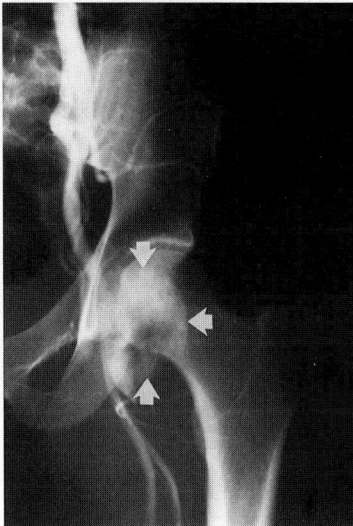

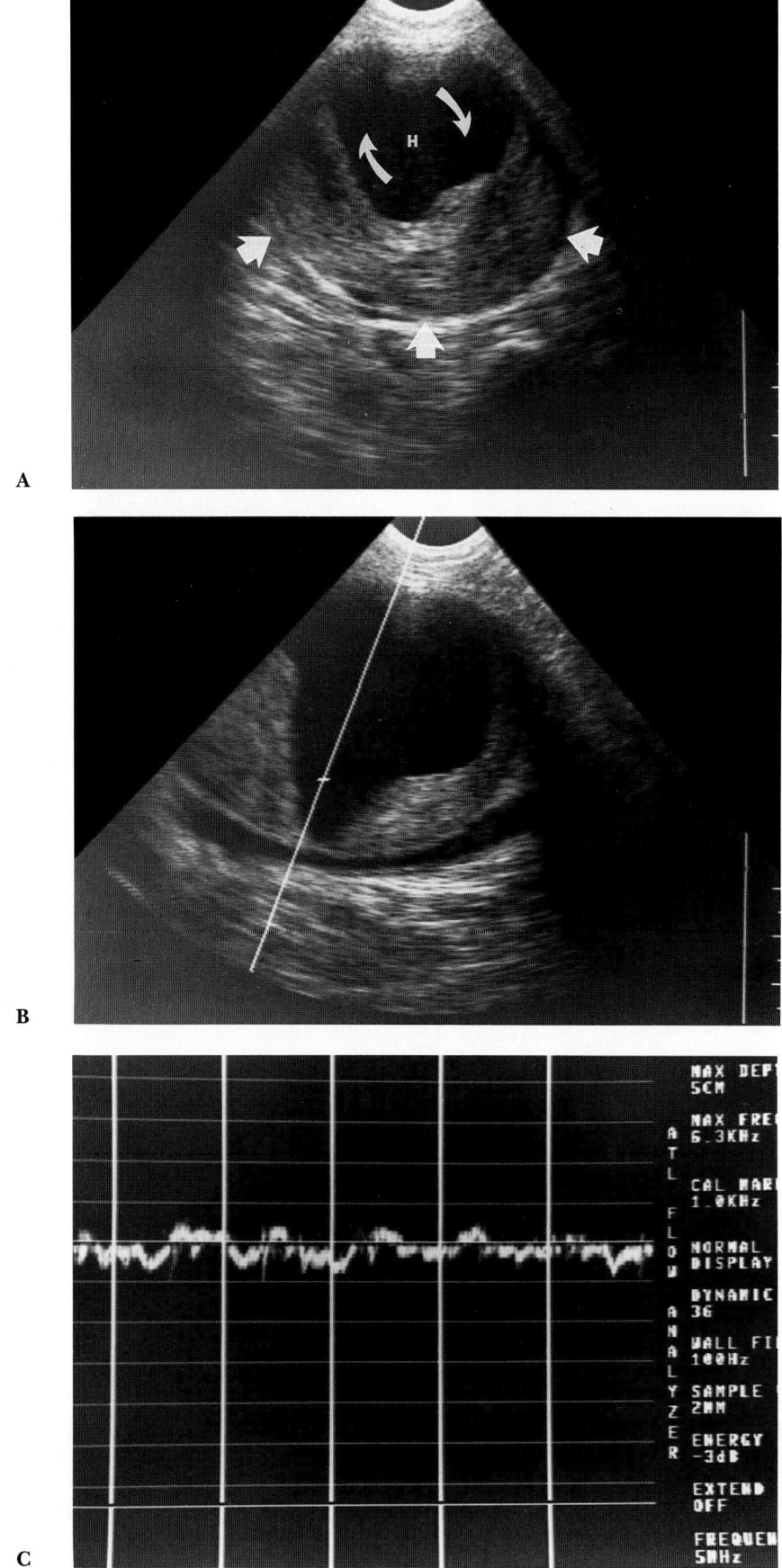

Fig. 6.14.

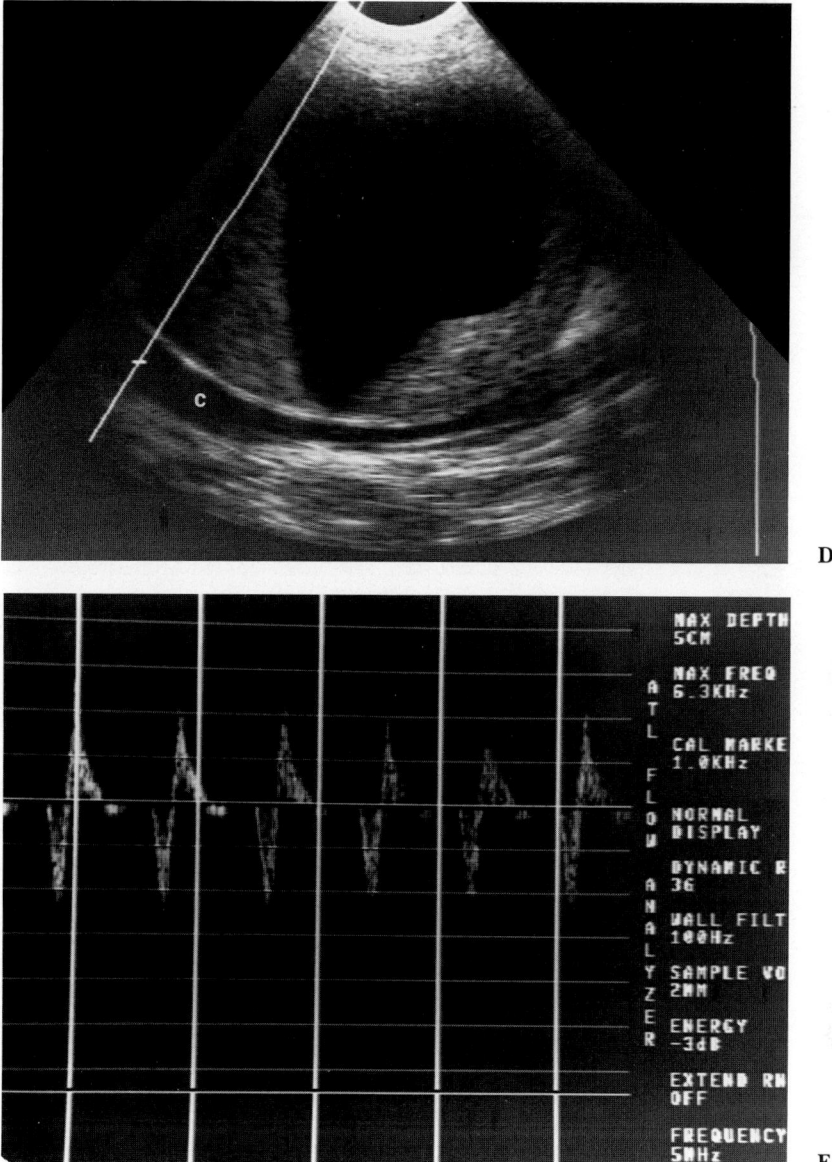

Fig. 6.14A–G. Pseudoaneurysm. Painless swelling in left groin is noted by patient 1 month after cardiac catheterization. A well-defined mass with an echogenic rind *(arrows)* and a hypoechoic center (H) (**A**) is present. Real-time evaluation showed systolic swirling of low-level echogenicity, which is characteristic of pseudoaneurysm. Doppler evaluation of the mass (**B,C**) shows unusual choppy flow pattern. Normal triphasic flow is preserved in the common femoral artery (C) posterior to the mass (**D,E**). Because of swelling of the affected leg, the femoral vein also was evaluated. The vein (**F**) (V) compressed normally yet exhibited no flow by duplex evaluation. Thrombosis is excluded with augmentation procedure (**G**). Patient's calf is squeezed, forcing blood through femoral vein, causing Doppler deflections as shown. *(See next page.)*

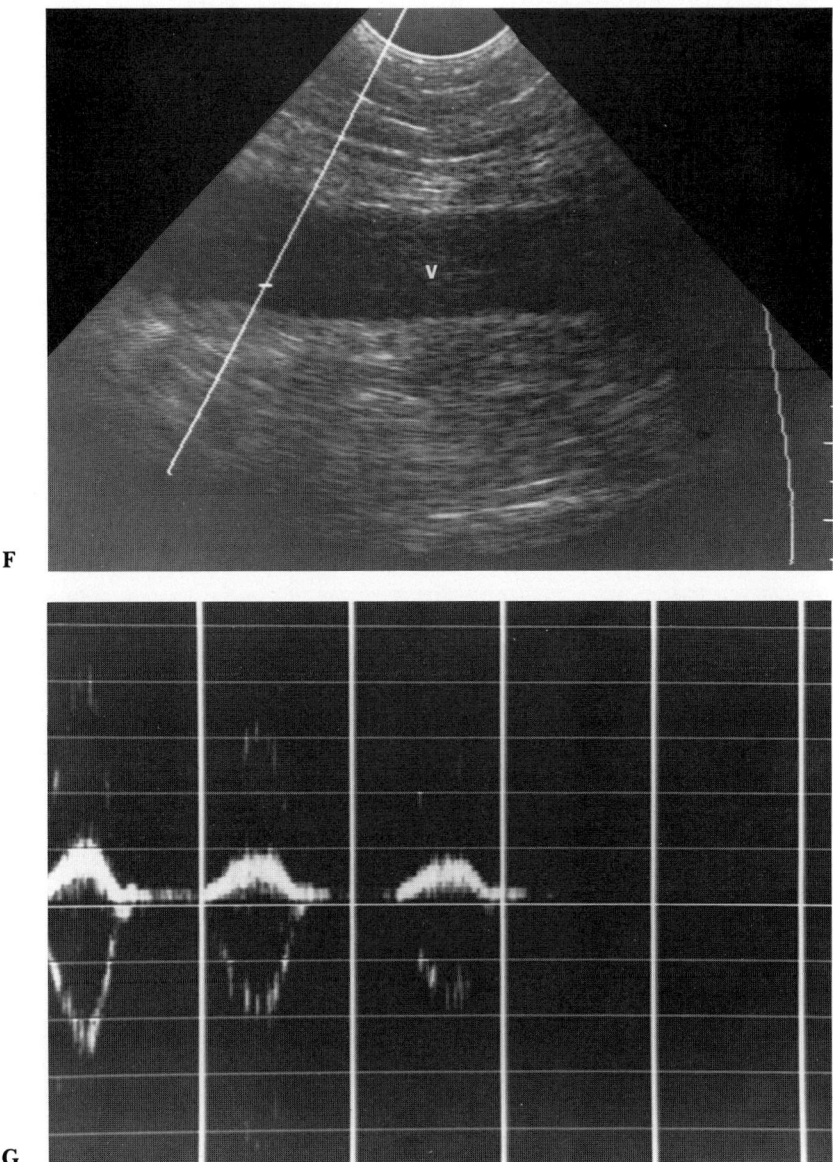

Fig. 6.14.

Fig. 6.15A–F. Arteriovenous malformation. Ten-year-old girl with left leg larger than right. Duplex evaluation of the larger leg was undertaken to evaluate for suspected deep venous thrombosis. Evaluation of the proximal calf veins (*arrrows*) (**A**) shows dilatation of the vessels and a pulsatile flow pattern (**B**). In mid-calf, a focal collection of cystic spaces (*arrowheads*) (**C**) is identified and confirmed to be vascular by Doppler evaluation (**D**). Early (**E**) and later phase (**F**) of selective arteriogram confirms arteriovenous malformation (**E,F**). *(See next page.)*

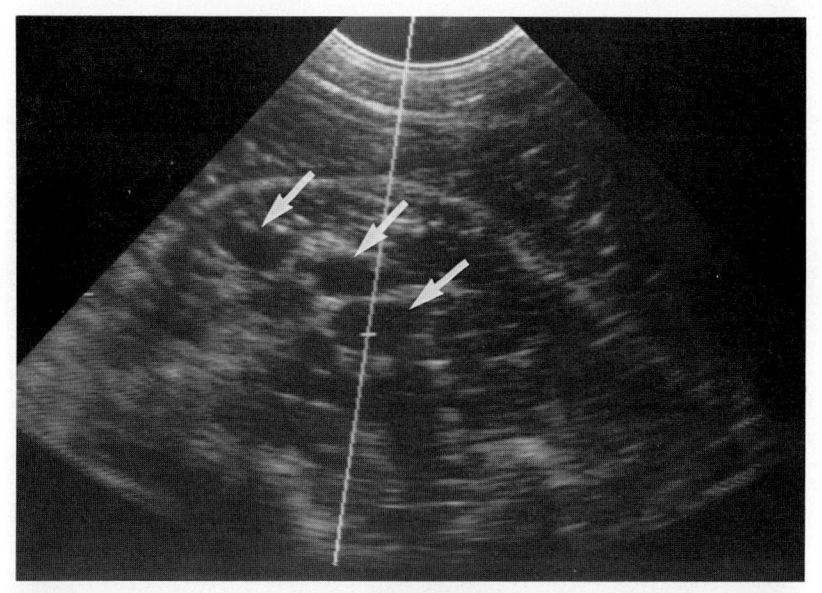

A

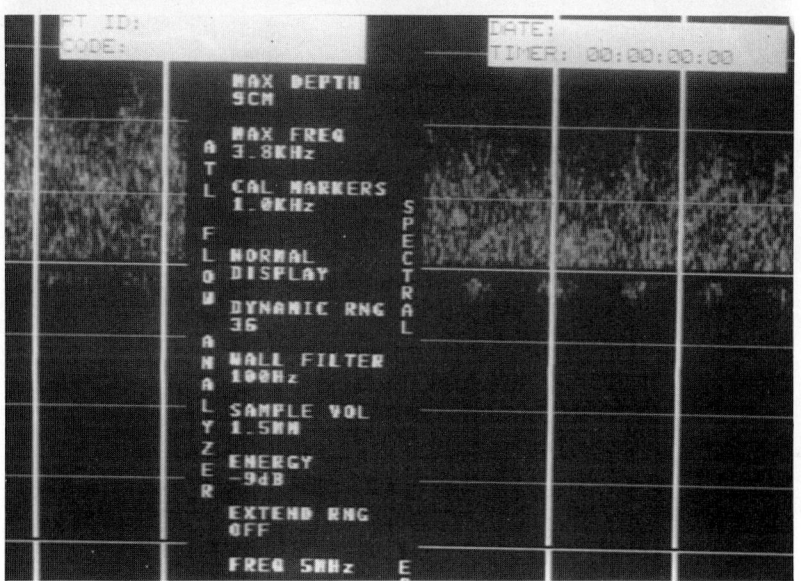

B

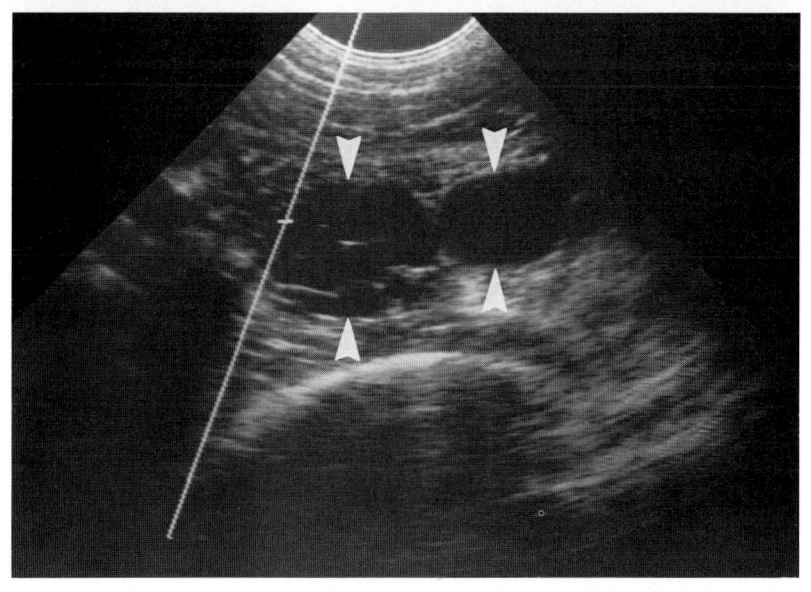

C

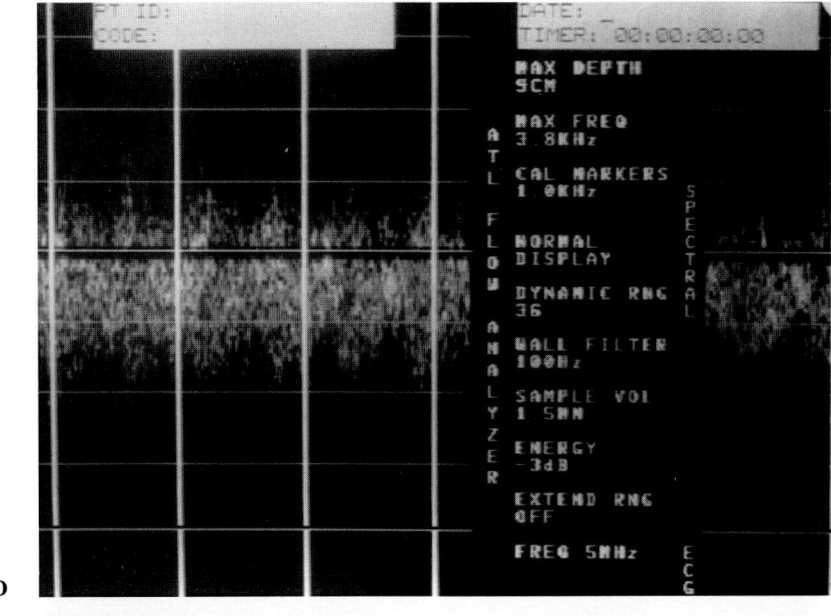

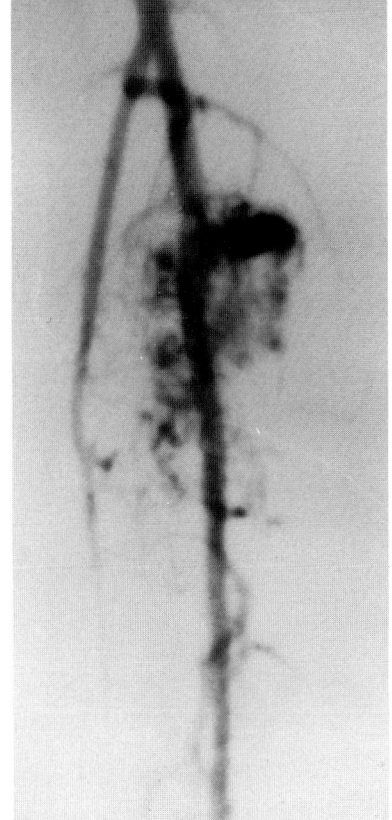

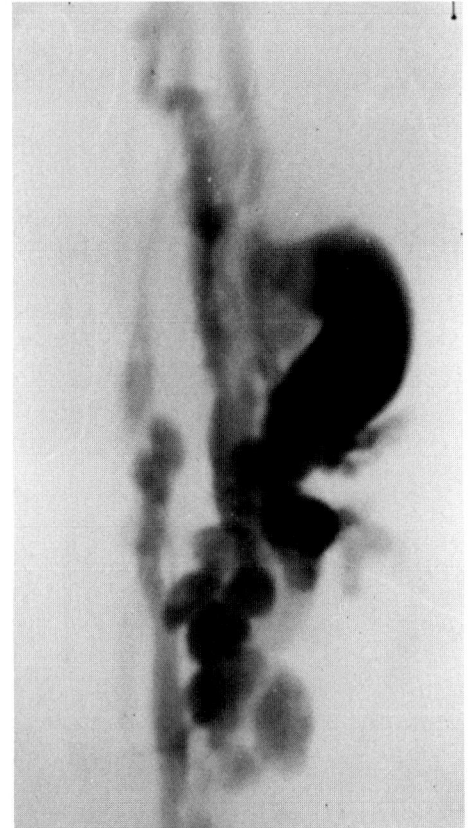

Fig. 6.15.

References

1. Imparato AM, Riles TS: Peripheral arterial disease. *In* Schwartz SI (ed): Principles of Surgery. New York, McGraw-Hill, 1984, pp 901–910.
2. DeBakey ME: The current status of Leriche syndrome. Surg Rounds 20, 1980.
3. Puylaert JBCM: Acute appendicitis: US evaluation using graded compression. Radiology 158:355, 1986.
4. Jager KA, Phillips DJ, Martin RL, et al: Noninvasive mapping of lower limb arterial lesions. Ultrasound Med Biol 11:515, 1985.
5. Evans DD, Mertens MA, Richardson J, et al: Comparative evaluation of iliac and femoral artery stenosis before and after angioplasty of duplex US, angiography, and arterial pressure measurements. Presented at Radiologic Society of North America, November 20, 1985, Chicago, IL.
6. Queral LA, Flinn WR, Yao JS, et al: Management of peripheral arterial aneurysms. Surg Clin North Am 59:693, 1979.
7. Gooding GAW: Aneurysms of the abdominal aorta, iliac and femoral arteries. Semin Ultrasound 3:170, 1982.
8. Choyke PL, White EM, Grant EG, et al: Duplex sonography of abdominal aortic aneurysms. Presented at the Radiologic Society of North America, December 5, 1986, Chicago, IL.
9. Jones AF, Kempczinski RF: Autofemoral bypass grafting. Arch Surg 11:301, 1981.
10. Wetzner SM, Kiser LC, Bezreh JS: Duplex ultrasound imaging: Vascular applications. Radiology 150:507, 1984.

7
Duplex Sonography of the Lower Extremity Venous System

E. MAUREEN WHITE

Radiographic evaluation of the lower extremity deep venous system has, until recently, been primarily accomplished by ascending contrast venography, which represents the accepted diagnostic standard. Although this is a sensitive and reliable means for detecting venous disease, lower extremity phlebography is not innocuous. Several potential complications to its use are well known and may suffice to preclude the examination in certain patients. These adverse sequela to intravenous contrast administration include severe allergic reaction, exacerbation of underlying azotemia or congestive heart failure, local tissue irritation, and toxic effect on the venous endothelium which may induce clinically significant phlebitis.

Due to these risks, a noninvasive test is desirable for assessment of the lower extremity veins, particularly in screening a large population of individuals. During the past 20 years or more, a variety of studies have been described. Most of these methods, such as impedance plethysmography (IPG), phleborheography (PRG), and radionuclide scintigraphy, have had variable success in the diagnosis of venous disease (1–4). High-resolution ultrasound is increasingly recognized as an excellent alternative technique (5–10). At several medical centers, this has become the primary initial screening modality for evaluating the lower extremity venous system (9,10). Although real-time imaging accompanied with various maneuvers generally provides for diagnostic examination, Doppler analysis has been shown to contribute useful adjunctive information. Technique of examination, anatomic considerations, and potential pitfalls are discussed in this chapter. Sonographic assessment for deep venous thrombosis, which represents one of the most common diseases to affect the lower extremity vasculature, is reviewed. Finally, duplex ultrasound evaluation of other pathologic processes that may involve the lower extremity deep venous system is described.

Lower Extremity Deep Venous Anatomy

Basic knowledge of the lower extremity deep venous anatomy is mandatory in both performing and interpreting these ultrasound studies (Fig. 7.1). The pertinent anatomy is described from the common femoral vein through the calf. This order is used to correspond with the usual sonographic approach to examination of the deep venous system in the lower extremities.

In the inguinal region, the common femoral vein is the major venous structure draining blood from the lower extremity into the external iliac vein, which takes origin at the level of the inguinal ligament. Through its course from the inguinal ligament to approximately the level of the lesser trochanter, the common femoral vein is located medial to the femoral artery. The common femoral vein is formed in the uppermost thigh by confluence of several vessels. Within the deep venous system, these vessels include the medially located superficial femoral vein, the more laterally positioned profunda femoris vein, and other smaller vessels. Several superficial veins also drain into the common femoral vein, including the greater saphenous vein and the lateral cutaneous vein.

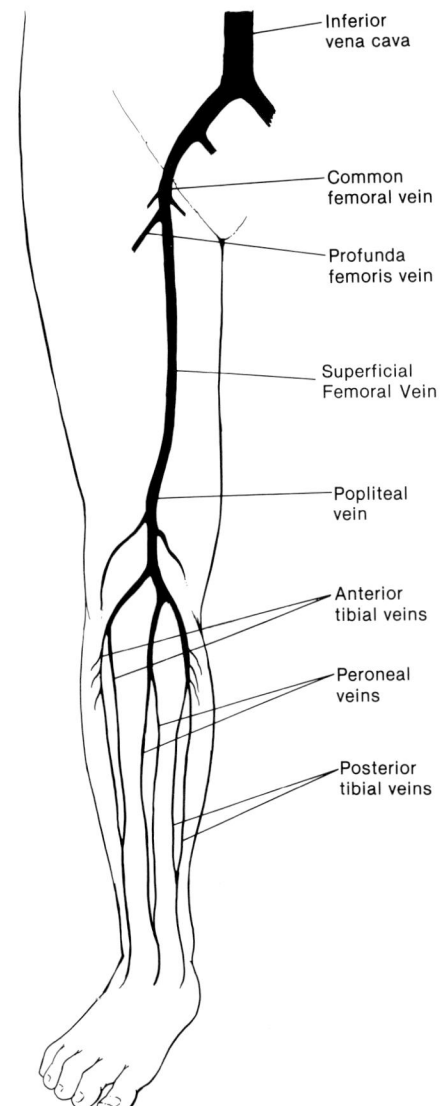

Fig. 7.1. Diagram of lower extremity deep venous anatomy.

The superficial femoral vein courses inferomedially along the proximal and midthigh, posterior to the femoral artery. At the adductor (Hunter's) canal, the vein passes posteromedially around the distal femur, to become the popliteal vein. Along the posterior aspect of the knee, the popliteal vein is located posteromedially to the popliteal artery. Within the proximal calf, the popliteal vein takes origin from three major vessels. The uppermost branch is usually the anterior tibial vein, which has a lateral course through the calf. The other two branches that converge slightly inferiorly include the posterior tibial vein, oriented medially, and the peroneal vein, interposed between the two tibial veins. Each of these venous trunks in the calf is generally composed of a set of two vessels. These veins and numerous branches course through the calf and into the foot. At the level of the metatarsal heads, the vessels usually interconnect through the plantar arch.

Ultrasound Evaluation of the Lower Extremity Deep Venous System

Because ultrasound demonstrates both arteries and veins as adjacent, tubular, branching structures, consideration must be given to various means for distinguishing these vessels. This may be accomplished by knowledge of anatomic relationships, by use of various maneuvers, and, finally, by application of Doppler technique. The anatomy of the lower extremity arteries and veins is fairly constant and application of these relationships greatly facilitates the examination. For example, in the region of the femoral triangle, the common femoral vein is located medial to the femoral artery. During real-time imaging the pulsatile quality of arteries may also be apparent, although it is sometimes transmitted to adjacent venous structures.

Various maneuvers may help to identify normal veins. Compressibility upon gentle application of external pressure is typical of normal veins, in contrast to arteries. Gentle compression transiently obliterates the normal venous lumen. With release of pressure, the vessel will immediately return to a normal caliber. The only exception to this finding is in a short segment of the superficial femoral vein which courses through the adductor (Hunter's) canal (6). This lumen is not normally obliterated upon application of pressure with the transducer.

The Valsalva maneuver may also be used to interrogate the iliofemoral veins (7–9, 11). In the supine patient, the Valsalva maneuver increases intrathoracic pressure and peripheral venous pressure, resulting in decreased venous blood return to the heart. This distends the extrathoracic veins, including the iliac and common femoral veins, which normally increase in diameter with the Valsalva maneuver. The

Fig. 7.2. Sonographic examination of the common femoral vein.

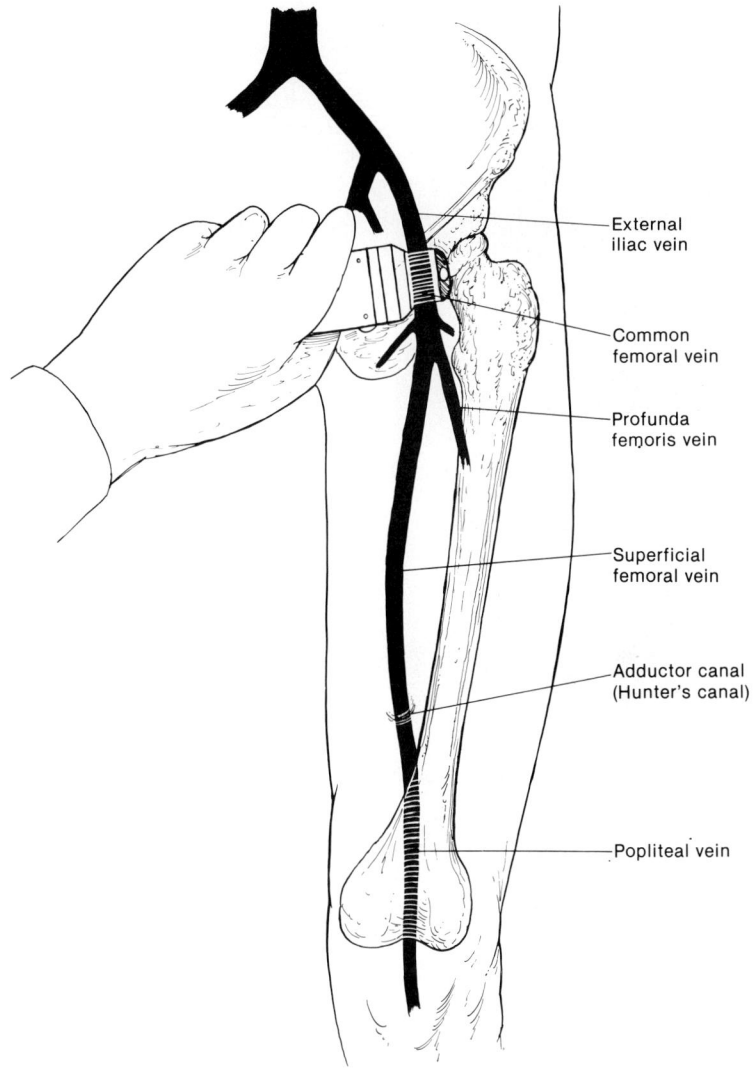

increase in diameter of the common femoral vein has been variably reported between 50 to 200% in one study (11) and 10 to 230% in another series (8). On cessation of this respiratory maneuver, the vessel initially collapses and then promptly resumes a normal caliber with normal breathing. More distally in the lower extremity, this maneuver is not helpful.

Finally, a facile and reliable means to distinguish arterial and venous structures is through the use of Doppler analysis. By placing the sample volume centrally within the vascular lumen, a normal vein will show continuous low-velocity flow. This venous waveform has a significantly different configuration than a lower extremity artery, which has a pulsatile quality, with a sharp systolic peak and little or no antegrade flow in diastole. Doppler analysis may be used not only to distinguish arteries and veins, but also to assess vascular patency.

Technique of Lower Extremity Venous Sonography

Sonographic examination of the lower extremity veins is generally performed using either a 5-, 7.5-, or 10-MHz transducer. Images of these veins are obtained in both transverse and longitudinal orientations. To confirm vascular patency, gentle compression is transiently applied along the vessel at intervals of approx-

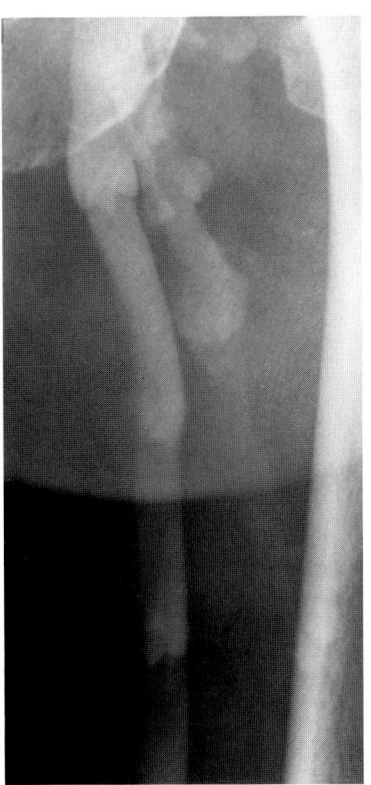

Fig. 7.3A–C. Normal venogram and duplex ultrasound examination of the deep venous system in the proximal thigh. **A**. Normal venogram of a segment of the superficial femoral vein and profunda femoris vein. **B**. Normal sagittal duplex sonogram of the deep venous system in the proximal thigh. **C**. Doppler sampling reveals a normal venous flow pattern.

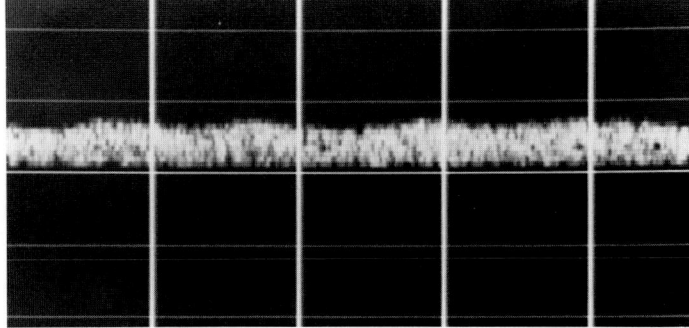

Fig. 7.4. Sonographic examination of the popliteal vein.

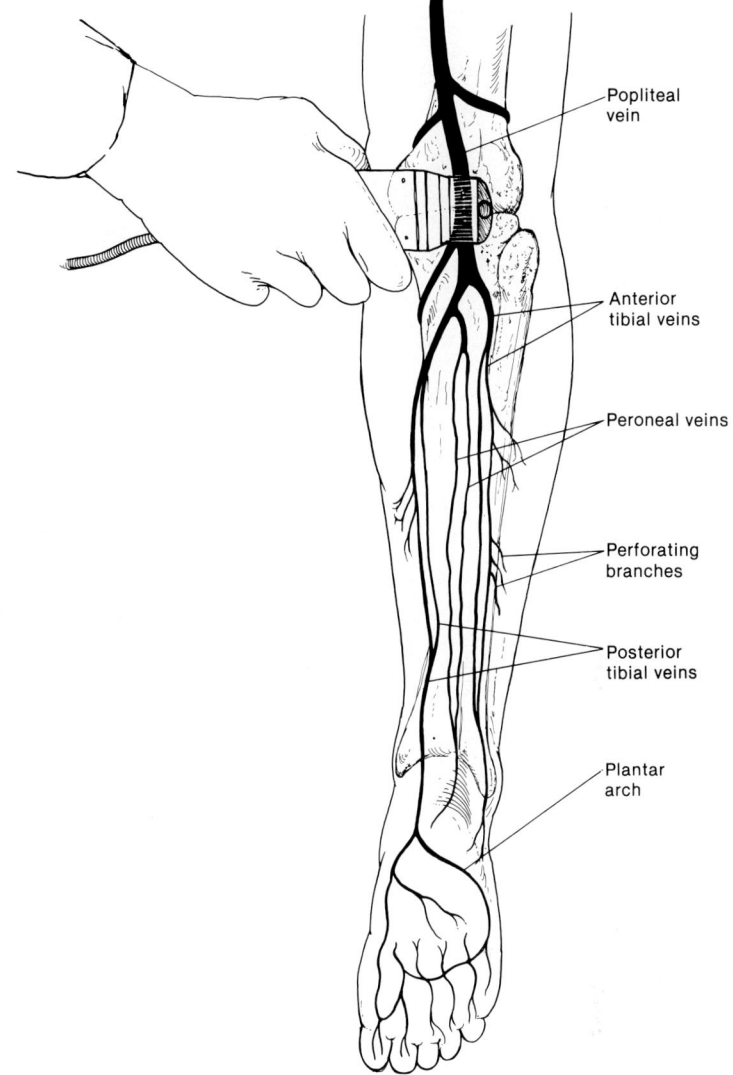

imately one inch or so. When applying compression to a longitudinally oriented vessel, the transducer must be maintained directly over the vessel. This is to avoid a false impression of compressibility which may result from the transducer becoming displaced off center. As a consequence, some sonographers only apply compression with the vessel oriented in the transaxial plane. The Valsalva maneuver also is used to assess venous patency. This is accomplished by demonstrating normal venous distension in the iliofemoral region. Doppler analysis, if available, may be used as a substitute or in conjunction with these maneuvers. This technique enables immediate differentiation between arteries and veins and documents vascular patency or occlusion.

Venous structures that are sonographically examined include the common femoral vein, the superficial femoral vein (in the proximal and midthigh), the popliteal vein, and whenever possible the upper trunks of the calf veins. With the patient in a supine position, the ultrasound study is typically begun by interrogation of the venous structures in the femoral triangle (Fig. 7.2). In this region, the common femoral vein courses medial to the femoral artery. Moving the probe into the proximal thigh, the common femoral vein is followed into the superficial femoral vein (Fig. 7.3). This vessel

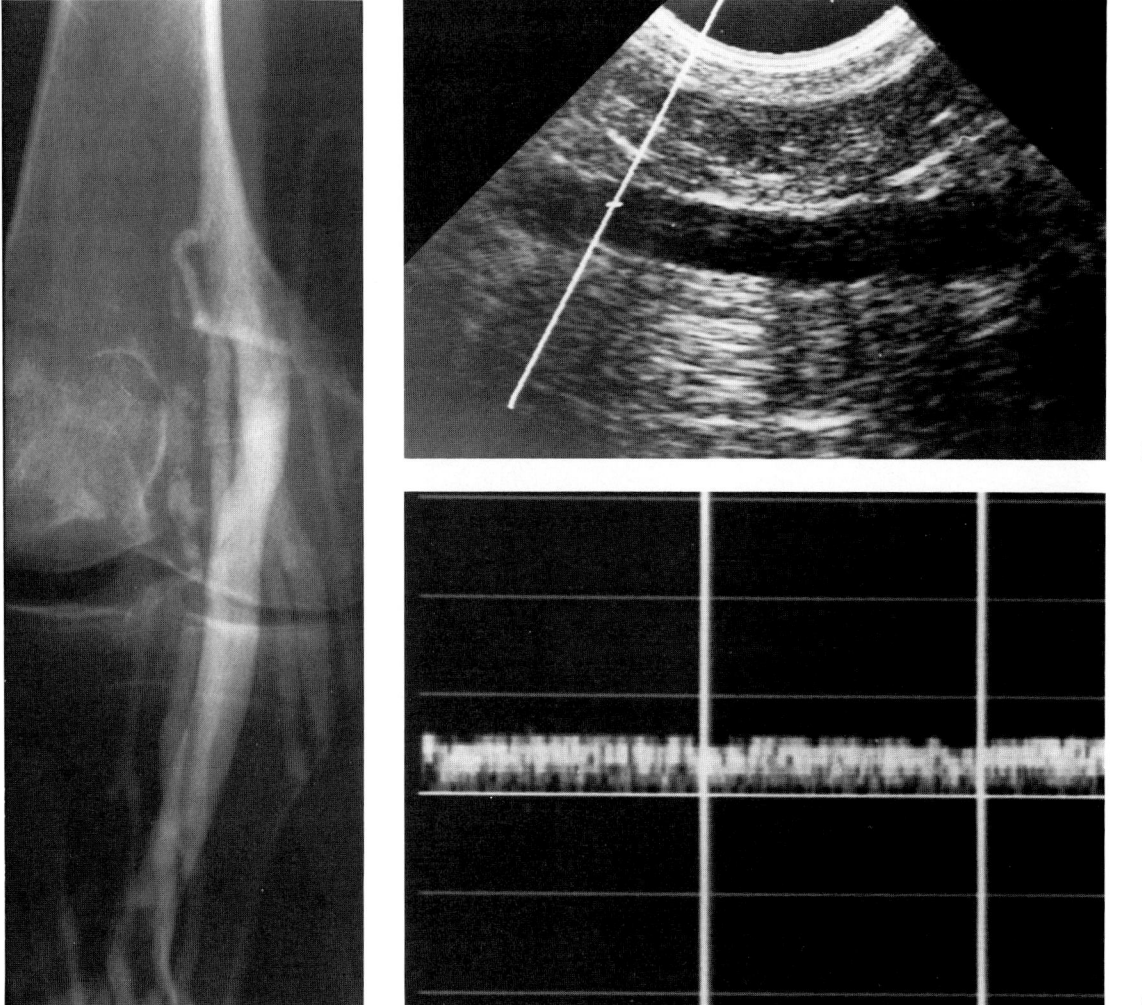

Fig. 7.5A–C. Normal venogram and duplex ultrasound of the deep venous system in the popliteal fossa. **A.** Normal venogram in the region of the popliteal fossa. **B.** Longitudinal duplex ultrasound showing low-level internal echoes within the popliteal vein, which result from artifact. **C.** Doppler analysis confirms a normal, patent vascular lumen.

is located anteriorly and medially within the thigh. At the level of the midthigh, the superficial femoral vein is oriented posteromedial with respect to the femoral artery. In the distal thigh, this vessel cannot usually be followed sonographically as it courses posterior to the femur.

The study is then continued by examining the popliteal vein posterior to the knee (Fig. 7.4). This is most easily accomplished by repositioning the patient prone or in a lateral decubitus orientation (Fig. 7.5). If the patient is immobile the popliteal area can be studied with the patient in a supine position, maintaining the hip and knee flexed. However, this is technically more difficult to perform than in the other positions. Anatomically, the popliteal vein is located posterior and medial to the popliteal artery at the knee. The popliteal vein takes origin in the upper calf from the confluence of three venous structures: the anterior tibial, posterior tibial, and peroneal veins. Occasionally, the upper and mid-portions of the calf veins may be sonographically visualized with sufficient clarity for diagnostic assessment. However, this often requires considerable technical expertise and patience.

Fig. 7.6. Intraluminal thrombus: longitudinal scan of a lower extremity vein. Thrombus extends along the vascular lumen (*arrows*), appearing as a discontinuous soft tissue mass.

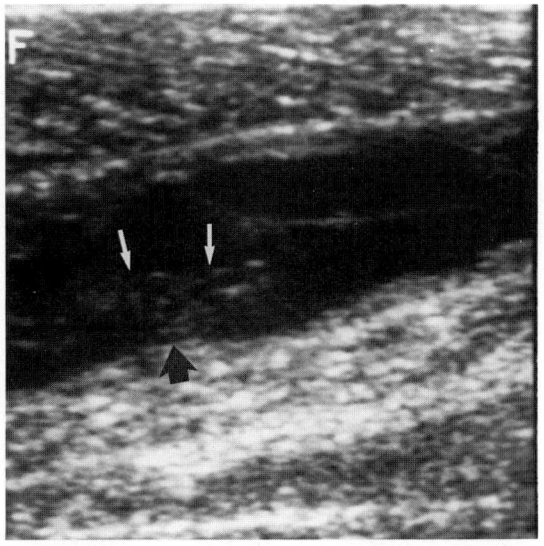

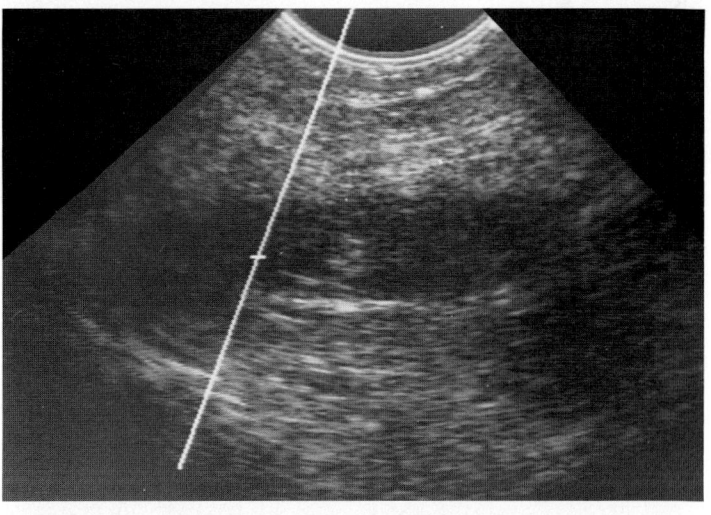

Fig. 7.7A,B. Intraluminal thrombus. **A.** The vascular lumen is filled with medium-level echogenic material on this longitudinal scan. **B.** Doppler sampling verifies the absence of detectable flow in this occluded vessel.

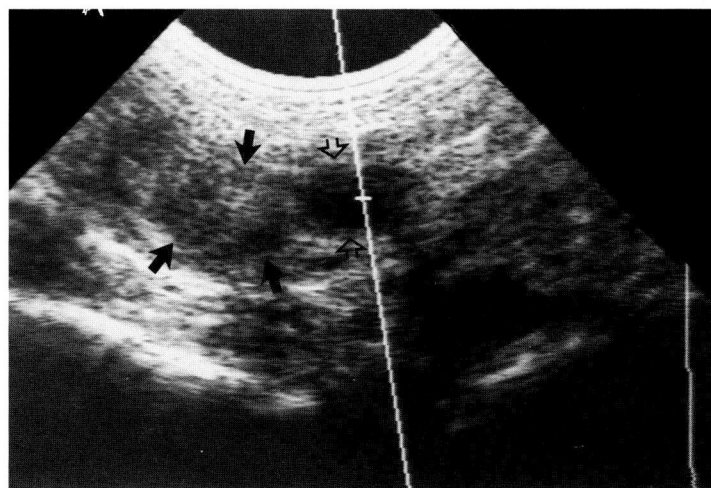

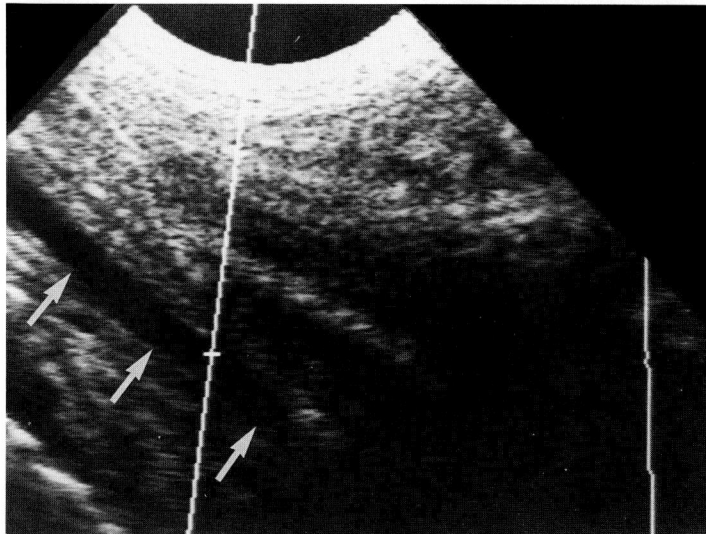

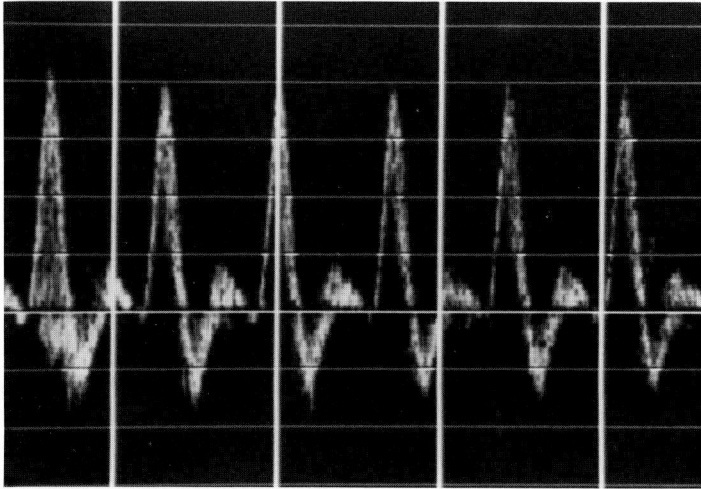

Fig. 7.8A–F. Intraluminal thrombus. **A.** Transverse image of the left inguinal region demonstrates the more medially located femoral vein (*solid arrows*) and the laterally situated femoral artery (*open arrows*). The cursor is positioned in the femoral artery. The gain settings have been standardized so that the femoral artery appears anechoic. Note medium-amplitude echoes filling the femoral vein lumen. **B.** Longitudinal scan of the femoral artery (*arrows*) in the inguinal region. **C.** Normal Doppler waveform in the femoral artery. **D.** Transverse sonogram of the left inguinal region, with the Doppler sample volume repositioned in the femoral vein (*solid arrows*). The femoral artery (*open arrows*) has again been standardized to appear relatively echo-free. **E.** Longitudinal scan of the femoral vein (*arrows*) in the inguinal region, containing medium-level echoes. **F.** No Doppler flow is detected on sampling of the femoral vein, confirming obstruction by thrombus.

7. Sonography of the Lower Extremity Venous System

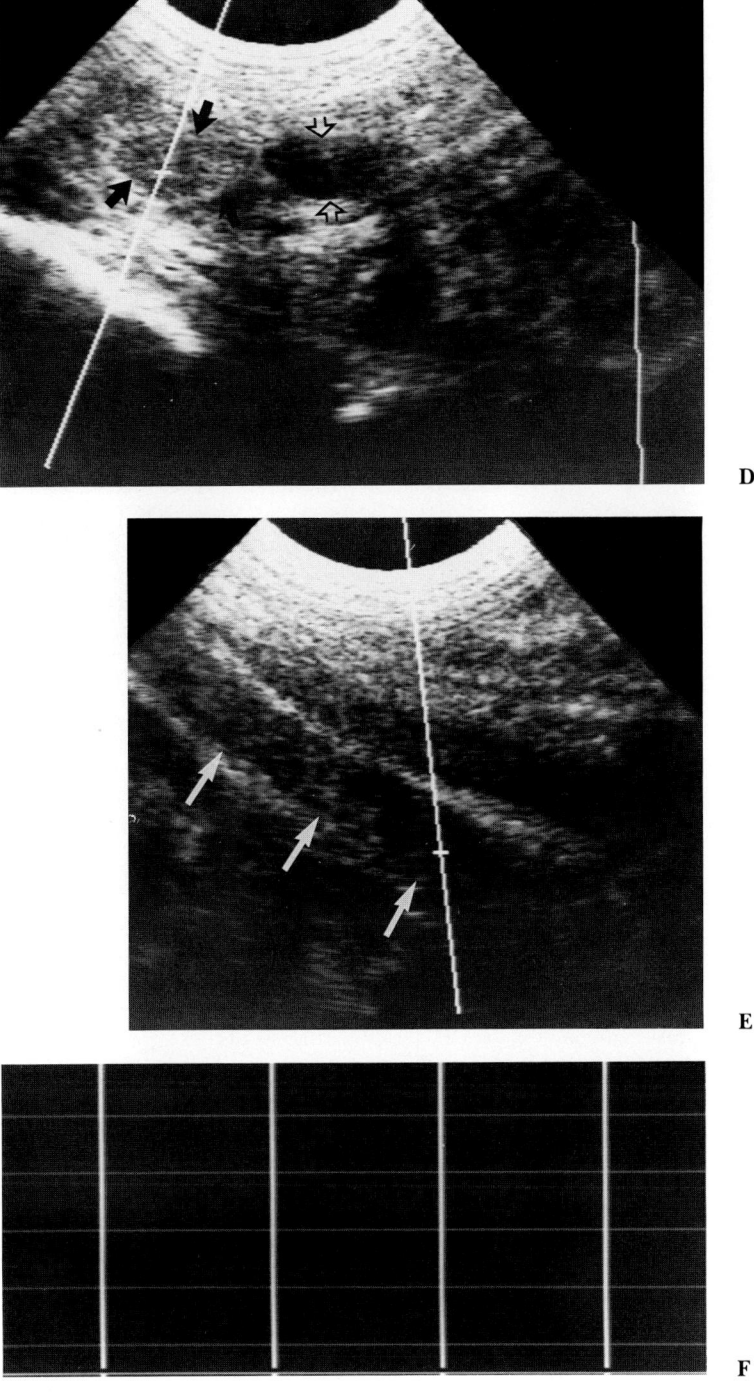

Fig. 7.8.

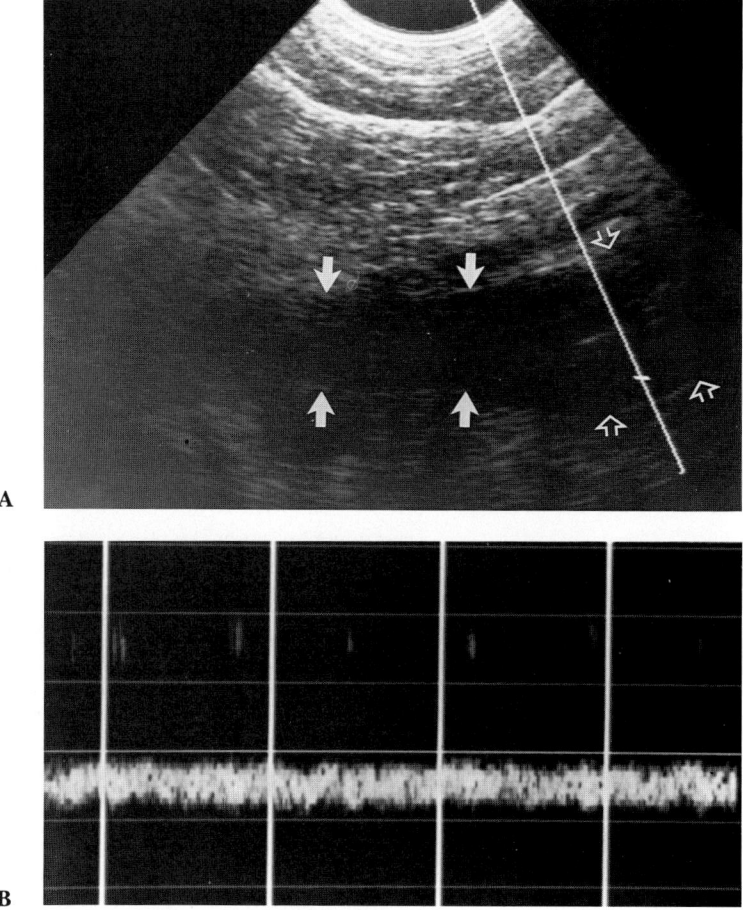

Fig. 7.9A–E. Calf vein thrombus. **A.** Longitudinal sonogram in the popliteal region and proximal calf. The lower portion of the popliteal vein (*solid arrows*) and two large branches in the proximal calf (*open arrows*) appear echo-free. **B.** Doppler analysis of these vessels shows normal flow. **C.** Following these vessels more inferiorly into the calf, echogenic material is present within some venous lumens (*arrows*) on this longitudinal scan. **D.** No flow is detected within the calf vein shown in **C**. **E.** Venogram in this patient confirms that thrombus is limited to the calf veins.

Lower Extremity Deep Venous Thrombosis

Deep venous thrombosis (DVT) of the lower extremities and pelvis is a common and serious medical problem. This is the primary source of pulmonary emboli, which represents a leading cause of morbidity and mortality, particularly among hospitalized patients. Fatal pulmonary embolism is estimated to account for approximately 100,000 to 200,000 deaths annually in the United States (12,13). The vast majority of venous thrombi are clinically silent. The difficulty in clinical diagnosis of deep venous thrombosis is underscored by the fact that approximately two-thirds of lower extremity thrombi occur in asymptomatic patients (12). When present, clinical findings that suggest deep venous thrombosis include unilateral lower extremity edema, pain on palpation over the affected veins, and a positive Homan's sign (upper calf pain on forced dorsiflexion of the foot).

Six primary sites of formation of lower extremity venous thrombi include the iliac vein, the common femoral vein, the profunda femoris (deep femoral) vein, the popliteal vein, the posterior tibial veins, and the intramuscular veins of the calf, particularly the soleal sinuses

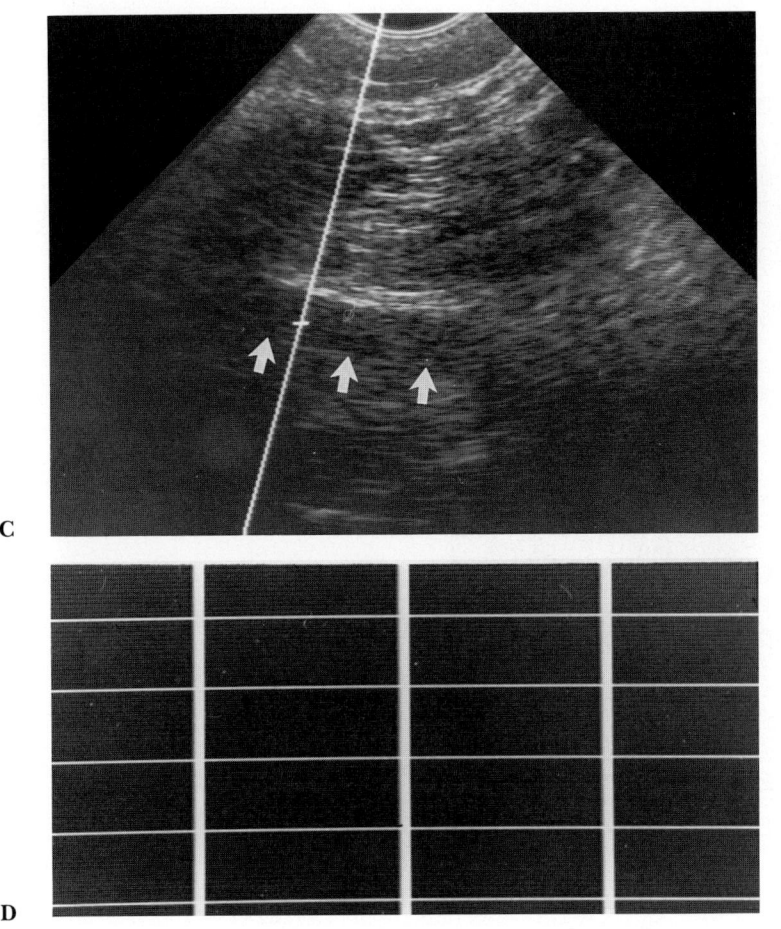
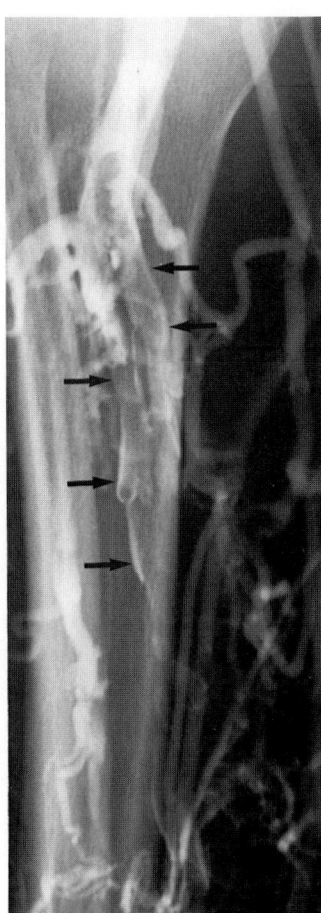

Fig. 7.9.

(14). Deep venous thrombi are often multiple and discontinuous. The earliest thrombi tend to appear below the knee. When localized to the calf, thrombi are usually self-limited, without significant risk of embolic sequela in most instances (15,16). Thrombi in the deep venous system above the knee, however, carry a more serious risk of significant pulmonary embolism. This probably relates to their tendency to be larger and more extensive than calf thrombi. It is known that thrombi may progressively propagate from small calf veins into the larger popliteal and femoral veins.

Ultrasound Findings in Deep Venous Thrombosis

Several published reports have described the application of ultrasound for assessment of deep venous thrombosis (5–8). Using real-time imaging, sonographic criteria have been established to allow this diagnosis. Ultrasound demonstration of flowing blood within the lumen documents patency in the vascular segment. Visualization of a discrete soft tissue mass within the venous lumen assumes the diagnosis of deep venous thrombosis (Fig. 7.6). Thrombi may show variable degrees of echogenicity, but they most often demonstrate a medium amplitude echotexture (Fig. 7.7). Potential pitfalls exist in using this finding alone. For instance, echoes may be artifactually introduced into a vascular lumen by the gain settings used. This is particularly difficult in patients who are extremely muscular, obese, or have marked lower extremity edema. This artifact may be minimized by standardizing the time gain compensation curve so that the adjacent artery is

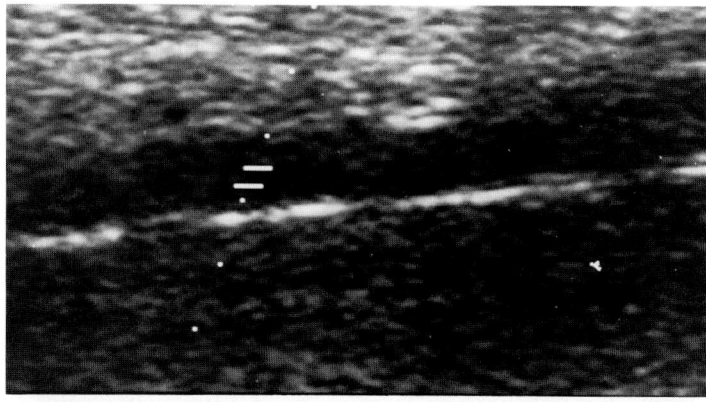
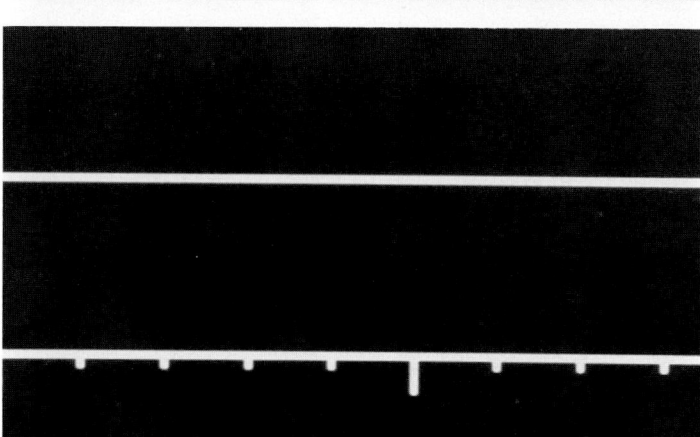

Fig. 7.10A,B. Occlusion of venous limb of dialysis access graft. **A.** Longitudinal sonogram of the venous limb of the graft. Low-level echoes are seen within the lumen. **B.** Doppler sampling through the lumen reveals no detectable flow.

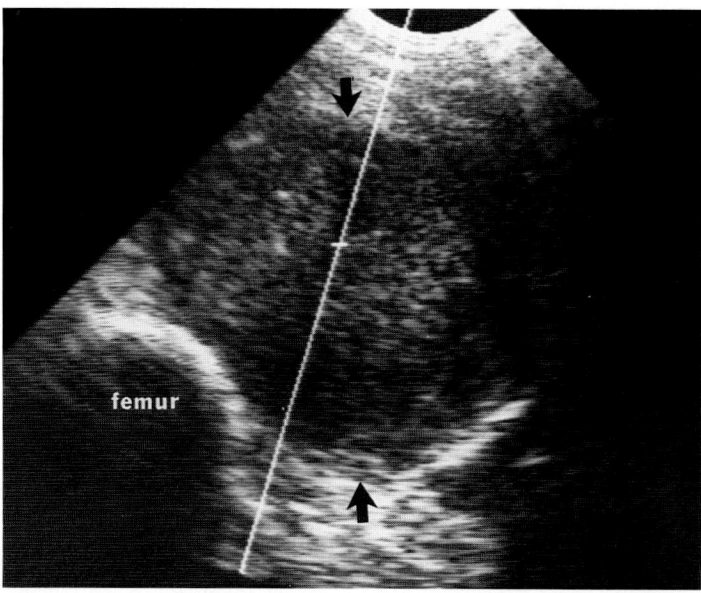

Fig. 7.11A–D. Soft tissue sarcoma adjacent to the distal femur. **A.** Transverse image demonstrating the large neoplastic mass (*arrows*) adjacent to the femur. **B.** Doppler analysis through the mass reveals scattered areas of venous flow. **C.** Longitudinal image of the superficial femoral and popliteal veins (*white arrows*), which are displaced by the tumor (*black arrows*). **D.** Patency of these major veins is documented by Doppler examination.

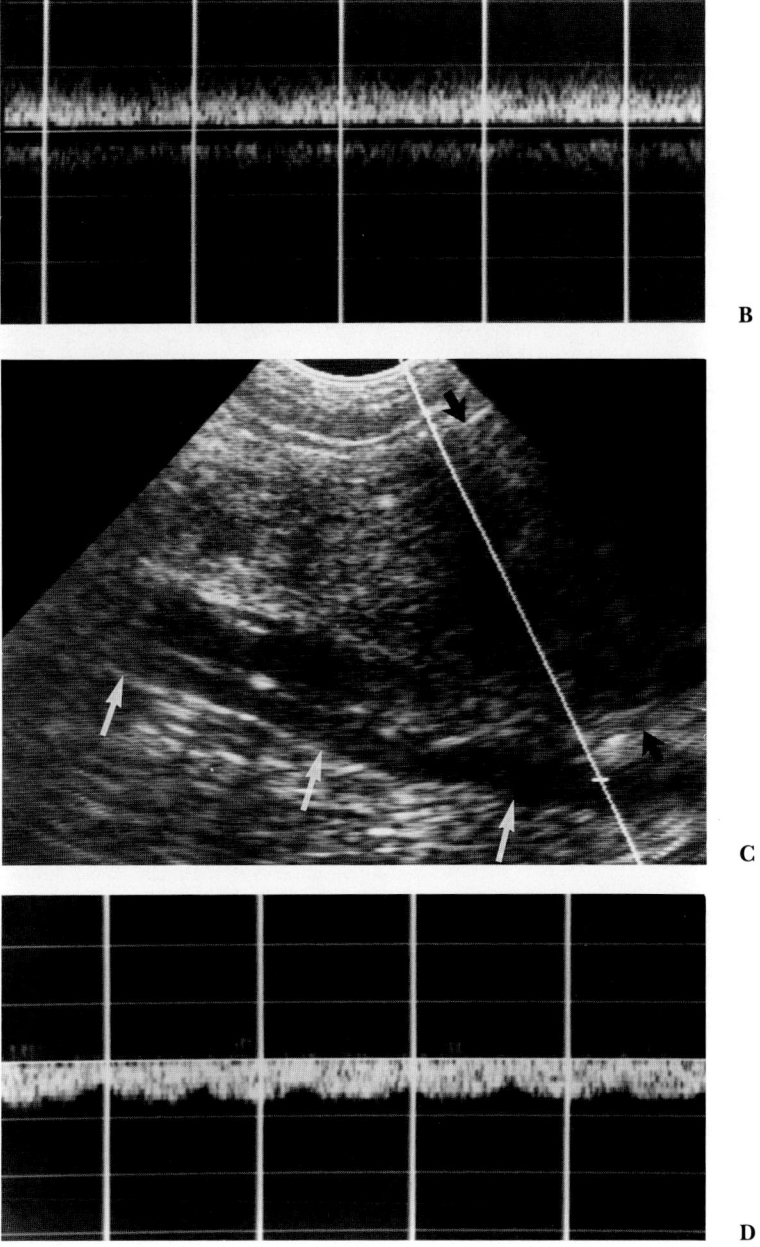

Fig. 7.11.

echo free (Fig. 7.8). The finding of low-level intraluminal echoes also may result from slowly flowing blood, which mimicks thrombus. Various maneuvers previously described or Doppler sampling will allow for this distinction. Conversely, the absence of echogenic material within a vascular lumen does not exclude the presence of clot. This is because fresh clot may appear virtually anechoic and therefore may not be recognized within the vascular lumen by real-time imaging alone.

As a consequence of ambiguities that may arise from visual inspection alone, various maneuvers such as vascular compression have become an extremely important part of the ultrasound diagnosis of deep venous thrombosis. Whether acute or remote venous thrombus is present, the diseased vessels will be noncompressible, whereas a normal venous lumen is easily obliterated with gentle application of external pressure. The only exception to this occurs in the adductor canal, a site where the

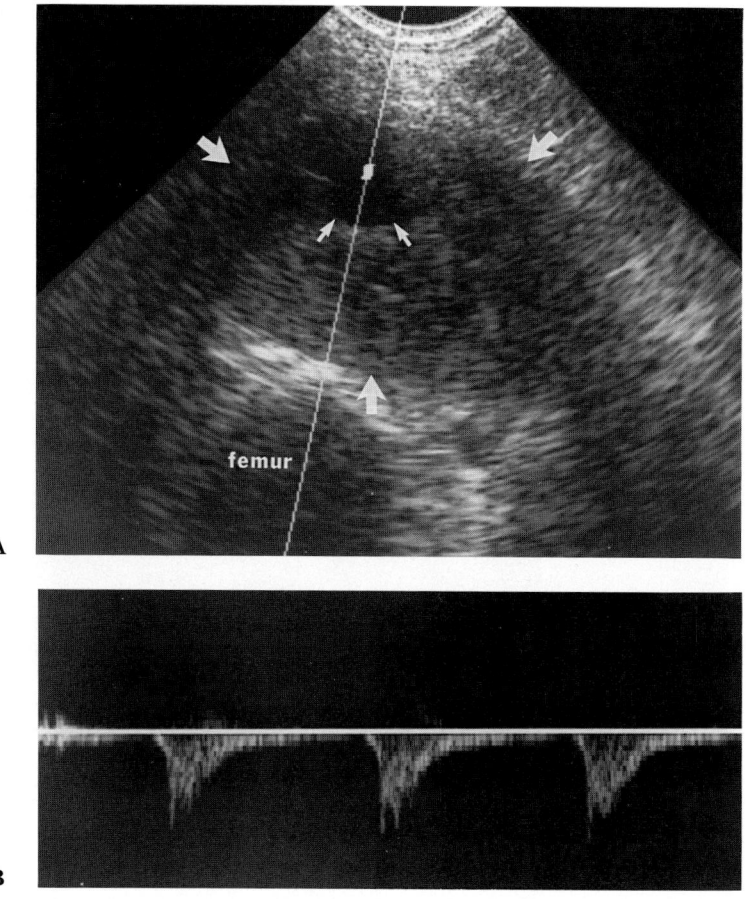

Fig. 7.12A–E. Hemangiosarcoma of the distal left thigh. **A.** Longitudinal sonogram shows a sizable mass (*large arrows*) in the distal thigh. This mass contains several anechoic cavities (*small arrows*). **B.** Doppler sampling of these anechoic areas reveals arterial flow. **C.** Contrast-enhanced computed tomographic (CT) scan in the distal thigh shows marked peripheral (*arrows*) and central hypervascularity. The irregular areas of central enhancement correspond to the sonographically anechoic regions which demonstrated arterial flow on Doppler examination. **D.** Magnetic resonance (MR) scan of the left thigh mass (*arrows*) shows signal void in the hypervascular areas on contrast enhanced CT examination. **E.** Arteriogram in the lateral projection shows the abnormal vascularity around the tumor as well as centrally within it (*arrows*).

normal superficial femoral vein is noncompressible. Because of the additional diagnostic information that compression provides, it should be used as an integral part of lower extremity venous sonography. Four published reports that independently evaluated sonographic diagnosis of deep venous thrombosis each emphasized the importance of compressibility in identifying thrombus (6–9). These clinical investigations documented sensitivities between 89 to 100% and specificities between 97 to 100% in the diagnosis of deep venous thrombosis using compression (6–9).

The Valsalva maneuver also has been used to evaluate the iliofemoral venous system, although variable results have been found (6,8,9,11). One publication describes a normal increase in the common femoral venous diameter of approximately 50 to 200%, and an abnormal dampened response ranging between a 10 to 50% diameter increase. However, in more recent literature, it has been stated that the normal diameter increases in the common femoral vein vary between 10 to 230%, with a mean increase of 52% (8). This wide range of response among individuals without

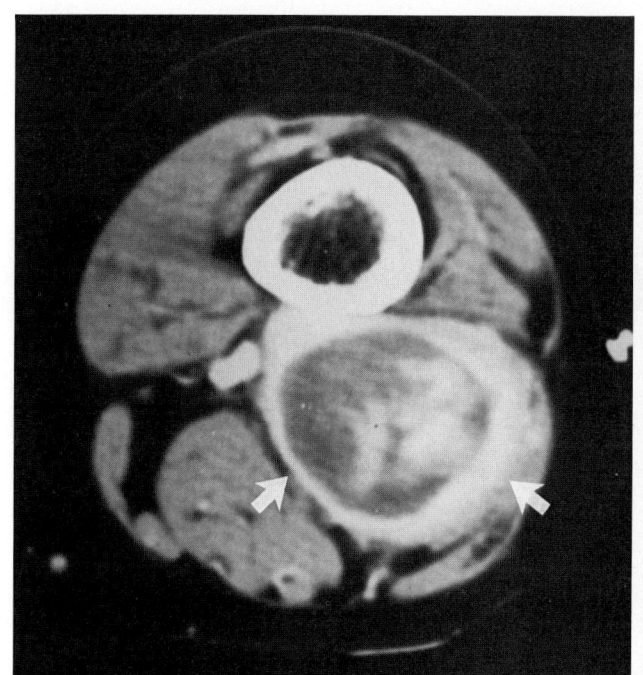
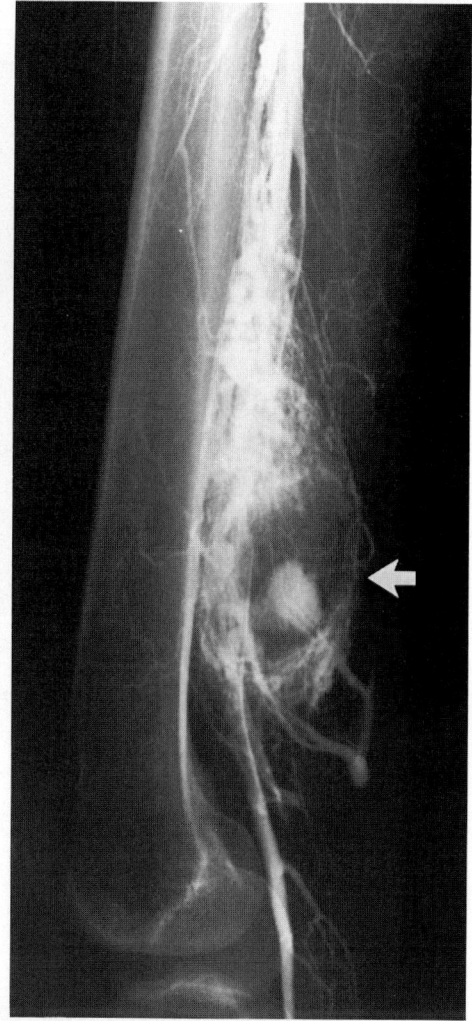
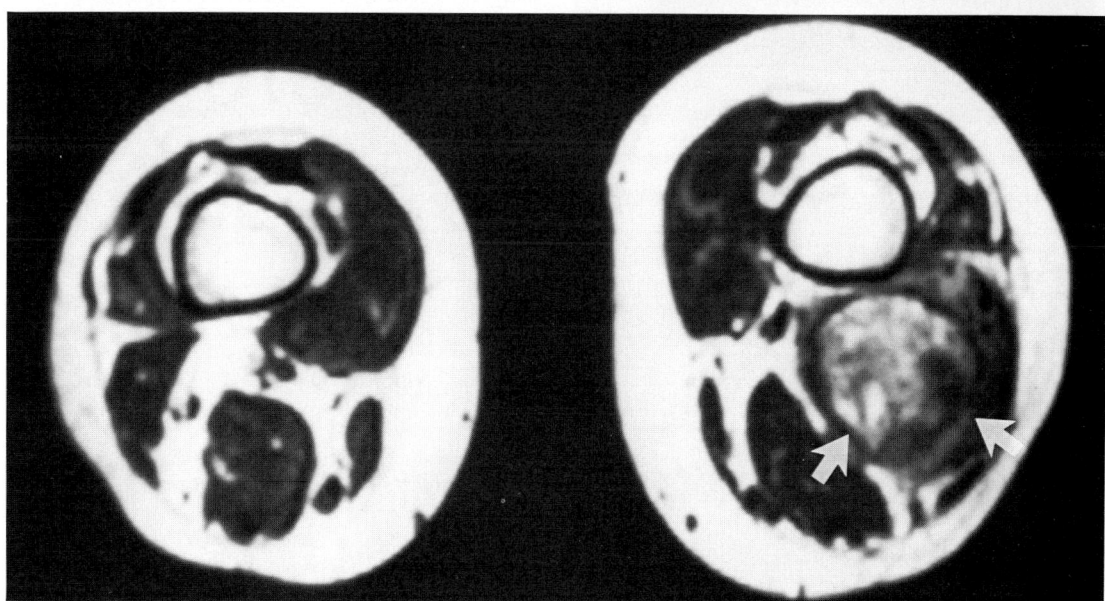

Fig. 7.12.

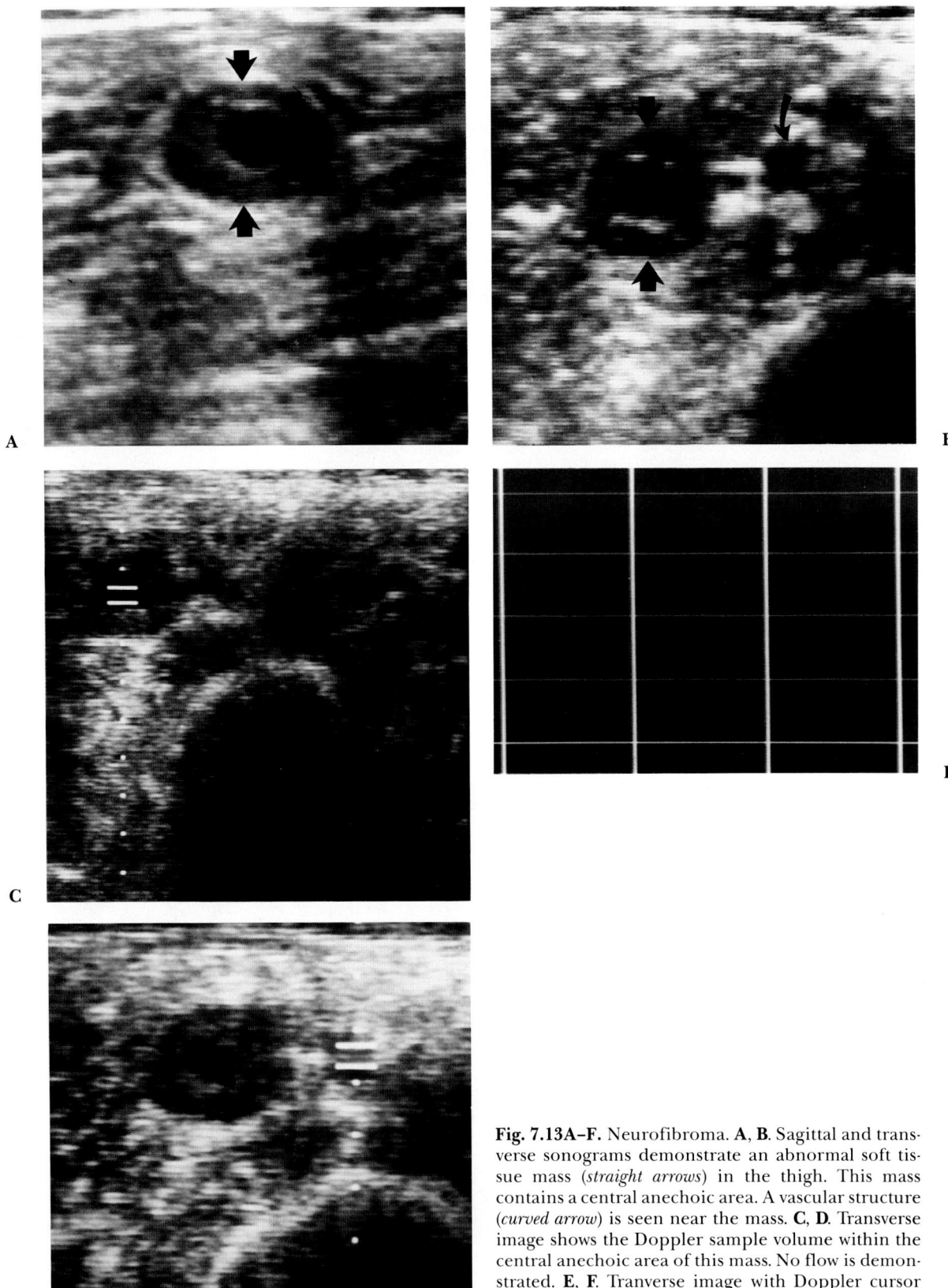

Fig. 7.13A–F. Neurofibroma. **A, B.** Sagittal and transverse sonograms demonstrate an abnormal soft tissue mass (*straight arrows*) in the thigh. This mass contains a central anechoic area. A vascular structure (*curved arrow*) is seen near the mass. **C, D.** Transverse image shows the Doppler sample volume within the central anechoic area of this mass. No flow is demonstrated. **E, F.** Tranverse image with Doppler cursor repositioned in an adjacent vessel, which proves to be a vein.

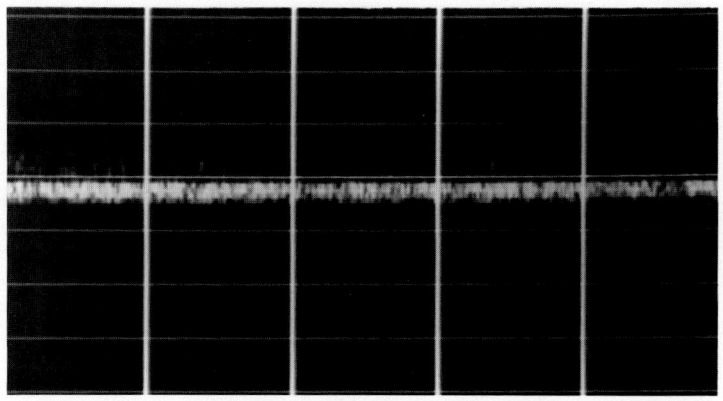

Fig. 7.13.

deep venous thrombosis likely results in part from differences in effort during the Valsalva maneuver, which some patients are unable to perform adequately. Furthermore, overlapping responses in patients with and without disease appear to preclude use of the Valsalva maneuver as an indicator of thrombosis distal to the common femoral vein (6,9). However, when little (less than 10% diameter increase) or no response to Valsalva maneuver is demonstrated, this correlates well with the presence of thrombus at or above the level of the common femoral vein. The sensitivity and specificity of this finding for common femoral vein thrombosis have been reported as 93 and 100%, respectively (8). Again, this criteria does not apply to deep venous thrombosis distal to the common femoral vein.

Until recently, most work in sonographic evaluation of the deep venous system has concentrated on findings and maneuvers during real-time imaging. Duplex examination has been included in one recent report that describes abnormal flow patterns in the common femoral and iliac veins with deep venous thrombosis (9). The sensitivity of this finding was 100%. However, these investigators were limited in assessing other lower extremity veins, because their equipment was reportedly insufficient for deep pulsed-Doppler analysis. With increasing availability of duplex scanners, Doppler analysis will likely assume an important adjunctive role in ultrasound examination of the lower extremity venous system. In our laboratory, it has proven extremely useful for confirmation of either patency or occlusion of the distal external iliac veins, common and superficial femoral veins, popliteal veins, and on occasion, the trifurcating trunks of the major calf veins (anterior tibial, posterior tibial, and peroneal veins). Documentation of absent flow within a vein is usually sufficient to preclude performance of other maneuvers. On one recent patient examination, duplex sonography allowed for diagnosis of isolated thrombus within calf veins near the trifurcation (Fig. 7.9). It is expected that greater availability and familiarity with duplex sonography will allow this technique to become a routine part of lower extremity venous ultrasound examinations, particularly in evaluation of difficult areas such as the calf.

Duplex Sonography of Other Diseases Affecting the Lower Extremity Venous System

There are several other clinical scenarios in which Doppler analysis may provide useful diagnostic information with regard to the lower extremity venous system. These include evaluation of arteriovenous graft patency among dialysis patients, diagnosis of arteriovenous malformations, and assessment of tumor vascularity. Furthermore, the affect on the venous system from adjacent masses such as hematomas and Baker's cysts may be evaluated.

When clinical suspicion of dialysis graft occlusion arises, duplex sonography is

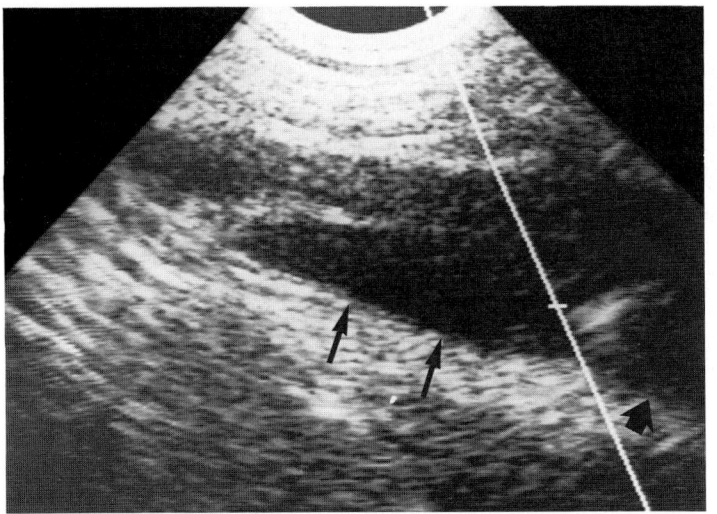

Fig. 7.14A–E. Metastatic implant compromising venous lumen. **A.** Longitudinal scan in the proximal thigh reveals a soft tissue mass (*short arrow*) within the lumen of the superficial femoral vein (*long arrows*). **B.** Doppler analysis around the mass confirms intraluminal venous flow. **C.** The cursor is repositioned within the intraluminal soft tissue mass (*short arrow*). The patent proximal venous lumen is indicated by the long arrows. **D.** No flow is present within this mass. **E.** Venography demonstrates an abnormal soft tissue mass narrowing the venous lumen (*arrow*). This was subsequently confirmed to result from adjacent neoplastic lymphadenopathy.

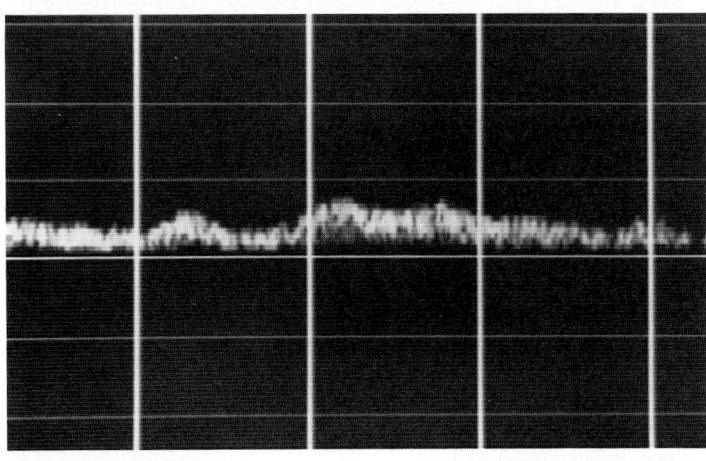

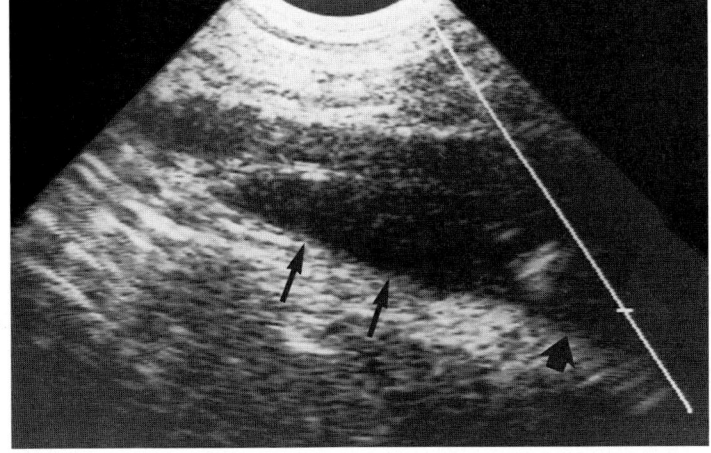

D

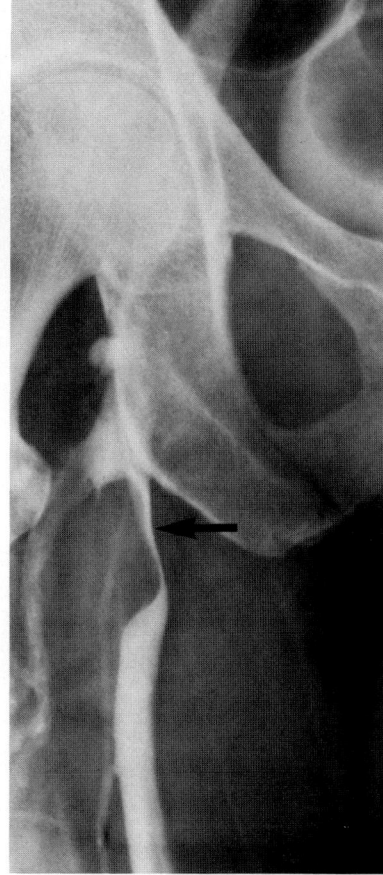

E

Fig. 7.14.

extremely helpful as a noninvasive means to assess vascular patency. Both arterial and venous limbs of the graft may be examined by Doppler analysis (Fig. 7.10). Congenital or acquired arteriovenous malformations also may be suspected or diagnosed by duplex ultrasound. This is accomplished by demonstrating markedly turbulent, distorted flow within a mass of convoluted, tubular channels. On occasion, this appearance may be difficult to distinguish from vascular masses of neoplastic origin. In the latter instance, however, more solid soft tissue is usually present, unless the vascular malformation has undergone a large bleed. Within tumors, arterial or venous waveforms may be detected (Figs. 7.11, 7.12), or no flow may be observed on Doppler sampling (Fig. 7.13). Duplex sonography also may be used to assess for neoplastic invasion or thrombosis of the venous structures adjacent to a tumor (Fig. 7.14).

Ultrasound has been extremely helpful in the evaluation of other masses that may occur in the lower extremities, such as hematomas and Baker's cysts. These nonvascular masses are important to recognize, as they may produce clinical symptoms that resemble deep venous thrombosis. No blood flow will be demonstrated in these masses. The displaced venous structures may be confirmed to be patent. However, when the mass is large, patent deep venous structures may be sufficiently compressed to preclude either visualization or detection of Doppler signal (Fig. 7.15).

Conclusion

Ultrasound has shown several advantages over standard lower extremity phlebography. It represents a noninvasive test without known complication, which may serve for screening and for follow-up studies of the lower extremity venous system. It is relatively inexpensive and may be performed portably. Recent reports indicate promising results in the songraphic evaluation of deep venous thrombosis. It deserves emphasis, however, that the reliability of this examination is extremely operator dependent, with several potential pitfalls if not properly performed. Nonetheless, several studies recommend sonography as the initial examination of choice for evaluation of possible deep venous thrombosis. Furthermore, ultrasound may demonstrate other pathologic

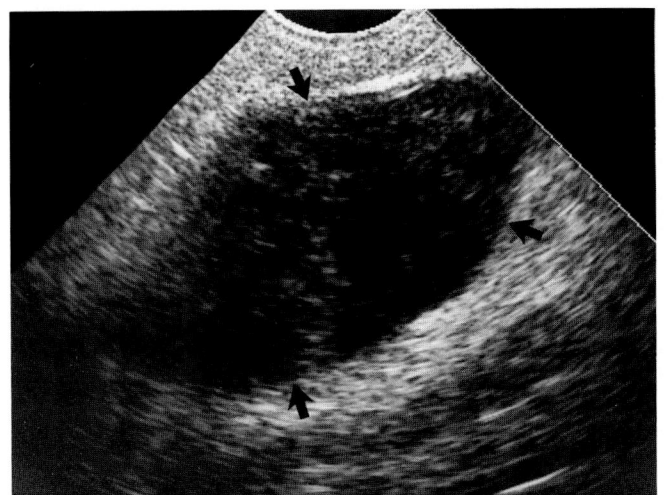

Fig. 7.15A–D. Hematoma extrinsically compressing the patent venous lumen. **A.** Longitudinal sonogram shows a large hypoechoic mass in the distal thigh and proximal calf resulting from a hematoma (*arrows*). **B.** Sonographic identification of the compressed veins was extremely difficult. **C.** Doppler sampling failed to detect the slow flow in these compressed but patent veins. **D.** Venogram demonstrates marked extrinsic compression of the popliteal vein (*arrows*).

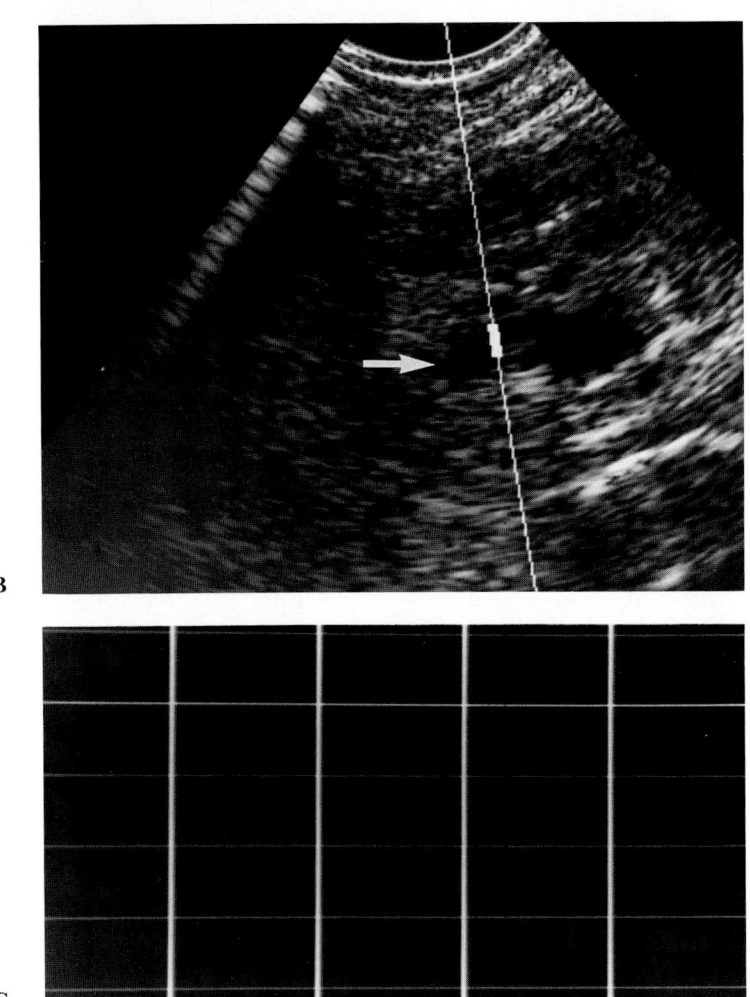

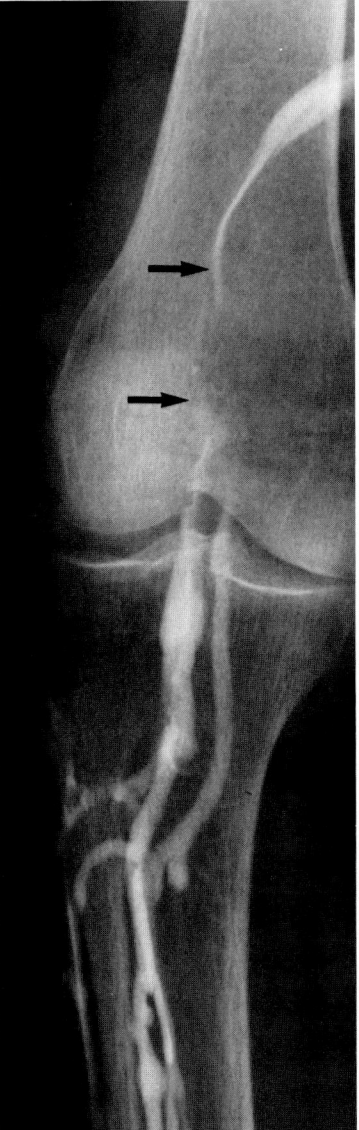

processes that share clinical similarities to deep venous thrombosis, such as hematomas and Baker's cysts. The application of Doppler sampling to these examinations has proven extremely useful in assessing the lower extremity venous system. With increasing availability of duplex scanners, Doppler analysis will likely become an integral part of ultrasound examination for deep venous thrombosis and other forms of lower extremity venous pathology.

References

1. Ramchandani P, Soulen RL, Fedullo LM, et al: Deep vein thrombosis: Significant limitations of noninvasive tests. Radiology 156:47, 1985.
2. Hanel KC, Abbott WM, Reidy NC, et al: The role of two noninvasive tests in deep venous thrombosis. Ann Surg 194:725, 1981.
3. Russell JC, Becker DR: The noninvasive venous vascular laboratory. Arch Surg 118:1024, 1983.
4. Sufian S: Noninvasive vascular laboratory diagnosis of deep venous thrombosis. Am Surg 47:254, 1981.
5. Raghavendra BN, Rosen RJ, Lam S, et al: Deep venous thrombosis: Detection by high-resolution real-time ultrasonography. Radiology 152:789, 1984.
6. Raghavendra BN, Horii SC, Hilton S, et al: Deep venous thrombosis: Detection by probe compression of veins. J Ultrasound Med 5:89, 1986.
7. Cronan JJ, Dorfman GS, Scola FH, et al: Deep venous thrombosis: US assessment using vein compression. Radiology 162:191, 1987.
8. Appelman PT, DeJong TE, Lampmann LE: Deep venous thrombosis of the leg: US findings. Radiology 163:743, 1987.
9. Vogel P, Laing FC, Jeffrey RB, et al: Deep venous thrombosis of the lower extremity: US evaluation. Radiology 163:747, 1987.
10. Langsfeld M, Hershey FB, Thorpe L, et al: Duplex B-mode imaging for the diagnosis of deep venous thrombosis. Arch Surg 122:587, 1987.
11. Effeney DJ, Friedman MB, Gooding GAW: Iliofemoral venous thrombosis: Real-time ultrasound diagnosis, normal criteria, and clinical application. Radiology.150:787, 1984.
12. Hirsh J: Thromboembolic disease. Hosp Prac 17:77, 1982.
13. Dalen JE, Alper JS: Natural history of pulmonary embolism. *In* Sasahara A, Sonnenblick EH, Lesch M (eds): Pulmonary Emboli. New York, Grune & Stratton, 1974, pp 77–88.
14. Sevitt S: Pathology and pathogenesis of deep vein thrombi. *In* Bergan JJ, Yoa JST (eds): Venous Problems. Chicago, Year Book Medical Publishers, Inc., 1978, pp 257–279
15. Moser KM, LeMoine JR: Is embolic risk conditioned by location of deep venous thrombosis? Ann Intern Med 94:439, 1981.
16. Kakkar V, Howe C, Hank C, et al: Natural history of postoperative deep vein thrombosis. Lancet 2:230, 1967.

Index

A

A/B ratio, 195
  increased, 202, 203, 204
Abdomen, color-flow imaging in, 187
Abdominal aorta, 132-133, 134
Abdominal aortic aneurysms, 146-147
Abdominal aortic dissection, 144, 148-153
Abdominal aortic pathology, 142-144, 146-147
Abdominal blood flow, diseases affecting, 142-176
Abdominal duplex sonography, 129-188
  in diseases affecting abdominal blood flow, 142-176
Aliased diastolic flow, 100
Aliasing, 4-5, 38
  with pulsed-Doppler, 71, 72
Amaurosis fugax, 7
Anemia, maternal, 206
Aneurysms, 143-144
  abdominal aortic, 146-147
  hepatic artery, 153
  iliac artery, 223
  intrahepatic portohepatic venous, 176
  mycotic, 226, 231
  peripheral, 218, 221-222
  popliteal artery, 224
  splenic artery, 171
Angiography, Doppler, 8
Angioplasty, 221-222
Aortic blood flow, 81
  fetal, 196-197
Aortic coarctation (COA), 120
Aortic insufficiency, 92, 96, 97-99
  mapping degree of, 100-101

Aortic stenosis, 92, 95, 96-97
Aortic valve, flow velocity curves in, 84, 85-86, 89
Aortic valve pathology, 92, 96-99
Aortic valve prostheses, 118
Aortic waveform analysis, fetal, 197
Apical four-chamber view, 83
Apical long-axis view, 82
Arterial bypass graft occlusion, 226-228
Arterial bypass grafts, 224-226
Arterial flow, 4
Arteriography, 8, 9, 34
Arterioportal fistulas, 175-176
Arteriovenous fistulas, 171
Arteriovenous malformations, 257
  congenital, 228, 230, 234-236
ASD (atrial septal defect), 118, 120
Atherosclerosis, 7-9, 211
  in legs, 211-214
Atherosclerotic plaque, see Plaque
ATN (acute tubular necrosis), 183
Atrial myxoma, left, 122, 125-127
Atrial septal defect (ASD), 118, 120
Azygous-hemiazygous veins, 147

B

Baker's cysts, 257, 259
Bernoulli equation, 93
Bifurcation turbulence, 40
Bile duct, 157

Biparietal diameter (PBD) measurements, 202
Blood flow
  abdominal, diseases affecting, 142-176
  aortic, see Aortic blood flow
  in fetoplacental circulation, 194-199
  plaque and, 35
  portal venous, 164-166
  turbulent, 79, 129
  umbilical, 195
  umbilical vein, 197
Blood flow direction indicator, 5
Blood flow profile, 4
Blood flow reversal, 11
Blood flow velocity, 81
Blood flow velocity curves
  in aortic valve, 84, 85-86, 89
  in left ventricle, 84-88
  in pulmonary valve, 88, 90, 91
  in right ventricle, 86, 89
Boundary separation zone, 39-41
Budd-Chiari syndrome, 169, 170

C

Calcific plaque, 28
Calcification, vascular, 180
Calf vein thrombus, 248-249
Cardiac abnormalities, Doppler assessment of, 91-96
Cardiac arrhythmia, fetal, 204
Cardiac catheterization, 69
Cardiac cycle, 4
Cardiac Doppler, 69-127
  technical aspects of, 69-73, 91
Cardiac lesions, 91-96
  miscellaneous, 122-127

Cardiac output, 118, 120
Cardiomyopathy, hypertrophic, 122–125
Carotid arteriography, 8
Carotid artery, 23–24
  common, *see* Common carotid artery
  external, *see* External carotid artery
  internal, *see* Internal carotid artery
Carotid bifurcation, 7
  evaluation of, 211
  normal, 18–20
Carotid bulb, 13, 18
Carotid disease, 7
Carotid examinations, 8
Catastrophic rupture, 147
CCA, *see* Common carotid artery
Celiac artery, 130, 133–134, 136
Cerebrovascular accidents, 7
Cerebrovascular atherosclerosis, 7–9
Cerebrovascular duplex sonography, 7–66
  criteria for stenosis, 37
  Doppler, 32–57
  real-time imaging, 23–32
  technical aspects of, 9–23
  vertebral artery, 57, 59, 61–66
Chorionic villi, 193
CI (congestion index), 166
Coarctation of aorta (COA), 120
Color flow mapping, 73–74, 77–79, 91
  in abdomen, 187
Common carotid artery (CCA), 10
  moderate narrowing of, 16–18
  normal, 15
  -subclavian junction, 12–13
  -subclavian stenosis, 14
  total occlusion of, 57, 60–61
  velocity compared to ICA velocity, 57
Common femoral artery, 211–214
  stenosis, 217, 221–222
Common femoral vein, 212–214, 239–241
Congestion index (CI), 166
Continuous-wave Doppler (CW), 5, 73, 76, 91
Coronary artery disease, 7
CW (continuous-wave Doppler), 5, 73, 76, 91

D
Deep venous thrombosis (DVT) of lower extremities, 248–255
Diastole, 4
Diastolic descent, 11
Diastolic flow, aliased, 100
Dicrotic notch, 11
Diphasic wave, low-resistance, 11, 12
Direct examinations, 8
Doppler
  cardiac, *see* Cardiac Doppler
  cerebrovascular, 32–57
  in complicated pregnancy, 199, 201–206
  continuous wave, 5, 73, 76, 91
  periorbital, 8
Doppler angiography, 8
Doppler angle, 1, 2
Doppler assessment of cardiac abnormalities, 91–96
Doppler beam alignment, 80
Doppler display, 78–81
Doppler effect, 1–2
Doppler equation, 1
Doppler examination, 81–83
Doppler flow patterns, 83–91
  abnormal, 96–127
Doppler physics, 1–3
Doppler shift, positive and negative, 74
Doppler shift frequency, 1–5
Doppler transducers, *see* Transducers
Doppler ultrasound, pulsed-, 1
  aliasing with, 71, 72
  block diagram for, 2
  in cardiac examination, 69–73, 91
  two-dimensional guided, 71
Duplex sonography, 1
  of abdomen, *see* Abdominal duplex sonography
  abnormalities, 34
  of atherosclerosis in legs, 211–224
  cardiac, *see* Cardiac Doppler
  of cerebrovascular system, *see* Cerebrovascular duplex sonography
  diagnostic success of, 9
  of diseases affecting lower extremity venous system, 255–257
  display, 3
  equipment of, 3–5
  of fetoplacental circulation, 192–194
  of lower extremity venous system, 239–260
  of peripheral arteries, 211–236
  technical considerations of, 1–5
  of uteroplacental circulation, 191–192
DVT (deep venous thrombosis) of lower extremities, 248–255

E
Ebstein's anomaly, 113, 117, 118
ECA, *see* External carotid artery
ECG (echocardiogram), 82–83
Echo arrival time, 3
Echo frequency, 1
Echocardiogram (ECG), 82–83
Echocardiography, two-dimensional, 69
Endarterectomy, 8
External carotid artery (ECA), 10
  differentiation from ICA, 21
  -MCA bypass, 58–59
  stenosis of, 21, 23

F
Femoral artery
  common, *see* Common femoral artery
  superficial, *see* Superficial femoral artery
Femoral vein
  common, 212–214, 239–241
  superficial, 240, 243–244
Femur, sarcoma adjacent to, 250–251
Fetal anomalies, congenital, 204–205
Fetal aortic blood flow, 196–197
Fetal aortic waveform analysis, 197
Fetal cardiac arrhythmia, 204
Fetal cotyledon, 194
Fetal death, intrauterine, 202–203
Fetal growth, 191
Fetoplacental circulation, 192–194
  blood flow in, 194–199
Fetoplacental waveform analysis, 195–199

Index

Fibrofatty plaque, 27, 29
Frequency
 Doppler shift, 1–5
 echo, 1
 generator, 2
 Nyquist limit, 71–73
 pulse repetition (PRF), 5, 70–71, 73
 transmitted pulse, 1

G
Gastric artery, left, 130, 136, 137
Gastroduodenal artery (GDA), 130, 133, 136
Gate lengths, 3
GDA (gastroduodenal artery), 130, 133, 136
Generator frequency, 2
Gray-scale imaging, *see* Imaging, real time pulse-echo gray-scale ultrasound

H
Heart failure, moderate-to-severe right, 166
Hemangiosarcoma of thigh, 252–253
Hematomas, 257, 258
Hemodialysis shunts, 226, 229–230
Hemorrhage
 intraplaque, 28, 32
 maternal, 205
Hepatic artery, 147, 153
 common, 131, 133, 135
 enlarged, 162
 proper, 130, 133
 right, 133, 157
Hepatic artery aneurysms, 153
Hepatic artery pseudo-aneurysms, 153, 157, 159–161
Hepatic circulation, 147
Hepatic vein, 131, 140, 144
Hepatic venous thrombosis, 170
Heterogeneous plaque, 32, 33
High-grade stenosis, 45–47
High-resistance triphasic wave, 11, 12
High-resistance vessels, 10
Hypernephroma, 178
Hypertension, 176
 maternal, 202, 205–206
 pregnancy-induced, 202, 205–206

Hypertrophic subaortic stenosis, idiopathic (IHSS), 122–125
Hypoxia, 201

I
Iatrogenic vascular lesions, 222, 224–234
ICA, *see* Internal carotid artery
Iliac artery, 214
Iliac artery aneurysm, 223
Iliac artery stenosis, 213
Imaging, real time, 23–32
 pulse-echo gray-scale ultrasound, 1
 physics of, 1–3
Indirect examinations, 8
Inferior vena cava (IVC), 131, 132, 140, 144
 anomalies, 144, 147, 154–158
 displacement/compression, 158
 duplication of, 147
 filters, 144
 thrombus, 155–157
 transposition of, 147
Internal carotid artery (ICA), 9
 differentiation from ECA, 21
 moderate stenosis, 42–45
 stenosis, 34
 total occlusion, 47, 49, 50–53, 56–57
 velocity compared to CCA velocity, 57
Intracardiac shunts, 120–122
Intrahepatic arterial branches, 131
Intrahepatic portohepatic venous aneurysm, 176
Intrahepatic shunts, 175
Intraluminal echoes, 154
Intraluminal thrombus, 245–247
Intraplaque hemorrhage, 28, 32
Intrarenal vessels, 143
Intrauterine fetal death, 202–203
Intrauterine growth retardation (IUGR), 201–202
Isoimmunization, rhesus, 205
IUGR (intrauterine growth retardation), 201–202
IVC, *see* Inferior vena cava

J
Jet effect, 157

L
Laminar flow, 79
Legs, atherosclerosis in, 211–224
Linear array transducers, 3
Low-resistance diphasic wave, 11, 12
Low-resistance vascular beds, 10
Lower extremity deep venous system, 239–240
 ultrasound evaluation of, 240–260
Lower extremity deep venous thrombosis, 248–255
Lower extremity phlebography, 239

M
Maternal anemia, 206
Maternal complications, 205–206
Maternal hemorrhage, 205
Maternal hypertension, 202, 205–206
Maternal smoking, 206
Mechanical transducers, 3
Mesenteric circulation, 174–176
Mitral insufficiency, 96, 102, 104–110
Mitral pressure half-time, 93–94
Mitral regurgitation, 104, 108–109
Mitral stenosis, 93, 94, 99, 102–104
Mitral valve, 81
Mitral valve area (MVA), 93, 94
Mitral valve pathology, 99, 102–110
Mitral valve prostheses, 118
Multiple sampling depths, 70, 74–75
Multivalvular disease, 97
MVA (mitral valve area), 93, 94
Mycotic aneurysms, 226, 231
Myxoma, left atrial, 122, 125–127

N
Neoplastic invasion of venous structures, 256, 257
Neurofibroma in thigh, 254–255
Nonrate-limiting lesions, 9
Nyquist frequency limit, 71–73

O
"O" diastolic flow, 11

Occlusion
  arterial bypass graft, 226–228
  portal vein, 157, 162
  superficial femoral artery, 219–220
  total CCA, 57, 60–61
  total ICA, 47, 49, 50–53, 56–57
Oculoplethysmography (OPG), 8
Orientation, transducer, 18, 82

P

Parasternal long-axis view, 82
Parasternal short-axis view, 83
Patent ductus arteriosus (PDA), 120
PBD (biparietal diameter) measurements, 202
PDA (patent ductus arteriosus), 120
Periorbital Doppler, 8
Peripheral arterial aneurysms, 218, 221–222
Peripheral arteries, duplex sonography of, 211–236
Phased array transducers, 3
Phlebography, lower extremity, 239
Physics, Doppler, 1–3
PI, see Pulsatility index
Plaque, 25
  blood flow and, 35
  calcific, 28
  fibrofatty, 27, 29
  heterogeneous, 32, 33
  soft, 25
  ulcerated, 28, 30, 31
Polyhydramnios, 201
Popliteal artery, 214, 216
Popliteal artery aneurysm, 224
Popliteal vein, 240, 243, 244
Porta hepatis, 157
Portal hypertension, 166–168
  splenic vein in, 172
Portal vein, 131, 140, 157
Portal vein occlusion, 157, 162
Portal vein thrombosis, 162–164
Portal venous blood flow, 164–166
Portal venous patency, 163–164
Portal venous system, 162–168
Portocaval shunts, 173, 175
Portohepatic vein shunts, sinusoidal, 176
Portosystemic shunts, 166, 172–176

Pregnancy, complicated
  Doppler in, 199, 201–206
  twin, 203–204
Pregnancy-induced hypertension, 202, 205–206
Pressure gradient, 93
Pressure half-time, 93
PRF (pulse repetition frequency), 5, 70–71, 73
Profunda femoris, 214, 215
Prosthetic valves, 118
  leaking, 119
Pseudoaneurysms, 226, 228, 232–234
  hepatic artery, 153, 157, 159–161
  splenic artery, 170
Pulmonary emboli, 248
Pulmonary valve, flow velocity curves in, 88, 90, 91
Pulmonic insufficiency, 109, 112–113
  trace, 114
Pulmonic stenosis, 104, 109, 111
Pulmonic valve pathology, 104, 109, 111–113
Pulsatility index (PI), 129, 183, 195, 205
  mean resting, 137–138
Pulsations, transmitted, 55
Pulse-echo imaging, see Imaging, real time pulse-echo gray-scale ultrasound
Pulse frequency, transmitted, 1
Pulse repetition frequency (PRF), 5, 70–71, 73
Pulsed-Doppler ultrasound, see Doppler ultrasound, pulsed-

R

Range ambiguity, 5, 71
Range gate, 70
Rate-limiting stenosis, 34
Real time imaging, see Imaging, real time
Red cell velocity, 9–10
Reflector speed, 1, 2
Regurgitant lesion, 92
Regurgitation, 97
Renal allografts, 182–187
Renal arcuate arteries, 132, 138
Renal artery, 132, 138, 140–143
  main right, 138, 141
  in pelvic sinus, 132
Renal artery stenosis, 176–177

Renal circulation, 176–182
Renal hilar vessels, 177, 180
Renal transplant artery stenosis, 183, 185, 186, 187
Renal vein, 132, 138, 140–143
  main, 132, 138, 142
  retroaortic left, 179–182
Resistance index (RI), 195
Rhesus isoimmunization, 205
RI (resistance index), 195

S

Sarcoma adjacent to femur, 250–251
Serpiginous structures, 164, 168
SFA, see Superficial femoral artery
Shift frequency, Doppler, 1–5
SMA (superior mesenteric artery), 130, 136–137, 139, 140
Smoking, maternal, 206
SMV (superior mesenteric venous) thrombosis, 174–175, 176
Soft plaque, 25
Sonic window, 11
Sonography, duplex, see Duplex sonography
Spectral broadening
  artifactual, 36–37, 43
  true, 42–45
Spiral arteries, 191
Splenic artery, 130, 136, 138
Splenic artery aneurysms, 171
Splenic artery pseudoaneurysms, 170
Splenic circulation, 170–172
Splenic vein, 131, 145
  in portal hypertension, 172
Splenic vein thrombus, 172
Splenoportal venous system, 140, 142, 145
Stenosis, 9
  aortic, 92, 95, 96–97
  common femoral artery, 217, 221–222
  criteria for, 37
  ECA, 21, 23
  high-grade, 45–47
  ICA, 34
    moderate, 42–45
  idiopathic hypertrophic subaortic (IHSS), 122–125
  iliac artery, 213
  mitral, 93, 94, 99, 102–104

nonrate-limiting, 9
pulmonic, 104, 109, 111
rate-limiting, 34
renal artery, 176–177
renal transplant artery, 183, 185, 186, 187
subtotal, 45, 47–49
superior mesenteric arterial, 176
tricuspid, 113
vertebral artery, 61, 63, 65
Stroke, 7
"Stump flow," 49, 54–55
Subaortic stenosis, idiopathic hypertrophic (IHSS), 122–125
Subclavian artery, 10
Subclavian steal syndrome, 61, 64–66
Subcostal four-chamber view, 83
Subcostal short-axis view, 83
Subtotal stenosis, 45, 47–49
Superficial femoral artery (SFA), 214, 215
  occlusion, 219–220
Superficial femoral vein, 240, 243–244
Superior mesenteric arterial stenosis, 176
Superior mesenteric artery (SMA), 130, 136–137, 139, 140
Superior mesenteric vein, 131, 140, 142
Superior mesenteric venous (SMV) thrombosis, 174–175, 176
Superior thyroid artery, 21, 22
Suprasternal long-axis view, 82
Systole, 4
Systolic peak, 11
Systolic rise, 11
Systolic velocities, 37
  maximum, 34

T

Thigh
  hemangiosarcoma of, 252–253
  neurofibroma in, 254–255
Thyroid artery, superior, 21, 22
TIAs (transient ischemic attacks), 7

Transducers
  blood flow measurement and, 194–195
  index mark, 82
  orientation of, 18, 82
Transient ischemic attacks (TIAs), 7
Transmitted pulsations, 55
Transmitted pulse frequency, 1
Traumatic vascular lesions, 222, 224–234
Tricuspid flow, 86, 89
Tricuspid insufficiency, 113, 115–118
Tricuspid regurgitation, 117, 165
Tricuspid stenosis, 113
Tricuspid valve, 81
Tricuspid valve pathology, 113, 115–118
Triphasic wave, high-resistance, 11, 12
Tubular necrosis, acute (ATN), 183
Turbulence, severe, 143
Turbulent blood flow, 79, 129
Twin pregnancy, complicated, 203–204
Twin-to-twin transfusion syndrome, 204
Two-dimensional echocardiography, 69

U

Ulcer, giant, 30
Ulcerated plaque, 28, 30, 31
Ultrasound
  pulsed-Doppler, *see* Doppler ultrasound, pulsed-
Ultrasound imaging, *see* Imaging, real time pulse-echo gray-scale ultrasound
Ultrasound pulse, 1–2
Umbilical artery, 193
Umbilical artery waveform analysis, 197–199
Umbilical blood flow, 195
Umbilical vein blood flow, 197
Umbilical vein waveform analysis, 199, 200
Uterine arteries, 191
Uteroplacental circulation, 191–192

Uteroplacental waveform analysis, 199, 200–201

V

Valsalva maneuver, 140, 175, 240–241, 252, 255
Valve motion, 79, 81
Vascular beds, low-resistance, 10
Vascular calcification, 180
Vascular compression, 251–252
Vascular lesions, iatrogenic/traumatic, 222, 224–234
Vascular patency, 129
Venograms, 242, 244
Venous flow, 4
Venous structures, neoplastic invasion of, 256, 257
Ventricle
  left, flow velocity curves in, 84–88
  right, flow velocity curves in, 86, 89
Ventricular septal defect (VSD), 120–122
Vertebral artery, 23, 28
  cerebrovascular duplex sonography, 57, 59, 61–66
  normal variations of, 62–63
Vertebral artery stenosis, 61, 63, 65
Vertebral artery-vein, 26–27
Vertebrobasilar insufficiency, 59
Vertebrobasilar system, normal, 62–63
VICA-VCCA (ratio of ICA velocity to CCA velocity), 57
Volume flow, 5
VSD (ventricular septal defect), 120–122

W

Waveform analysis
  fetal aortic, 197
  fetoplacental, 195–199
  umbilical artery, 197–199
  umbilical vein, 199, 200
  uteroplacental, 199, 200–201

Z

Zero line, shifting, 78, 79